HYDROTHERAPY

in

NATUROPATHIC MEDICINE

HYDROTHERAPY

in

NATUROPATHIC MEDICINE

in their own words

Edited by Sussanna Czeranko, ND, BBE
Foreword by André Saine, ND

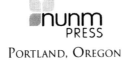

nunm
PRESS

PORTLAND, OREGON

Front cover: Vincent Priessnitz [1799-1851] center
and Father Sebastian Kneipp [1821-1897] seated on the chair.

NUNM Press
National University of Natural Medicine
049 SW Porter Street
Portland, Oregon 97201, USA
www.nunm.edu

Managing Editor: MiKayla Ryan
Production: Fourth Lloyd Productions, LLC.
Design: Richard Stodart

NUNM Press gratefully acknowledges the generous and prescient financial support of HEVERT USA which has made possible the creation and distribution of the *In Their Own Words* historical series.
The HEVERT COLLECTION comprises twelve historical compilations which preserve for the healing professions significant and representational works from contributors to the historical Benedict Lust journals.

Printed in the United States of America

ISBN: 978-1-945785-12-2
Library of Congress Control Number: 2018933551

Water is the sacred element which makes life
possible for the exquisite variety of all species;
human, animal, plant, and insect alike.

Water is the universal elixir.
Using water as a healing agent is sanctified
and embedded in our traditions and in
the accumulated wisdom of the centuries,
unequal to anything reductionist medical
science can conjure.

In celebration of water,
we honor with much deserved gratitude
the brilliance, wisdom, and prescience
of Vincent Priessnitz, Sebastian Kneipp and
those who followed in their footsteps.

TABLE OF CONTENTS

FOREWORD

The Hevert collection is a colossal work that sorts and edits the best writings of some of the pioneers of naturopathic medicine. This painstaking labor was necessary to develop tools for understanding this part of our past. I have always believed that in order to master one's discipline one must know its history. From that perspective, the Hevert collection serves its purpose admirably.

Sussanna Czeranko, whom I have known close to twenty-five years, has always shown a keen interest in nature cure, which is at the very core of naturopathic medicine. With a masterly hand and scholarly approach, she has been able to give a new lease of life to some the most valuable experiences reported by many of the pioneers of our profession.

Hydrotherapy, the subject of this tenth volume, is at the core of the nature cure movement of naturopathic medicine, which emphasizes living and healing according to the nature of human beings and their environment.

The ideal way of practicing naturopathic medicine is through a systematic application of the fundamental principles of medicine. Above all, the physician seeks to guide the person to live a life that is conducive to good health; however, despite the best prevention, people will fall sick and a comprehensive approach to intervention is called for, which seeks, first, to address the fundamental causes of sickness and, second, when necessary, to encourage, support or trigger the innate healing process by using various forces, agencies and influences of nature.

One of the most important of those agencies is water. The science of using water for health and healing is called hydrotherapy; hence the importance of this volume. Hydrotherapy could also be called thermotherapy, for warm and cold applications are used to enhance function and can thus play an important role in the preservation and restoration of health. Hydrotherapy is as old as humanity, however, the use of heat for healing, such as during fever, is found throughout the animal kingdom, and even in the plant kingdom and down to unicellular organisms; thus it has evolved over billions of years as a part of a complex of general and nonspecific defense and remedial measures.

The use of hot and cold applications for healing is thus a brilliant and powerful way of imitating nature. By the time he or she graduates, every naturopathic student should have made a point of acquiring a thorough understanding of the fundamentals of hydrotherapy and its application in health and disease. Hydrotherapy is simple to use and can be applied universally to people of all ages for the preservation of health and the recovery of health from acute and chronic diseases.

For instance, let us examine the outcomes in mixed populations of ambulatory and hospitalized pneumonia patients with five different therapeutic interventions, namely pre-antibiotic allopathy (PAA), contemporary conventional care (CCC), unqualified* homeopathy, Hahnemannian homeopathy and hydrotherapy. Since pneumonia is today divided into two main categories, community-acquired pneumonia (CAP) and health-care-acquired pneumonia (HCAP), and since morbidity and mortality are much higher in HCAP than in CAP, I have limited the mortality comparison of CCC to CAP.

The data show that hydrotherapy, homeopathy in general and especially Hahnemannian homeopathy unequivocally offer the safest and best outcomes for patients with pneumonia and, therefore, from the perspective of evidence-based medicine, would receive the highest possible recommendation of any intervention for these patients (1A/strong recommendation with high-quality evidence). The results of this comparison can be better appreciated in the following table:

Treatment	Number of Patients	Number of Recoveries	Survival Rate (%)	Number of Deaths	Mortality Rate (%)
Unqualified Homeopathy	25,216	24,350	96.6	866	3.4
Hahnemannian Homeopathy	960	956	99.6	4	0.4
Hydrotherapy	568	559	98.4	9	1.6
Pre-antibiotic Allopathy (PAA)	148,345	112,272	75.7	36,073	24.3
Conventional Contemporary Care (CCC)	33,148	28,607	86.3	4,541	13.7

Sources: André Saine, "The American School of Homeopathy and the International Hahnemannian Association: The High Point of Homeopathy, Part III," *Liga News*, no. 17 (April 2016): 17–23; and Simon Baruch, *The Principles and Practice of Hydrotherapy* (New York: William Wood, 1908).

---

*By "unqualified" is meant that it included genuine homeopathy as well as other practices considered to be homeopathic by their practitioners, such as pathological prescribing and polypharmacy.

The results obtained by hydrotherapy are not too far behind those of genuine Hahnemannian homeopathy. However, the genius of naturopathic medicine is its capacity to combine different approaches to create a synergetic effect. Not only should no one ever die from pneumonia, whatever its severity, under the combined application of hydrotherapy and homeopathy, together with water-only fasting, but also the recovery should be remarkably quick.

By affecting the fundamental causes of disease and by using the different forces and influences of nature to heal in a gentle manner, such as hydrotherapy, naturopathic medicine is a most wise approach to health care, because it is rational, scientific, safe, effective and inexpensive.

Our literature on hydrotherapy is vast but has been largely unexplored. In the introduction to this volume, Dr. Czeranko surveys some of the history of hydrotherapy since Vincenz Priessnitz, and thus opens a window to the richness of our past. Here is a treasure trove of information, which has unfortunately been long forgotten, on how best to use hydrotherapy in all types of situation.

Generations of naturopathic students to come will owe a debt of gratitude to Dr. Sussanna Czeranko and her team, as well as to my alma mater, NUNM, and the Hevert family, for having made possible the realization of such an invaluable project.

André Saine, ND
Co-author with Dr. Wade Boyle,
Lectures in Naturopathic Hydrotherapy (1988)

PREFACE

Hydrotherapy in Naturopathic Medicine is the tenth book in the twelve-volume Hevert Collection. It records the early use of water applications that were used by the men and women who championed safe healing methods in the early 20th century. The use of water as a primary and primordial healing medium is as old as time. The historical events that accompany Benedict Lust and his colleagues provide the context showing how Hydrotherapy was the healing platform from which Naturopathy sprang.

It was very natural for water to be a major element in Naturopathy's first medical tool box. Vincent Priessnitz used water to heal mercury poisoned patients lethally dosed with calomel by their medical doctors. His widely known successes were documented by doctors curious to understand how Priessnitz cured the incurable. Simple cold water was his weapon against harmful treatments and disease. Priessnitz opened the flood gates for medical doctors to emulate his water cures and what ensued was the first wave of Hydrotherapy in America in the mid-19th century. Father Sebastian Kneipp followed Priessnitz a half a century later, using water as his primary healing agent successfully curing the poor as well as Europe's aristocracy.

Over the years, though, water has been eclipsed from its inaugural, prominent place in the naturopathic armamentarium. Water applications and therapies have almost been relegated to the old fashioned and out dated, dismissed as archaic, inferior treatments not scientific enough to be seriously included as essential, important elements in health care. After all, how could water be contemplated as a powerful healing agent when it is so ubiquitous and harmless?

Having observed numerous naturopathic clinics over the years, I have often been told that Hydrotherapy is too labour intensive, takes up too much space and besides, it requires a sink and water. Consequently, Hydrotherapy is not common in the contemporary Naturopath's office. There are so many new powerful tools that are at our disposal and our attention is distracted from those early roots. Although, every naturopathic school teaches the Constitutional Hydrotherapy protocol and perhaps includes the virtues of a throat "warming compress" and cold wet socks, using other water applications is a rarity within a naturopathic family practice.

The main objective for this book is to make available a compilation of seminal articles on the topic of Hydrotherapy. They were transcribed in their entirety and appear as they were first published by Benedict Lust in his various magazines. A few of the articles come from Benedict Lust's very first publishing efforts, a German magazine called *Amerikanischen Kneipp-Blätter* (1896-1899) extoling the wonders of Father Sebastian Kneipp's Water Cure therapies. In 1896, Lust was 24 years old and he had found a new purpose and direction, giving meaning for his life: to spread the word about Kneipp. His venture into publishing was a brand new experience for this young man. Lust continued to publish magazines on health and eventually Hydrotherapy expanded to include many other different therapies.

This book captures the relevant Hydrotherapy materials found in Lust's publications from 1897 to 1923. The Benedict Lust publications span 50 years, from 1896 until his death in 1945. At National University of Natural Medicine's library, almost all of the publications with the exception of the first year of his publication can be found in the university's Rare Book Room. In previous books of *The Hevert Collection,* articles found in Benedict Lust's publications appear from 1900 to 1923. In *Hydrotherapy in Naturopathic Medicine,* 66 articles have been selected from NUNM's library's earliest books that Lust published, 1897–1899 and although German was the principle language used, Lust also included a few English articles in *Amerikanischen Kneipp-Blätter.*

There are many reasons why I have taken such pleasure in creating *Hydrotherapy in Naturopathic Medicine.* For one, this new volume gathers together all of the Water Cure and Hydrotherapies used from Naturopathy's inception by those long forgotten pioneers such as Vincent Priessnitz, Father Sebastian Kneipp, Louis Kuhne, Friedrich Bilz, Adolf Just, Alfred Baumgarten, Carl Schultz, Simon Baruch and others. These men left behind pearls of wisdom that are not to be forgotten. Reading their contributions to Hydrotherapy *in their own words* provides understanding and a richer appreciation for the precious, valuable gift that Hydrotherapy brings to Naturopathy.

Water is a timeless healing, life-sustaining wonder that others in the contemporary era, such as Drs. André Saine and the late, Wade Boyle's, described eloquently in their monumental book, *Lectures in Naturopathic Hydrotherapy* (1988) which is a cornerstone for all students immersed in naturopathic programs all across North America. Their book kept alive the Water Cure traditions that "Drs. John Bastyr, Harold Dick and Leo Scott passed to a new generation of naturopathic physicians". (Wade, Saine, 1988) Generation after generation, Wade and Saine's book will continue to be a wellspring of inspiration for naturopathic students yearning to practice traditional naturopathic methods. I am indebted to these two men whose love of history has had such an incredible impact on my journey into naturopathic history.

A second reason why this present volume, *Hydrotherapy in Naturopathic Medicine,* has imprinted upon my soul is that learning directly from the pioneers of Hydrotherapy sheds invaluable insights enabling us to implement the various hydrotherapies with confidence. The voices of those who championed Hydrotherapy in late 19ᵗʰ and early 20ᵗʰ centuries leave their echoes of clinical pearls for us to grasp and implement. Many of the earliest articles were written by Sebastian Kneipp and these Lust faithfully included in his mission to advance Kneipp's work in America. Lust utilized parts of chapters taken from Kneipp's books and included these as articles in his publications. Kneipp books are still readily available in reprint form, and so I used some discretion to not replicate all of the articles in Lust's earlier publications which were entirely devoted to Kneipp's writings. Kneipp's voice was quickly replaced with other Hydrotherapists and the passion for water as a therapeutic agent was widely embraced. You will discover, though, that despite Hydrotherapy's being the indisputable foundation for the early Naturopaths, with time the introduction of new treatment options changed how Hydrotherapy was used.

As a naturopathic student at CCNM, my initiation to Hydrotherapy was scheduled as a single lecture on Constitutional Hydrotherapy treatment that was developed by Dr. O. G. Carroll from Spokane, Washington in 1923. At the time, elective courses, such as Constitutional Hydrotherapy, were sometimes relegated to a Saturday because of insufficient time within the curriculum's weekly class schedule. On this particular Saturday, the lecture was disappointingly cut short because of weather. Sadly, it was not inclement weather that truncated the Hydrotherapy classes; rather, it was the sun shining. The weather was warm and the teacher was an avid bicyclist and wanted to go cycling. My much later exposure to the Lust publications have made me realize now more than ever that on that sunny day, Hydrotherapy as a precious tool never took root with our cohort at CCNM for the remarkable potential of Hydrotherapy did not get adequate or even fair space in our learning. On that sunny day, Hydrotherapy as a modality receded for me until many years later when I rediscovered the power of water on my own terms. I needed to personally use water to heal myself after a near death automobile accident. In healing myself, I re-discovered a forgotten yet immensely powerful tool from Naturopathy's origins.

In this collection, there are unfortunately no articles written by O. G. Carroll on Constitutional Hydro in Lust's journals, nor was I able to find one written after 1923 in any of Lust's publications. In most of the naturopathic colleges and universities, Hydrotherapy has been by and large inadvertently reduced to one water application, benefitting from Carroll's Constitutional Hydro work. Certainly, as the profession was evolving, sustaining one water application was better than losing them all.

The completion of this book brings with it immense awe and reverence for the men and women skilled in the use of water to restore health. The art of naturopathic medicine is truly the providence of the early Hydrotherapists who understood implicitly how to use water as one of the supreme healing tools in our repertoire. What a precious tradition and what powerful tools the early Hydrotherapists passed to us. This book is a collection of articles that chronicle the Water Cure therapies they used and which evolved into Hydrotherapy and forward into an even bigger platform, Naturopathy itself.

When beginning to shape this tenth volume, I felt daunted by the sheer scope and importance of this central element of our medicine. There is just so much history and terminology that come with this subject. The journey through, however, has been immensely rewarding and *Hydrotherapy in Naturopathic Medicine* is now resting in your hands. To aid those not familiar with Hydrotherapy, there is a glossary at the end of the book defining the various water applications and the terminology used in Hydrotherapy. I hope that you find this useful.

I have been often in Dr. André Saine's classes dazzled by the vivid, living details he provided about people from the past, so engaging that one would have thought they were his personal friends. He brought history alive for us and I remain to this day personally grateful for the tireless, incalculable work he continually produces to advance Naturopathy and Homeopathy through his writing, lectures and preceptorship. When I was a young student attending Canadian College of Naturopathic Medicine [CCNM], Dr. Saine's work was already legendary. My classmates and I all vied to preceptor with him in his clinic. His love of traditional naturopathic practices and devoted passion for Homeopathy were steeped in profound understanding, knowledge and clinical experience. We all wanted to be like him, to be able to harness the wisdom of the elders.

Dr. Saine has been a mentor to naturopathic students as long as I have known him. His passion for Hydrotherapy and Homeopathy is contagious and deeply needed more than ever as Naturopaths continue to cope with the dominant, orthodox medical terrain. The allure of drugs and biomedical dogma is indeed incubating alliances and divisions within our profession in the form of new labels such as "integrative" and "functional" medicine.

Dr. Saine has an extraordinary personal library that encompasses centuries of homeopathic and early naturopathic literature. Recently, he shared that one of his favourite books is *How to Treat the Sick Without Medicine*, (1874) written by James C. Jackson, whose entire personal library eventually found its way into Dr. Saine's own magnificent library collection. Jackson operated one of the largest sanatoriums in

Dansville, New York in 19th century, before the inception of Naturopathy. He practiced highly successful health care without the use of drugs, employing the true materia medica of "first, air; second, food; third, water; fourth, sunlight; fifth, dress; sixth, exercise; seventh, sleep; eighth, rest; ninth, social influences; tenth, mental and moral forces". (Jackson, 1874, 26)

I am truly grateful to everyone who has made this book possible. This book stands on the shoulders of luminaries who dared to make a difference. To the students at National University of Natural Medicine, no words can express my gratitude for the work that you have done to see this book to the end. The number of articles discarded are more than what made it through to the final version. I want to acknowledge every NUNM student who typed articles while navigating her or his intense course loads and juggling personal lives. I bow with gratitude to **Aaron Potts, Adam Dombrowski, Alla Nicolulis, Allison Brumley, Ashley Benson, Cadence Wong, Cody Strodtman, Delia Sewell, Erin Conlon, January Bourassa, Karis Tressel, Katie Clements, Kristen Carle, Lacy Nuckols, Laura Weldon, Lauren Geyman, Lucy-Kate Reeve, Mackenzie Clark, Meagan Hammel, Megan Danz, Meredith Trump, Michelle Brown-Echerd, Misty Story, Node Smith, Rebecca Jennings, Renae Rogers, Rhesa Napoli, Stephanie Woods, Susan Manongi, Tiffany Bloomingdale, Tiny Dreisbach, Tristian Rowe,** and all those whom I am inadvertently missing here. I especially applaud **Adam Dombrowski and Aaron Potts** for the scanning of images for this book. There were hundreds of images needed to be scanned and this painstaking work was done exceptionally.

And, as this book project moves into the last quarter of our work and production plan, my appreciation for the invaluable organizational help that I had received from **Dr. Karis Tressel** during the early stages is not forgotten. I am deeply grateful for her profound love of the traditions and history of Naturopathy and for her inspiring, loving tenacity with this project.

The schedule of a student is packed with studying, never ending tests, and the fearsome final exams leaving little room for anything else. It is a wonder that our naturopathic medical students at the end of four or even six years of study can still stand and know their own names. Yet, one day will arrive when your grueling days at NUNM will come to an end and you will be walking across the stage to accept your diploma. The skills and gifts that you have worked so diligently to acquire will be exactly what patients are searching for. You have so much to offer as Naturopaths. You have chosen a path of sacred work steeped with a valiant and honourable history. You will be truly loved and cherished by your patients because you listen and truly care. Remember to trust

Nature's power of healing, the *Vis medicatrix naturae*! Listen carefully to your patients and they will feel enlivened and grateful to have found their way to you.

I am very thankful for the encouraging support of the Hevert Corporation in Germany. Thank you and my most gracious accolades to Mathias and Marcus Hevert for your generous contributions allowing this book series to become a reality. Much gratitude, as well, to the unwavering, behind-the-scenes support of the Board of NUNM, MiKayla Ryan, Susan Hunter, and Jerry Bores who understood from the beginning the importance of this project.

Oh, where would this amazing book be without the fastidious and meticulous excellence that Fourth Lloyd Productions, Nancy and Richard Stodart, my designers and mentors, bring to this latest book! Books are cumbersome beasts and working with Nancy and Richard whose alacrity and superlative skills make the whole process seem relatively simplistic and easy. You both make my journey into the twilight zone of history an absolute joy. Thank you both for the exquisite care that you took with every minute detail! Nancy, I applaud your wisdom and Richard your artistic sensibilities is simply outstanding. I am always dazzled and awed by the book covers and this one is breathtaking.

I save the best for the last. I am forever indebted to my dear husband, David Schleich, who knows exactly how to pick me up when I have lost my *Vis* in the midst of incalculable details. I love that we both share a passion for history and am so awed by his patience to listen to my stories of dead and forgotten people whom I have bonded with for life. To share the history of Naturopathy brings me closer to Nature's truths. Thank you David for your unwavering support and love.

Lastly, I am so indebted to the men and women who live in these pages, and who occupy almost every minute of my day. They may have lived a hundred years ago, but they have left a legacy of wisdom and passion that fills me with confidence and gratitude for their contributions to a literature that I can read and implement in my own practice and, along with my wonderful collaborators, with you. The conviction and experiences of our elders of healing incurable diseases with simply using water should not be forgotten. Innocent and available water was the secret weapon of Priessnitz, Kneipp and those who followed. Using water is the way to know its powerful healing magic.

Blue sky blessings,
Sussanna Czeranko, ND, BBE
Portland, Oregon
February 2018

Whoever has a knowledge of the effects of water, and knows how to use it in its extremely manifold ways, is in possession of a remedy which cannot be surpassed by any other, whatever its name may be.

—Sebastian Kneipp, 1897, 186

Let me once more repeat the fundamental and universal rule to be strictly observed without exception in every one of my water [applications]. No one whose body is not sufficiently warm, who is shivering with cold, should take any cold water application.

—Sebastian Kneipp, 1898, 115

Yes, back to nature and a proper mode of living, mentally, morally and physically, and a rational usage of water, was the magnetic doctrine which seemed to electrify the entire world and was re-echoed from one end of the globe to the other.

—N. Tally, Jr., M.D., 1898, 227

While the public in general is under the impression that walking in the grass is the principal means of healing in the Kneipp cure, there is a little more to understand, a little more to know for the practitioner of the Kneipp Water Cure than simply the how and when to take a walk in the grass.

—Benedict Lust, 6, 1900

This latter end is easily effected by water cure. I recommend for your study these books on water as a curative agent: The True Healing Art, by Russell Thacher Trall; My Water Cure, by Sebastian Kneipp; New Science of Healing, by Louis Kuhne, and The Natural Healing System, by Friedrich Eduard Bilz.

—August F. Reinhold, 1900, 206

As we, horror-struck, contemplate the outrages perpetrated during the dark Middle Ages against dissenters and witches, I doubt that in the years to come people will fail to understand how we could authorize a class of men—the medical doctors to undermine our health with thousands of deathly drugs, and to hack, slash and saw us all to pieces.

—August F. Reinhold, 1900, 206

Kneipp's theory is that the cause of all disease lies in the blood—either from the fact of the blood being vitiated by the presence in it of morbid matter can be expelled by water. For the purposes of his cure he employs water in the form of wraps, compresses, packs, steaming, washings, and affusions.

—Friedrich Eduard Bilz, 1901, 212

As Father Kneipp never examined a patient by auscultation or percussion, and yet achieved such remarkable results in the cure of disease, it is worthwhile to enquire how he arrived at his diagnosis, and arranged his plans to treatment.

—Friedrich Eduard Bilz, 1901, 212

Whoever understands Nature, and knows that everything which is in the spirit of Nature and according to her dictates must result in the greatest blessing for mankind, will welcome this bath, and to him it will bring blessing and happiness in abundance.

—Adolf Just, 1901, 316

Let no one say that he does not need the natural bath, because he is well. For it is plainly not the first intention of Nature to cure diseases by the bath, but rather to keep her creatures well, bright and happy.

—Adolf Just, 1901, 316

If the physician will tell you that your blood is poor, that you have bad blood, scrofulous blood, in short that you are predisposed to all the diseases of the blood that are known, what is to be done? A campaign against the accumulation of foreign matter in the system must be instituted at once.

—Dr. Alfred Baumgarten, 1903, 124

I want to say right here that the knee douche is as good in its place as any of the larger applications, and to despise it evidences a lack of insight and appreciation for what it has done to others.

—Dr. Alfred Baumgarten, 1904, V (1)

I am sorry to add that many naturopathic physicians have abandoned Hydrotherapy. Sometimes the physician has not money enough, or thinks he has not money enough, to equip his treatment rooms with the suitable arrangements and appliances. Expensive equipment is not necessary.

—Carl Schultz, 1914, 345

I believe that in this country the hydropathic treatment has not been understood enough. I think the time will come when all our hospitals will have appliances to use the Water Cure treatment in all its forms.

—A. H. Meisenbach, M.D, 1904

Priessnitz was one of the first to organize the use of water into a system, for which he deserves great credit. Winternitz, of Vienna, did much in bringing and establishing Hydrotherapy upon a sound and scientific basis.

—Joseph A. Hoegen, N.D., 1917, 311

After the first shock of the chill is over, the pack is very soothing, pleasant and refreshing, and proof that the pack has a beneficial and quieting effecting upon the whole nervous system is, that nearly every patient falls asleep while in it.

—Joseph A. Hoegen, N.D., 1917, 315

When we have once grasped the way in which Nature works, there can be no difficulty in our understanding how, as may occur in chronic disease, the momentary disturbances (curative crises) called forth by the sun bath, may be counteracted immediately by cooling water baths.

—Louis Kuhne, 1917, 363

As I have already remarked, I can cure all disease but not all patients. For where the bodily vitality and therefore, the digestive power, is already broken down, these remedies will afford relief, such indeed as no other means will, but they cannot in such case effect a complete cure.

—Louis Kuhne, 1917, 368

Vincent Priessnitz' principle, expressed in his own words, is: "Not the cold but the body heat, produced by the reaction to cold water, is the healing factor."

—Benedict Lust, 1918, 223

However, no lecture, review, book, treatise or compendium on Water Cure is complete, or can in any way be authoritative without giving honor to the man who is justly called the Father of Modern Hydrotherapy. The monumental work which elevated Water Cure once for all above suspicion, and placed it beyond the scope of charlatanry is the live work of William Winternitz.

—Robert C. Biéri, 1921, 224

Spread three blankets, one on top of the other, on the bed. Over these spread a sheet which has been dipped in cool water and wrung out.

—William Freeman Havard, 1921, 325

INTRODUCTION

Hydrotherapy and Naturopathy share a synergy well known in the naturopathic community. That connection begins when the young German immigrant, Benedict Lust, became very sick back in 1894 when he was 22 years old. He chose New York City to live in and quickly translated skills he had acquired in Germany, France, Switzerland, and England to becoming an exceptional, world class waiter in the prestigious Savoy Hotel. He dove into the American dream of working hard to build a prosperous future, putting in inordinately long hours, saving money, making connections, and building a reputation for reliability. However, while on a short break at the World Expo in Chicago in 1893, he suffered an accident descending from a tram. A downward health spiral ensued, including a diagnosis of tuberculosis and exhaustion, arising from his habit of putting in grueling hours. Unable to resume his work, and desperate for a path to recovery, Lust returned to Germany where he sought out Sebastian Kneipp about whose remarkable water therapies he had heard. At Wörishofen, the site of Kneipp's Water Cure establishment, Lust spent eight months to get well. His treatment, though, morphed into an apprenticeship because he found himself not only getting well, but also studying purposely with the master of Water Cure. Lust restored his health and found himself infused with a zeal that opened unimaginable doors that would persist throughout his life.

Even though water therapies were already present in America when Benedict Lust first returned to New York City in 1896, he was all fired up to launch his mission to promote Father Sebastian Kneipp's method of healing. As part of his industriousness in this mission, and still a youthful 24, he began spreading the word, launching his first magazine, *Amerikanischen Kneipp Blätter* that same year. Fulfilling his promise to Father Sebastian Kneipp to raise awareness of Water Cure in America, Lust wrote, edited and translated many widely read articles in his early publications. There were numerous excerpts from Kneipp's books and from other German authors writing about Kneipp Water Cure, with occasional English translations from Kneippian books. As the name of his magazine indicated, Kneipp's name and water cure therapies were exclusively targeted to an audience composed mostly of German immigrants who would be very familiar with Kneipp's contribution to health and Hydrotherapy. As a precursor of what was to come, there were even in the earliest issues of *Amerikanischen Kneipp Blätter* English translations from Kneipp resources. Some of these treasures have been included in this collection. Many of these early articles would be reprinted and reappear in later publications.

Benedict Lust is synonymous with Naturopathy, both as its founder but also as its architect. He watched over Naturopathy for 50 years, cultivating, nurturing and guiding the formation of the profession in America. Without Hydrotherapy and the contributions made by Kneipp, and I might add, Priessnitz, one can wonder how Naturopathy would have manifested without Lust. To say that Naturopathy evolved from Hydrotherapy is a given, and indeed a well- accepted fact. Lust essentially planted Kneipp's Water Cure methods in America and then nurtured the seeds with every nutrient he could find. Benedict Lust began with the foundational Water Cure healing protocols and philosophy of Priessnitz and Kneipp and it grew from there. Water Cure was the foundation and from it a new profession began to evolve which introduced the best principles of its European origins and generated a brand new healing paradigm.

So, what you will experience in *Hydrotherapy in Naturopathic Medicine* is this first blush of exuberance for water therapies and then you will discern a gradual and progressive shift. The passion for water was allocated to other modalities which were, perhaps for the newly forming profession of Naturopathy more electrifying, more scientific, or more lucrative; or so it seemed. In the beginning Naturopathy took its directive from Kneipp's method of Water Cure with all the therapeutic interventions revolving around water. The record shows that as the years tumbled by, there was less Hydrotherapy in Naturopathy, but not because Hydrotherapy was ineffective or defective. In fact, the opposite is true; the literature demonstrates that no therapeutic agent, with the exception of Homeopathy, ever surpassed the clinical successes of Hydrotherapy. Pointedly representative of the enduring triumph of Hydrotherapy in this era was the impact its treatments brought to battling the Spanish Flu epidemic of 1918.

At no time in history was Hydrotherapy more depended upon to exact a cure in an extreme epidemic situation as this world-wide flu. The Naturopaths, using wet sheet packs and dietary counsel, saved lives when the Allopaths using calomel and aspirin could not. In Volumes I and II of the Hevert Collection title, *Clinical Pearls in Naturopathic Medicine,* you will encounter accounts of myriad cases and protocols extolling the use of Hydrotherapy for various diseases. In previous books in the Hevert series, such as *Vaccination and Naturopathic Medicine,* there is much evidence of Hydrotherapy as the chief agent safely restoring health in circumstances of rampant contagious and life threatening diseases. Henry Lindlahr, for example, presents cases of small pox and scarlet fever with astounding cures using cold water applications.

Prior to Lust's publishing endeavours to give Kneipp's water therapies a place in America, we encounter an abundance of writings from Joel Shew (1816-1855). He published numerous titles based on Priessnitz' work. He had studied medicine in New York and then went to Gräefenberg to study with Priessnitz. His books include: *The Water-cure Manual (1847, 288 pp)*, *Hydrotherapy or the Water Cure* (1849 3rd Edition, 360 pp), *Consumption: its Prevention and Cure by the Water Treatment* (1851, 286 pp), and *The Water-cure in Pregnancy and Childbirth* (1851, 122 pp).

Fowler and Wells were publishers based in New York City who specialized in Water Cure and Phrenology as well as in other alternative medical topics. In the mid-19th century, they published a seven volume series called *The Water-cure Library* and featured one or more writers in each volume. Joel Shew was prominent in this collection of work, writing entire treaties and adding to others with his shorter manuscripts. Joel Shew lived 39 years and his contributions to Water Cure were phenomenal, although now largely forgotten. After having studied with Priessnitz, Shew returned to America where he was instrumental in raising the caliber of Priessnitz' work with his objective medical writings. He documented cases and meticulously described the various Priessnitz therapies. I would like to think that Shew was the incubator and catalyst for this first wave of Hydrotherapy in America, work which Lust carried on some decades later.

Another book written in 1850 by John Bell, M.D., was an historically relevant book that presented within its 658 pages all of the existing hydrotherapies used at the time globally. Its long, full title is most illuminating: *Dietetical and Medical Hydrology. A Treatise on Baths; Including Cold, Sea, Warm Hot, Vapour, Gas, and Mud Baths: also, on the Watery Regime, Hydropathy, and Pulmonary Inhalation; with a Description of Bathing in Ancient and Modern Times* (Barrington and Haswell, Philadelphia, 1850). There were many other books written in the 1850's by medical doctors such as J. H. Rausse, C. C. Schieferdecker, F. A. Gräeter and others. Their teacher often was the none other, Vincent Priessnitz who is largely responsible for water becoming noticed and used as a therapeutic modality.

The second wave of writers on water would come forward in the early 20th century. In 1901, for example, John Harvey Kellogg's book, *Rational Hydrotherapy* (F. A. Davis Company, Philadelphia) and its 1193 pages mark a colossal shift in the American Hydrotherapy landscape. The book contains 293 illustrations, 18 of which were in colour (unique at the time). We can grasp the monumental scope of this book by reading Kellogg's dedication: "To his friend, Dr. Wilhelm W. Winternitz, Professor of nervous diseases in the Royal and Imperial University of Vienna, and founder of the first hydriatic clinic, the author respectfully dedicates this volume." (Kellogg, 1901, iii) Kellogg brings the rigor of Winternitz' scientific work into print in English. The lexicon that we are introduced to in Kellogg's work is striking and there is a sense that Hydrotherapy had finally arrived confidently within the medical paradigm. Winternitz was a student of Priessnitz, and we in his work see the continuity of Priessnitz moving into the 20th century.

There are numerous Hydrotherapists who in the late 19th and early 20th century added their voices to strengthen Hydrotherapy within medicine. All of these men were medical doctors and they wrote one or more books to strengthen water's place, challenging the forces of vaccines, and drugs. Let us review this remarkable landscape of literature to absorb its sheer volume and value to this history of Hydrotherapy in North America. Very often, the author would indicate on the title page, his affiliation, place of work and accomplishments. Many of these books are readily available to this day as re-prints.

George Knapp Abbott, A.B., M.D., Dean of Faculty and Professor of Physiologic Therapy and Practice of Medicine in the College of Medical Evangelists of the Loma Linda Hospital wrote several books, *Technique of Hydrotherapy* (1908, 128 pp), *Elements of Hydrotherapy for Nurses* (1912, 275), *Principles and Practice of Hydrotherapy for Students and Practitioners of Medicine* (1914, 521 pp, The College Press, Loma Linda).

Simon Baruch, M.D.'s affiliations and responsibilities were vast across his remarkable career. He was the attending physician to the Manhattan General Hospital and New York Juvenile Asylum; consulting physician to the Knickerbocker, Montefiori and Bellevue Hospitals, hydrotherapeutist to Sea View Hospital for tuberculosis, formerly professor of Hydrotherapy, College of Physicians and Surgeons, Columbia University, and Honorary member of the South Carolina Medical Association. His three books include: *The Uses of Water in Modern Medicine* (1892, 228 pp), *The Principles and Practice of Hydrotherapy, A Guide to the Application of Water in Disease for Students and Practitioners of Medicine* (1898, 435 pp), *An Epitome of Hydrotherapy for Physicians, Architects and Nurses* (1920, 205 pp)

William H. Dieffenbach, M.D., was Benedict Lust's professor when he had attended New York Medical College in 1901. Dieffenbach was also a professor at New York Homeopathic Medical College, physical therapist to Volunteer St. Gregory's Hospital, and electro-therapist to Flower and Hahnemann Hospitals. His book includes images of various therapies and concludes with treatment protocols for many diseases. The title of his book is *Hydrotherapy, a Brief Summary of the Practical Value of Water in Disease for Students and Practicians of Medicine* (1909, 267 pp).

Guy Hinsdale, A.M., M.D., wrote *Hydrotherapy, a Work on*

Hydrotherapy in General, its Application to Special Affections, the Technic or Processes Employed and the Use of Waters Internally (1910, 466 pp). His dedication is to "Dr. William Osler, *Regius* professor of medicine and student of Christ Church, Oxford, as a token, of the Author's regard." (Hinsdale, 1910, 5)

Curran Pope, M.D. was a professor of numerous subjects at the University of Louisville Medical Department. He had many posts as associate editor of many medical journals. He wrote the impressively large 646 page book, *Practical Hydrotherapy, a Manual for Students and Practitioners* in 1909. His book is replete with photographs and beautiful graphics. He draws from Kellogg and Winternitz and writes in his Preface that he "offers no apology for another work upon hydrotherapy, as there are at present very few works in the English language." (Pope, 1909, v)

There are so many more who wrote on Hydrotherapy. I have included here reference to the more prominent writers found in National University of Natural Medicine's Rare Book Room. Each of these men, who were also medical doctors, had no doubts of the efficacy and merit of Hydrotherapy. Winternitz was one of the first to establish a scientific paradigm that included a lexicon to accompany the scientific investigation and conclusions.

Notwithstanding this rich tradition of scholarship and literature, we are faced squarely from our early 21st century perspective with the question, *Who is to blame for the demise of Hydrotherapy within Naturopathy?* I have found in my professional encounters that more than a few contemporary Naturopathic Physicians are not familiar with this development in their history; that is, the diminishing of hydrotherapy in clinical practice. This question begs an answer and the only clues provided by all of those men and women pioneers are the writings that they left behind. The answer is unsettling and has jarred my longing to restore Hydrotherapy to its rightful location in the Naturopathic armamentarium. I yearn some days for a nostalgic, albeit impossible outcome to this dilemma in modern naturopathic practice. When I think of the world of Hydrotherapy that existed for those early practitioners of Naturopathy, I sometimes experience a sadness arising from the inexplicable loss of water cure, evaporated, so to speak, from the tool box of Naturopathy. I encourage you to read along with me and gather in the abundant clues that lie in the literature. You may concur with my nostalgia and lament about Hydrotherapy in our profession.

Among the insights or clues to why Hydrotherapy declined is that the literature documents how suspicious and even contemptuous orthodox medicine was of water therapies. For example, during the ravages of those epidemics which plagued the American population in 19th and early

20th centuries, the positive impact of water therapies on these diseases presentations rapidly generated backlash from the Regulars. Their assault on Hydrotherapy was deliberate, sustained and effective. We may well have forgotten how politically and legally brutal these determined Allopaths were in protecting their turf from the early Naturopaths who were practicing Hydrotherapy. Benedict Lust himself was charged 18 times, attracting and receiving fines from $200 to $2,000 (a $500 fine would be the equivalent today of $12,000). Another way to understand what $500 meant in 1910 is to reverse the calculations. If I were to receive a $500 fine today, that sum would be less than $20 in 1910 dollars. A $12,000 fine for administering a bath seems preposterous and at the same time very serious. Even so, many of the early Naturopaths who practiced Hydrotherapy and who routinely employed air, light and water baths were persecuted and prosecuted in this way, the penalties imposed so hefty that they often bankrupted them, capsizing their lives and propelling them into a cascade of disaster. These men and women who chose Nature's healing methods such as Hydrotherapy were prosecuted as criminals and did not have the resources to fight the powerful AMA or its membership determined to put an end to Naturopathy.

It is not by accident that those men and women who rallied to natural healing methods chose water to restore health. Many had turned to the European Water Cure establishments to recover their health using water and it was quite natural for them to want to share their enthusiasm with others. Their lives were changed and there was no turning back.

On first glance, *Hydrotherapy in Naturopathic Medicine* may appear to be a book about Sebastian Kneipp (1821-1897) and indeed, Father Kneipp dominates the pages of this book simply because he wrote three books which propelled him as an international personality and celebrity recognized world-wide. Kneipp's own writings essentially formed the foundation for Lust's magazine, especially in the beginning. Benedict began publishing in 1896 and in the following year Sebastian Kneipp passed away, on June 17, 1897. Kneipp's life had influenced and touched thousands and thousands of patients who came to Wörishofen for his famed Water Cure. Even after the death of Kneipp, Lust continued to hail his praises for the Priest and his method of Water Cure.

Although Kneipp was the center of Lust's attention, there is a small thread of recognition for the man whom many consider to be the Father of Hydrotherapy, Vincent Priessnitz (1799-1851). The Who's Who of Hydrotherapy begins with Priessnitz who is, alas, blatantly understated in this book. Although many existed before him who used water, his combined astute observation and a gifted intuition opened the flood gates for Hydrotherapy. His name, though, does not resound with any fanfare, fireworks or medical credentials. He was long dead when those who were to shape the destiny of Naturopathy had begun their search for mentors and healers. There were no personal writings left behind by Priessnitz.

Unlike Kneipp who was literate, Priessnitz' childhood and schooling were abbreviated abruptly with the death of his older brother, forcing him to quit school at six years old so that he could help his poor blind father tend the farm. When Priessnitz was eight, his father also died leaving young Vincent to care for his mother and sisters and to run the operations of the small farm that provided their livelihood. There was no opportunity for Priessnitz to pursue education after the death of his father.

Because he was almost illiterate, Priessnitz' work would eventually be documented by many medical doctors who flocked in Gräefenberg to learn about and emulate his work. Priessnitz would eventually find his way into the Lust's publications via writers such as Richard Metcalfe, a British Hydrotherapist, who had personally experienced Priessnitz' Hydrotherapy at Gräefenberg.

In this way, then, much acclaim was attributed to Priessnitz as the one who "invented the sweating, not only in dry blankets, but also in wet sheets" (Metcalfe, 1898, 124) which had greatly influenced those who followed him in the practice of hydrotherapies. Priessnitz' contributions to Hydrotherapy are largely unparalleled. His bequeathing of water applications to future generations formed the foundation for those who followed. Priessnitz originated the wet sheet wrap, the sweating bath, wet bandages, the rubbing wet sheet, the friction bath, half baths, and the hip bath [sitz bath]. He also used prevailing treatments such as full baths, and local baths, such as foot baths and douches.

In any case, to fully appreciate the scope of Priessnitz' contributions, one must first recognize that Priessnitz could not read about these therapies; rather, he managed to learn them on his own. The therapies that he applied at Gräefenberg would eventually be modified and altered by those who followed in his footsteps, yet the principles of cold water would not change. The essence of Hydrotherapy is encapsulated by Priessnitz' wise observation, "Not the cold but the heat produced by the cold water is the healing factor". (Lust, 1900, 2)

Although Priessnitz and Kneipp lived in the 19th century, Kneipp only discovered Water Cure by reading Johann S. Hahn's small volume, *On the Power and Effect of Cold Water* (1737) three years before the death of Priessnitz. Their lifespans did not include much overlap or opportunity for collaboration. Even so, both men originated from humble and impoverished beginnings, both suffered ailments with little hope of recovery, and both made personal discoveries of healing that would become renowned throughout the world, bringing thousands of desperate patients to their doors. Neither of these men used any diagnostic equipment to arrive at uncannily accurate diagnosis, and both men developed remarkable gifts of observation that made them skilled diagnosticians, quite envied by medical professionals. Keeping modest and simple habits, both men maintained simplicity throughout their lives. Both attracted the attention of local medical fraternities who brought legal confrontations and criticisms against their clinical accomplishments. And yet, both also attracted doctors wanting to study with them.

Doctors, either jealous or eager to replicate Priessnitz' and Kneipp's successes, flocked to their doorsteps. The doctors who came to study with Priessnitz and Kneipp would leave convinced, and life-time converts to water therapies. They would be so impressed by what they saw in these water healing facilities that books would be written to enrich and advance Hydrotherapy. Priessnitz' advocates, such as Drs. Joel Shew, Christian Schieferdecker and Francis Græter articulated and provided comprehensive accounts of what Priessnitz' water cure entailed. From these writings, Priessnitz endured.

For example, Græter's *Hydriatics, Manual of the Water Cure* (1842) recorded his personal experiences at Græfenberg and he had the auspicious providence of actually receiving water treatments by Priessnitz. Græter's comprehension of Priessnitz' work was articulated in his book about this eminent Father of Hydrotherapy. Another small treasure found in NUNM's Rare Book Room, entitled *Vincenz Priessnitz: the wonderful power of water in healing the diseases of the human body,* was authored in 1844 by Dr. Christian Charles Schieferdecker and published in Philadelphia. My search did not end here, though; then I found yet another outstanding book describing in minute detail the work of Priessnitz. The book, *The Water Cure Manual,* was written in 1849 by Joel Shew, M.D. Shew, who I would soon learn, had written many books on Water Cure at Priessnitz' Græfenberg. Græter's, Schieferdecker's and Shew's books collectively offer us unusual and rare accounts, especially powerful because these men actually witnessed and experienced Hydrotherapy at the side of Priessnitz. They realized "the necessity of scientific observation [to establish] scientific and rational methods." (Græter, 1842, 61) On another note, these men who studied meticulously Priessnitz' work were in some ways committing career suicide as they mutinied from the medical orthodox views of their times.

Described as a humble man, Kneipp dedicated his life and his books as an offering to the common poor people of his remote little village of Wörishofen in Germany. Kneipp writes, "I have written my little book [*My Water Cure,* 1886] first of all for poor sick people, for whose benefit, keeping before my eyes the heavenly reward." (Kneipp, 1902, 384) His books were written to be accessible to everyone, especially those who did not have within their means to afford the expensive options of medical doctors. Those who were in need of healing were never turned away and so when Benedict Lust and Henry Lindlahr sought his help at Wörishofen, Kneipp's life work expanded to America with these two men as emissaries, like there was no tomorrow. It is because Kneipp personally touched the lives of men and women that Hydrotherapy became the foundation for Lust and Lindlahr as a new healing paradigm when they returned to America.

This introduction would be remiss without mentioning two exceptional and remarkable men for their tremendous foresight, wisdom and articulation of the core principles of Hydrotherapy. Although their names and stories are buried with time, their contributions were immortalized in books that they left in their wake. These books would be the galvanizing forces shaping and germinating Naturopathy during its infancy.

The first man is Louis Kuhne (1835-1901) who wrote, *The New Science of Healing* (1891) and *The Science of Facial Expression* (1897, English edition). His first book would re-direct the course of medicine, especially within the field of natural healing. Henry Lindlahr (1862-1924) was given a copy of *The New Science of Healing* at a time when his life was dangling on a thread. Faced with a diabetic prognosis, before the advent of insulin, Lindlahr was face to face with imminent death. He read Kuhne's entire book in one night, forever changing his life. He would never look back to his previous life of hedonistic excess.

The second man who left his fingerprints all over Naturopathy was Adolf Just (1859-1936). His book, *Return to Nature* (1896) was the keystone for the emerging Naturopaths in America in the beginning of the 20th century. Adolf Just, faced with ailments that left him desperate for respite, found healing by imitating Nature's methods. Just extolled the wonders of "earth cure" using earth compresses, and sleeping on the earth to imbibe the vibration of Mother Earth. He also introduced a simple bath called the "natural bath" that he had observed animals in the wild partake of. He called his center of healing, Jungborn, which would in time be replicated by others who visited Just in the Harz Mountains in Germany. One such man was Emanuel Felke, a pastor from an impoverished mining district in Germany. Felke visited Just's Jungborn and returned to his congregation and emulated the use of earth and the natural bath. Felke became a local legend for his use of Homeopathy, combined with clay baths and Just's famous natural bath. This bath takes a minute to do and has the restorative power to erase years of fatigue, and stress from the body. Having used the natural bath for the past two years, I can attest to its sublime power to alleviate adrenal fatigue and make the spirits soar.

Lust, with the help of his brother-in-law, Reverend Albert Stroebele, translated Just's book in 1901 and excerpts from *Return to Nature* would find their way into Benedict Lust's publications, securing within Naturopathy the laws of Nature and a solid foundation for healing. Lust always made space for advertisements for *Return to Nature* which certainly helped spread Adolf Just's work and also the emerging Naturopathic movement.

What becomes very obvious to me as I peruse the different views of Hydrotherapy presented in the many articles in Lust's publications is the dearth of defining words and terms to describe the physiological impact of Hydrotherapy. Without a viable and consistent lexicon and supporting evidence within the naturopathic community, Hydrotherapy seemed doomed. There is some evidence that a few Naturopaths were keen to elevate the stature of Hydrotherapy and they incorporated language in an effort to convey an exact message. However, this number was not large. So, by not systematically adopting more precision with terminology within Water Cure, the vague generalizations and cumbersome wording inherited from Kneipp's abhorrence of the nefarious German medical system and eschewing of its alienating terminology and jargon would ultimately contribute to the disempowering and exclusion of water as a medical agent, especially for the upcoming Naturopaths. The early Naturopaths may have used hydropathic terminology, but did not systematically strive to establish any reliable standardization to ensure its longevity and to mark its importance within Naturopathy.

The articles included in this book represent many points of view; let us begin with Sebastian Kneipp. In one of the first English articles found in *Amerikanischen Kneipp Blätter*, we learn that the water applications that Kneipp used included: "wet sheet packs, baths, vapors, gushes or douches, ablutions, localized compresses and drinking of water". (Kneipp, 1897, 186) The goal of using water as a therapeutic agent was "to dissolve and to evacuate the morbid matter and to strengthen the [body]". (Kneipp, 1897, 186) Kneipp's simplistic definition of the actions of water applications is consistent among his writings and of those written by his naturopathic followers. The signature features characterizing Kneipp treatments from others were the *brevity* of a cold water treatment, and not using a towel to dry afterwards. "The not-wiping helps to [establish] the most regular, most equal and most speedy return of natural warmth." (Kneipp, 1897, 187)

Although, "hardening", the process of exposing the body to cold applications in pursuit of strengthening the body, was associated with Kneipp in the Lust publications, I have found the use of the word, "hardening" used also by Priessnitz and his colleagues. A few of the treatments used by Kneipp to harden patients included walking or treading in cold water and/or snow. "The regular duration of such a walk in the snow is three to four minutes." (Kneipp, 1897, 279) Emphasis was put on *constant* movement when either walking in snow or in cold water.

Kneipp passed June 17th, 1897, and prior to his death, he had a succession plan in place to ensure the survival of the healing "Kurhaus" in Wörishofen. "The Order of the Brothers of St. John, who had many hospitals in Europe, accepted the offer to continue [Kneipp's water] cure." (Lust, 1897, 281) A young man, Prior Reile, who studied with Kneipp for several years, assumed the duty to continue Kneipp's work. Two medical doctors, Drs. Mahr and Albert Baumgarten also conducted their Hydrotherapy practice in W"rishofen. Despite the passing of Kneipp, people continued to flock to the Kurhaus for Kneipp treatments. There would be at any one time, over 2,500 patients receiving Water Cures. (Lust, 1897, 281)

The Kneipp version of the wet sheet is quite different from the wet sheet wrap conceived by Priessnitz. Kneipp adopted the wet sheet and had three versions which involved covering the patient with a wet sheet or having the patient lie on a wet sheet or both, being covered and lying on top of the wet sheet. The key point to the wet sheet was the number of times that the "coarse piece of linen would be folded; that is, 3, 4, 6, 8, or 10 times". (Kneipp, 1897, 310) Once the wet sheet was applied, then "a woolen blanket or a piece of linen doubled two or three times is laid upon it, in order to close the wet covering tightly and to thoroughly prevent the entering of the air." (Kneipp, 1897, 310)

Kneipp did not deny that he used the coldest of cold waters for his water applications, but never did he condone the use of ice cloths or ice bags directly on the body. He emphatically cautioned, "I repeat again that I oppose absolutely any application of ice, and I assert, on the contrary, that water applied in the right way, is to soften and to extinguish any heat, even the most violent in whatever part or organ of the body it may be raging." (Kneipp, 1898, 126) Kneipp also criticized the frequent practice of blood-letting which was 'utterly against God's eminent design'. He writes, "By every loss of blood, whether it be caused by a fall, an accident, or by bleeding, leeches, or scarifying, a particle or part of this stock of blood, of this essence of life, is lost and in the same measure the body's life is shortened." (Kneipp, 1898, 126)

Kneipp's books offered easy, understandable instruction on how to administer the simple water applications that he used in his *Kurhaus*. Throughout *Hydrotherapy in Naturopathic Medicine,* we encounter different methods to use water with instructions and an explanation for its benefits. Foot baths were very popular and were used concomitantly with the other water applications. Kneipp used both cold water and warm water. Kneipp was very clear that warm water was never used on its own, but with the addition of herbal decoctions and infusions, such as salt, wood ashes, hay flowers, oat straw, and malt in the warm or hot baths. Hay flowers, discovered by Kneipp, were the plant materials found at the bottom of a hay stack. Kneipp used hay flower infusions in warm foot baths to aid in evacuating waste matter. Salt and wood ashes, mixed together were used for weak and nervous patients, while warm oat straw decoctions were "unsurpassed dissolving every possible callous of the feet". (Kneipp, 1898, 137)

Kneipp liked the cold foot bath to help patients unable to sleep. He explains, "In diseases, the cold foot bath serves principally for leading the blood drawn from the head and chest." (Kneipp, 1898, 137)

Warm baths were also endorsed by Kneipp with one important difference: after a warm bath, a short one minute cold bath followed. A variation of this bath took 33 minutes, beginning with a warm bath of ten minutes duration, followed with one minute of cold bath and this cycle was repeated three times. One of the principle rules underlying Kneipp water treatments is that warm water was always followed with subsequent cold water applications.

By 1898, Kneipp's reach around the world was still evident with the numerous Water Cure establishments even a year after his death. Dr. A. N. Tally, M.D., contributed two articles for Lust's publications on "Kneipp Cure Institutes in America". Tally lists 13 different conditions that Hydrotherapy successfully treated. Europe had had a long tradition of two weeks or longer sojourns at Water Cure facilities. Tally encouraged the American readers of Lust's magazine to consider spending two or three weeks each year in one of these Kneipp facilities for detoxification and hardening rather than at the costly summer resorts. (Tally, 1898, 227)

One such place where people could obtain the full line of Kneipp water treatments was just 30 miles from New York City, at the Bellevue Sanitarium in Butler, New Jersey. Louisa Stroebele, the proprietress of this 60 acre oasis of natural beauty, had employed Benedict Lust as the Bellevue's Hydropathic Physician. The Bellevue was the perfect place to escape the hustle and bustle of city life. "Bellevue offers the advantage of having an open air swimming [pool] on its own grounds, Turkish-Russian baths in the building, and air and sun baths in tents specially arranged for the purpose." (Stroebele, 1899, 141) Air and sun baths were popularized by Arnold Rikli which we know as 'sun bathing' to acquire a sun tan.

When beginning his publications, Lust's primary objective was to further Kneipp's teachings in America. Most Americans associated Kneipp with people walking on wet grass in Central Park. To explain more fully Kneipp's work and to set the record straight, Lust would begin writing his own articles, rather than relying upon Kneipp's books for content for his publications. In 1900, Lust began publishing an English edition of his German magazine, *Amerikanischen Kneipp Blätter* and renamed it, *The Kneipp Water Cure Monthly.*

It seems fitting that Lust would begin his first English issue with his article on Kneipp's signature water application, the gush or *güsse*. Kneipp used a simple garden watering can to administer a steady stream of water that would flow like a sheet of glass over the skin. He created a gush for every part of the body including the full body gush and the most complicated of gushes: the lightening gush which used pressurized water. Lust essentially re-iterates Kneipp when listing the purpose of all of the gushes: to "dissolve morbid matter in the blood, evacuate what is dissolved, make the cleansed blood circulate [correctly] and harden and strengthen the enfeebled organism". (Lust, 1900, 7)

To really appreciate the value and the various uses of the knee gush, reading some of the treatment plans is most revealing. The best place to view these was in a new monthly column, "Hydropathic Medical Advisor" offering free hydropathic advice to the readers of *The Kneipp Water Cure Monthly* which Lust began in 1900. Its author was a young man, Ludwig Staden, an Hygienic Physician or 'Naturarzt'. In the debut issue, Staden received two letters from readers inquiring about asthma and headaches. His reply is revealing and comprehensive. Staden provides a hydrotherapy treatment plan indicating the frequency and duration of each of the water applications, along with dietary recommendations. For the asthma case, Staden prescribes cold sponge bath every morning followed with a friction rub. Then, he outlines a routine of various treatments that include bed steam baths, knee gush or douche, back and upper douches, alternate hot and cold foot baths, enemas, hot chest compresses, and alternate hot and cold baths for the hands. (Staden, 1900, 14) The knee gush was usually the first gush administered to a patient before using the larger gushes, such as the back or upper gushes.

Benedict Lust provided ample space in his magazine for the different kinds of water therapies in the first two years of his English publications (1900-1901). In the March 1990 issue, for example, Lust writes about the Spanish mantle, the half bath and vapor foot bath. The striking difference between Lust's articles and those he previously published is that we can see that he has gained much confidence using Hydrotherapies and is now adding his voice to his writings. Although the Kneipp excerpts still continue to be seen, there is distinctly a diminishing Kneipp presence.

The Spanish mantle consisted of a long shirt made of coarse linen that was dipped in cold water and wrung out. It was a patient-friendly application that resembled very much the wet sheet wrap. "The bed must be prepared beforehand. Woolen blankets are spread over it in such a way that the patient may lie down on them. He is then [snuggly] wrapped in the blankets." (Lust, 1900, 36)   The Spanish mantle helped eliminate morbid matter which it did superbly. "Father Kneipp experienced cases in which the white linen of the mantle seemed to be dyed yellow." (Lust, 1900, 37)

The half bath was taken in a bath tub with the water level reaching the patient's umbilicus when seated in the bath tub. "Of course, only cold water is used." (Lust, 1900, 37) The half bath was an excellent bath to initiate patients unaccustomed to cold water, before being introduced to the cold full bath. The half bath was also combined with other water therapies depending upon the disease being treated.

The vapor foot bath was used for all types of foot problems. The materials needed were a small tub for hot water, a chair for the patient to sit on, and a blanket to retain the steam. The feet rested on a plank placed on the tub. One important caveat regarding any kind of vapor bath: "the vapor bath must always be followed by a cooling application which has to extend over all parts which perspired." (Lust, 1900, 38)

In a two part series, Lust takes the pulse of the natural healing community in America and presents a survey of the various clubs, societies and associations related to Kneipp. Lust jokes: "Whenever a few Kneippians meet, a society is soon founded." (Lust, 1900, 55) In the second part, Lust lists the major sanitariums, clinics and water cure establishments. Many of these were key advertisers in Lust's publications and from these, a core group would eventually become a catalyst creating the next phase of natural healing in America. Viewing the advertisements placed in this article, "Natural Healing in America, Part II", we can catch a glimpse of the who's who of Hydrotherapy in Eastern America. For example, people such as Elsie Amend provided Kneippian treatments in New York City; Carola and Ludwig Staden operated Brooklyn's first Light and Water Cure Sanitarium; F. W. Rittmeier offered a whole gamut of therapies from Kneipp, Priessnitz and Louis Kuhne at his Water Cure Institute on East 82nd, one street from John Scheel's clinic. Some of these advertisers would form the core group who would in September, 1901 establish the first Naturopathic Society of New York.

John H. Scheel operated a sanitarium, the *Badekur,* not far from Lust's office. Scheel would be the first to coin the word, "Naturopathy" which would become the new branding for Hydrotherapy. Scheel's motto: "Study everything, keep the best and use it in the interest of suffering humanity." (Lust, 190, 79)

Kneipp's influence in the 19th and early 20th century on natural healing is quite understandable when we realize that his book, "*My Water Cure,*" was translated into 14 languages and was sold in every country. It was

published for the first time in 1886 and since then has had 73 [editions]".
(Lust, 1900, 67) No wonder Kneipp had become a household name at
the end of the 19th century. Lust had the perfect branding vehicle in his
own publication to promote and sell not only the books of Kneipp, but
also all sorts of health products for Americans to experience the Kneipp
Water Cure.

Kneipp's domination in *The Kneipp Water Cure Monthly* would continue for a very long time but not without some gentle modifications. For
example, in the October, 1900 issue, Lust published a letter to the editor
from an English Hydropath, Richard Metcalfe, who had over 40 years of
practice under his belt. In a fatherly and paternalistic manner, Metcalfe
sent to Lust a list of suggestions for his magazine. Acting with gracious
kindness, Metcalfe's letter is an offering of mentoring to young Lust. Metcalfe writes, "First, I should be careful in not making the Journal too much
of Father Kneipp's Water Cure; admit articles of every description bearing
upon hygienic remedial measures." (Metcalfe, 1900, 186) He also suggests that Lust include submissions on electricity and massage, exercise,
diet and the craze of air cure. Metcalfe's counsel would manifest over the
years and we witness an expansion of health topics with new therapies
replacing the water emptied from the Kneippian watering can.

August Reinhold's eclectic offerings from his Institute for Water Cure
at Lexington Avenue, New York City illustrated the trend of adopting a
wide variety of therapeutics to which Metcalfe alluded. Reinhold recommends a booklist of authors that include Russell Trall, Sebastian Kneipp,
Louis Kuhne and Friedrich Bilz. He credits "Vincent Priessnitz in the
beginning [of the 19th] century [with demonstrating] the curability of all
disease by plain water." (Reinhold, 1900, 206) What concerned Reinhold was the contempt of a medical fraternity towards Hydrotherapy.
He writes: "Even today the medical doctors selfishly try to suppress [the
methods of Kneipp and Kuhne] by sneering at it and calling it a humbug."
(Reinhold, 1900, 206)

As we saw earlier, Lust added a feature to his magazine in an attempt
to attract more readers by the inclusion of a free advice column. In 1901,
Staden's column was renamed to "Naturopathic Advice" and space allotted to it increased substantially. Rather than answer two or three letters,
as he did in 1900, Staden had tripled the number of letters in his advice
column. While the letters published in *The Kneipp Water Cure* offered
free advice, the demand for the free advice exceeded the allotted space,
generating an advice-for-fee service. At the bottom of the page appears,
"To whom it may concern. Patients who desire advice by mail have to
send $2 in advance for first letter, $1 for any additional service. Otherwise, no answer in future." (Staden, 1901, 170) Letters were fielded from
California to Illinois, to the eastern States. The gamut of queries included

sciatica, cold feet, appendicitis, enlarged tonsils, hay fever, skin eruptions, fatigue, indigestion, etc. His advice column illustrates the versatility of the various hydrotherapies and also leads us to an encyclopedic work by Friedrich Bilz (1842-1922).

The therapies and protocols used by Staden in his advice column followed similar protocols found in Bilz' books, *The Natural Method of Healing*, (1898), a two volume set expounding upon Kneipp's water cure methods. Bilz' 2 volume set contained 2065 pages with every page packed with detail and invaluable information for any Hydrotherapist. Bilz' books are a testament to the success and expansive reach of Hydrotherapy.

In the article, "The Kneipp Cure", Bilz gives an account of Kneipp's life and credits Kneipp's work in Water Cure as a revival of water as a healing agent. Bilz defines terms that are found throughout Lust's publications writing: "The expression, "The Kneipp Cure," refers to the curative system carried out by Father Kneipp at Wörishofen, in Bavaria." (Bilz, 1901, 211) The "Natural Method of Healing", the name of his book, also became associated with his method of using water and herbs. Bilz adopted most of Kneipp's methodology and expounded upon it while creating his own. Whenever, "Natural Method of Healing" is referred to in the early literature, it is an unspoken understanding that the author is referencing Friedrich Bilz' work.

Bilz did not sever his ties with Kneipp, but instead continuously paid homage by writing about the merits of Kneipp's work. He listed the fundamental rules of Kneipp cure to include shorter applications; the colder the water, the shorter the application; no use of towels to dry off; observe the signs of a reaction to monitor treatment. (Bilz, 1901, 212-213)

When Richard Metcalfe sent Lust his letter of guidance, he also sent Lust some of his personal writings to be used in any of Lust's magazine at his discretion. Lust did publish an article on "Vincent Priessnitz" which was an historical overview of Hydrotherapy from the ages from Hippocrates through to the 18th century. Metcalfe presents an European perspective of authors and titles of their books which adds to the richness of water as a therapy. Metcalfe had spent much time at Gräefenberg and even wrote a biography of Vincent Priessnitz, entitled *Vincent Priessnitz, the Founder of Hydrotherapy* (1898). Despite the number of doctors who wrote books on Hydrotherapy, Metcalfe credits Priessnitz as being the one person who truly understood the power of water. He writes: "It remained for one greater and more far-sighted to grasp at once the whole secret of water treatment, and to develop and systematize it in one short lifetime. That man was Vincent Priessnitz." (Metcalfe, 1901, 20)

Not all water treatments employed the coldest of waters. *Fomentations* were also used and were defined by Lust as "a simple and effective method of applying moist heat to any part of the body by means of flannel wrung out of boiling water, milk, or any medicated hot fluid". (Lust, 1901, 241) A guiding tip for fomentations was that they "ought to be applied as hot as the skin can bear, and although moist, the hot liquid should be thoroughly squeezed out of the flannel applied to the skin". (Lust, 1901, 241)

Of note is that the "temperature" viewed by the pioneers of Hydrotherapy established classifications that do not jive with our current concepts of hot and cold. For example, warm water at 90° F/32° C may for many of us feel actually tepid or cold. In the next article, "Baths and the Water Cure", Lust lays down some guidelines for temperatures used in water therapies. Lust classifies bath temperatures as follows: "The temperature of a cold bath may be from 33° to 70° F/0.5° to 21° C; a tepid bath from 80° to 96° F/27° to 36°; a hot bath from 100° to 112° F/38° to 44° C." (Lust, 1901, 241) He adds when cold baths are useful: "Cold baths are harmful when the powers of the body are too languid to bring on a reaction, but beneficial in cases of nervousness or general debility." (Lust, 1901, 241) In this early article in 1901, Lust favours the use of cold water. In time, we will see Lust warm up to the idea of using hot water in Hydrotherapy. But by this point, he had very little good to say about hot water. His caution to his readers: "Excessive use of the hot bath in any form is bad, as it tends to make the skin dry, harsh, and scaly, by diluting the secretions of the sebaceous glands, the oil of which is intended by Nature to keep the skin smooth, glossy, and soft." (Lust, 1901, 241) As we continue to read, though, we will discover that Lust's disdain for hot water did not last long.

Another guide to help us understand the temperature scale for the water therapies is given by Bilz who uses very specific temperatures for different conditions. In his article, "Bad Health", we are exposed to Bilz through the lens of "Natural Method of Healing". He lists various conditions and provides concise and clear instruction on how to use water to heal. For example, when treating a fever, he writes, "For it is an inviolable principle, when combating disease, not to apply treatment to a single part of the body only, but at the same time to the whole of it." (Bilz, 1901, 288) This article is a mouth-watering preview for the next book in the Hevert Collection, *Clinical Pearls in Naturopathic Medicine*. This article is worthy of your attention and I am sure you will want to make notes of Bilz' protocols for fever, violent abdominal pain, chronic constipation, headaches, etc.

While Bilz complied with many of Kneipp's water therapies, there is one man whose contributions to natural healing would follow another drum beat and echo across oceans and continents. Adolf Just published

Return to Nature (1896) which would become a guiding light and permeate the very core of Naturopathy. I am smitten with Just and his insights into the healing power of Nature. He writes, "Since I look only to Nature when I want to know the right thing to do for my health and my well-being, I always find that everything that I have recognized as strictly natural, that is, as thoroughly in the spirit of Nature, has on trial always proved itself to be the right thing entirely." (Just, 1901, 315) Nature is the guide, the message, and the Vis to the healing process.

The "natural bath" was the precious gift that Just left to us. In my early days of researching the Lust publications, I often encountered the term, "natural bath" and it slipped off the page as if I would of course know what a natural bath was except that I had no idea whatsoever. Taking a natural bath is a life changing and indelible experience that changes us always for the good. My first time having a natural bath was at Emanuel Felke's healing sanitarium in Bad Sobernheim, Germany. It is impossible to communicate the power of this one or two minute bath. After taking just only two of these baths over a period of two mornings, I felt like I had shed ten years-worth of stress and fatigue. I devoutly take my daily natural bath every morning, rain or shine. Adolf Just says, "Let no one say that he does not need the natural bath, because he is well. For it is plainly not the first intention of Nature to cure diseases by the bath, but rather to keep her creatures well, bright and happy." (Just, 1901, 316)

Lust abided the advice of Richard Metcalfe and brought many different subjects into his publications. In 1902, he changed the name of his magazine from *The Kneipp Water Cure Monthly* to *The Naturopath and Herald of Health*. We already saw a premonition that change was afoot in the 1900 December issue with an advertisement in which Lust listed his professional title as "Naturopathic Physician". It would take another full year before the metamorphosis of the Kneipp Water Cure to a broader and more inclusive healing paradigm would occur. With the new name of the health magazine, Lust was like a boy in a candy store: so many candies and what to choose? In any case, it is important to note that the inclusion of Naturopath in the name of the new magazine signaled that change was inevitable.

Periodically, Lust would publish a short excerpt from one of Kneipp's books or even borrow heavily from Kneipp. In the December issue, 1902, Lust wrote on the neck compress using much of his material from Kneipp. Kneipp applied the neck compress and never left it on for any length of time. Lust writes, "If you want cold to diminish heat, then you must renew your bandage every quarter of an hour and continue it for an hour or an hour and a half." (Lust, 1902, 493) Although the neck compress was an excellent means to cure a sore throat, leaving the throat compress in place for a long period was not wise, often causing more inflammation rather than less. Lust clarifies, "The neck bandage can and does draw the blood from the head to the throat, but it must not stay there, and the only way of getting rid of what has been drawn into it is by constantly renewing the bandage." (Lust, 1902, 493) Sometimes, distal compresses to relieve throat inflammation were favoured and more indicated than local throat compresses. Lust writes, "It would be still better to lay a six-fold cloth on the stomach which would rapidly develop increased warmth [and] so relieve the inflammation in the throat." (Lust, 1902, 493)

When Sebastian Kneipp passed away, Dr. Alfred Baumgarten became an important link in the Kneipp lineage. Fastidious in his research to corroborate Kneipp's observations with a scientific rigor, Baumgarten published *Die Kneipp'sche Hydrotherapie* (1909). In the article, "Drinking Cold Water", Baumgarten defends his beloved teacher's critics who accused Kneipp of merely laying on of hands or being an imposing personality and dismissing water as simply humbug. To these, Baumgarten says, "No man has ever been more systematic in his cold water application than Father Kneipp." (Baumgarten, 1903, 49) Baumgarten, having spent years studying with Kneipp, had developed a passion to understanding Water Cure. He explains the healing crisis during a water treatment: "In the first place severe colds, then diarrhea which appears suddenly after going over to symptoms of cholera. ... The symptom most in evidence, however, is insomnia." (Baumgarten, 1903, 50)

In a second article, "Water Applications", Baumgarten explains the importance of knowing how to interpret the effects of cold water seen on the skin and to correlate the reactions internally. Baumgarten spent years conducting experiments to confirm the physiological changes in the body during Hydrotherapy. The skin gives clues as to what is occurring internally. When cold is applied externally, the first response [or the primary reaction] is that the skin changes colour. In the case of Caucasians, there is a blanching or paleness that occurs almost immediately. *

When the skin blanches or the physiological response in the superficial blood vessels is a spasm or a constriction forcing the blood to the interior of the body. Baumgarten writes, "This spasm generally lasts but a short time, some 70 to 80 seconds according to the state and condition of the individual. Now then, after these 70 to 80 seconds have passed, these

---

*In darker skin, these changes and skin reactions are less perceptible. With the help of colleagues at NUNM, Dr. John Brons and NUNM students, principally Khaleed Alston (NUNM 2020), conducted a well-designed but small study of the changes in skin in people of colour in reaction to cold water applications. The primary or blanching process is not as distinctive as the secondary reaction where a reddening of the skin is clearly visible regardless of skin color. —Ed.

small capillary blood vessels, which before had contracted, again expand and the blood rushes to the surface."* (Baumgarten, 1903, 124)

Baumgarten is describing the physiological primary and secondary reactions that occur in the capillaries. The blanching is the primary reaction, and when the capillaries open up, the secondary reaction includes the return of colour to the skin. This was labelled as the reaction during a water treatment and indicated that the cold water had achieved its goal. Baumgarten comments: "The reaction so much spoken of in the Water Cure is nothing more than a rush of blood to and from the inner organs which in coming to the skin gives it the peculiar red coloration" (Baumgarten, 1903, 125)

Cold water had one significant response on warm bodies that surpassed all of the other effects and that was the movement of blood. Cold water placed on a body would be one of most efficient ways of improving blood circulation. Baumgarten writes,

> The mass of blood rushing and flowing to and from the organs displaces and mingles with greater masses of blood. The larger the displacement and the oftener it occurs, the more improved the circulation in general will be. When the heart has attained that condition in which it is able to supply with blood every part of the body from extremity to extremity, then we can say that the circulation is perfect. (Baumgarten, 1903, 126)

The marvelous benefits of cold water therapies were most convincing, especially to Baumgarten who saw first-hand how quickly patients restored their health. Kneipp's douche was an example "that even the weakest and most delicate can undergo treatment, and that we no longer need to call the Water Cure a "horse-cure" when we can achieve such great results with the most simple means". (Baumgarten, 1903, 184) He cites an example of the arm douche: "Under personal observation, study and experiments, I have found the arm douche to be very efficacious for heart failure." (Baumgarten, 1903, 184)

The simplicity of water can cause some to think that water applications can do no harm. Baumgarten counters:

> On the first glance, Water Cure seems very simple and many are tempted to boast that they can apply the water treatment as well and efficiently as the next man. This is a mistake. The order of the various applications is a potent factor and requires a close study and years of experience to be able to adopt them to individual cases. (Baumgarten, 1903, 184)

---

*What Baumgarten and fellow Hydrotherapists described as the reaction would be again labelled as the *Lewis or hunting reaction*, named after Thomas Lewis who in 1930, noted the alternation of vasoconstriction and vasodilation in extremities exposed to cold.

Lust concurs with Baumgarten and makes a list of diseases for which caution is paramount when treating with Hydrotherapy. Lust also recognized the limitations of water; he writes: "Let this be carefully noted, and let it not be believed that every disease can be cured by water, or only by water." (Lust, 1903, 286) In order that Water Cure be successful, the patient must be taken into account. "Water Cure unmitigatedly demands a robust constitution and a fairly vital condition. Water Cure modified appeals with infinite gentleness to the delicate child and the sensitive woman." (Lust, 1903, 286)

The use of cold applications to 'harden' the constitution and increase the body's resistance to cold was central to early naturopathic care. "Hardening", or making the body healthier and more resilient, was equivalent to preventative care. The early Naturopath believed fervently that hardening was one of the most important aids to health and strength because the body is able to resist injurious influences. In his article, "Means of Hardening for Children and Adults", Lust presents all of Kneipp's therapies as related to their purpose. For instance, vapors and warm baths dissolved morbid matter and the different compresses and bandages evacuated the dissolved morbid matter. The distinction between a compress and a bandage is that the compress is laid on a part of the body and a bandage is wrapped around the body or body part.

Hardening applications for blood circulation included showers, douches, gushes, cold affusions and baths. (Lust, 1903, 313-321) Another famous Kneipp hardening method is walking barefoot on wet grass or stone pavement, in the snow or in cold water. Lust's article is comprehensive and provides instructions and suggestions for modifications for all of Kneipp's water applications.

Although water may seem easy and completely harmless, Lust provides a list of 13 suggestions to make water safe and to prevent mistakes. His first suggestion is repeated by other authors: "Cold water should never touch cold flesh." (Lust, 1904, 4) Another principle with Hydrotherapy is that if warm water is used, cold water must end the treatment. Lust spends time elaborating on the importance of body warmth and provides another list of how to exercise correctly. This article is noteworthy because there is recognition of the importance of physical exercise which Lust called "Kinesitherapy" [sic] and included it as "the third factor in natural healing". (Lust, 1904, 6)

Kneipp was most famous for a small water application, the knee gush or knee douche. Baumgarten asks the obvious question, "Many will ask, only a knee douche? What effect can a knee douche have? I want to say right here that the knee douche is as good in its place as any of the larger applications, and to despise it evidences a lack of insight and appreciation for what it has done to others." (Baumgarten, 1904, 7) The maxim, "the bigger, the better", does not apply to Hydrotherapy. The knee gush is a perfect example of a small water application that has tremendous benefits.

The characteristic of a knee douche in Baumgarten's words is as follows: "An application of cold flowering water from the kneecap to the feet, applied in such a manner as to form a flowing sheet of water over the whole lower leg." (Baumgarten, 1904, 7) He continues, "The water must be applied evenly until, after sixty or one hundred seconds, the reaction will set in." (Baumgarten, 1904, 7) The reaction of the reddening of the skin is a clear indication that the knee gush is finished. The knee gush improves circulation and is a refreshing and strengthening tonic, relieves fatigue, nervousness, gout, rheumatism, etc. Lust cites the knee gush for insomnia. He writes, "[The knee gush] is very useful for drawing the blood from the head and strengthening nervous patients; also to induce sleep in cases of insomnia." (Lust, 1904, 147-148)

The knee gush, as small as it is, is not for the faint of heart, for it can be so intense that "you will find in the words of Kneipp that he repeatedly refers to the knee douche and states how men, strong, robust, have crouched like children, and have yelled when it was applied". (Baumgarten, 1904, 8) It is important to give attention to these small, innocuous water applications, because they are much more powerful than meets the eye.

Kneipp's fame spread worldwide and those who sought out his water therapies in desperation were given a second chance. As indicated earlier, Benedict Lust was such a person who at "22 years of age, went back to Germany to die of consumption, given up by all the medical men who had had anything to do with him". (Lust, 1904, 145) After eight months at Wörishofen, Lust was a picture of perfect health. In a lecture given in New York City, Lust loved to share stories of Kneipp. He described Kneipp as "a man of very simple life, but [who] possessed a large share of personal magnetism that created confidence and love and made people willing to obey him promptly and unquestioningly". (Lust, 1904, 145)

The literature shows that, not surprisingly, questions popped up regarding the credibility and the methodology of Kneipp's Hydrotherapy. For example, we are familiar with 'hormesis' in Naturopathy, meaning that small doses are stimulants, while large doses are either toxic or suppressive. In 1905, the question, "Does Hydrotherapy Require Reform?" was posed to address how to implement Hydrotherapy in line with the Arndt-Schultz law which was based upon the work of Professors Arndt and Schultz of Greifswald who conducted experimentation on dosage in 1888. Lust points out: "In Water Cure, it is also better to remain at slight and medium strong stimulants, in preference to more strong ones." (Lust,

1905, 70) Lust compares the short cold water gushes used by Kneipp with the long exposures to cold water advocated by the Priessnitz followers. In some ways, this article on the Arndt-Schultz exemplifies the methods used by Kneipp because of his very short cold water applications. The take away message is "It must be made a principle that a thorough reaction must take place before a new application is given; but this reaction does not come as soon as we are often apt to think it does." (Lust, 1905, 71)

Throughout Lust's publications, one comes to the realization that most of the authors of the articles on Hydrotherapy are essentially adherents of Kneipp. Nevertheless, it is interesting to note the slight variations from author to author when describing a particular water application. T. Hartmann is definitely a Kneippian disciple. He uses the same coarse linen compresses and the same hay flower concoctions that Kneipp used and reiterates Kneipp's logic. For example, in "The Compresses", Hartmann says, "In the case of hay flower packs, I make an exception because these are dissolving. I apply them for swollen hands and feet, or I make these packs of oat straw which always dissolve the most obdurate gouty swelling." (Hartmann, 1905, 372) The benefit of adding new voices to the dialogue of Hydrotherapy is that we learn more. Hartmann reveals why vinegar is so useful in the compresses: "Packs in which salt water or vinegar is used also produce good effect; they open the pores and produce warmth very quickly. There is scarcely any difference at all between vinegar or salt water." (Hartmann, 1905, 373)

In Hartmann's article, we can learn more about the different compresses and their uses. One compress is worth taking note of, the short pack or the short bandage. The short pack or bandage is similar to the wet sheet wrap except that a person can easily apply this pack on his or her own.

> The short pack begins under the arm, and reaches to the knees. Over the wet sheet a dry one is put and then the woolen blanket. … The dampness of the wet sheet passes over to the dry one; the morbid matter of the body is absorbed by the wet cloth, which has, then the same effect as a compound lead plaster. (Hartmann, 1905, 374)

The compound "lead" plaster that Hartmann is referring to is worrying. It is my hope that lead did not mean *plumbum*, but I fear it well may have. Hartmann also cites elsewhere the "pitch plaster", though, which was most likely a common treatment for the removal of slivers. There is whole discussion on sauerkraut as medicine and Hartmann shares the uses of a sauerkraut poultice:

Externally, sauerkraut can be usefully applied as a poultice, particularly for fresh wounds, old ulcerating cancers, inflammation, injuries, headaches and lumbago, as also for contusions and certain ear troubles. Applied in this way, it hastens the bringing of an ulcer to a head, reducing the pain during this time. (Hartmann, 1905, 375)

Kneipp's chief rationale for Hydrotherapy was purifying the blood. In an article by Lust, "The Effect of Kneipp's Treatment on Diseases", the quality of blood was discussed. There are many references in the Lust publications that speak of the supreme importance of oxygen; the more, the better. Air baths and skin hygiene spoke of the skin's ability to inhale oxygen to increase the body's oxygen levels. Lust attributes Kneipp's water treatments to affect the inhaling of the skin by increasing the blood circulation of the capillaries. Lust's explanation is plausible: "The more blood-waves [capillaries] appear on the surface of the skin, the more oxygen is imparted to the blood." (Lust, 1906, 74) However, what is lacking in Lust's writing is a scientific foundation to make his statement hold water, so to speak. It is true that when cold water is applied to the skin, that the blood circulation is put into motion; however, increasing oxygen via the skin requires a few steps that are missing in Lust's writings.

Lust spends a paragraph on the importance of Kneipp's water treatments on the blood and he finishes his article on how to use water applications for the treatment of an ulcer, fever, influenza and rheumatism. The cases that Lust presents are worthy of our attention because with simply using water, his patients were cured. "Kneipp's ablutions always produce soothing effects. The best illustration of this statement is that of acute articular rheumatism. When symptoms of typical swelling, and flush of the right knee joint, accompanied with a great deal of pain and high fever became apparent, I at once take the watering pot and pour ice-cold water over the knee of the patient." (Lust, 1906, 75) The patient cured in four weeks. How often do we hear of patients today ridding themselves of rheumatism in a month with drug therapies? The symptoms are alleviated, but not the disease.

Ablution, the simple washing of the body using a cloth or the hands, had many applications. Lust provides some tips on how to administer an ablution. He prefers using the hands rather than cloths or sponges. He writes, "The washing with the hand has many advantages. The first one is that a pressure is exercised by one human organism on the other; the second is that the humidity to be imparted can be fairly gauged." (Lust, 1907, 261) The time duration of an ablution is crucial. Lust writes, "When the ablution is finished, the patient is not wiped, but a warm shirt is put on and he is lightly covered. All this has to be done in a minute."

(Lust, 1907, 261) If the ablution fails to give "the expected and sooth-ing effect, the ablution has either been made too slow or too late in the evening". (Lust, 1907, 262) Lust provides variations of the ablution for bed-ridden patients, nervous patients and children.

Rules or guiding principles on how to practice using Kneipp's water treatments were the theme of many articles that appeared in Lust's publi-cations. Dr. Bauergmund wrote a list of ten commandments in the article, "How Should Kneipp's Treatment be Taken?" His first predictable rule, "Cold water is only to be applied if the body is warm." (Bauergmund, 1908, 69) Abiding this rule is an absolute necessity if water therapies are to be successful. His second rule: "Before each application of cold water, wet the chest and temples with water." (Bauergmund, 1908, 70) Cold water splashed onto the face initiates the "dive reflex" that causes brady-cardia and slows respiration, a very useful tool if one is faced with some-one panicked or anxious. The rules that Kneipp used were developed by the astute, cumulative, clinical observation of thousands of patients. The scientific language of the physiological and clinical basis for Kneipp's rules would be discovered long after his death.

Kneipp and Priessnitz' water treatments would be carried forward by the medical men who came to study with them. Dr. Bauergmund is a case in point. He was one of the doctors who studied with Kneipp and per-petuated Kneipp's work with his writings. Although water applications were such a good thing, Bauergmund writes that caution must be taken to not go to excess. He follows Kneipp's cue, "'Individualize and avoid excess' must be our motto." (Bauergmund, 1908, 73)

The literature exhibits the growing interest in Lust's publication from medical Hydrotherapists, such as Drs. Baumgarten and Bauergmund whose commitment was to see Kneipp therapies prosper. Another, Dr. L. Winternitz, grapples with the problem that water therapies work, but lack scientific justification. The article, "Is Kneipp's Hydrotherapeutic Treat-ment Unscientific?" addresses some of the opposition that Dr. Winternitz faced with fellow colleagues. The cold water used in Hydrotherapy is not exactly every body's cup of tea, nor does immersing one's self in freez-ing cold water elicit immediate motivation to take the plunge. To coun-ter misconceptions of cold water, Winternitz and others wrote to set the record straight. On the issue of cold versus warmer temperatures used in a tepid bath, he writes,

> Kneipp requires only five to six seconds for his half bath, while a half bath with tepid water requires several minutes to produce reaction, and demands the mechanical procedure of friction after the bath, if the patient is not to leave it in a shiver; whereas the reaction after a Kneipp half bath promptly ensues as soon as the

patient has emerged from it. He who has tried both forms of half bath on his own person, will be sure to prefer Kneipp's, on account of the more lasting reaction. (Winternitz, 1909, 222)

Winternitz provides an explanation of why the body feels warmer after a cold plunge or a cold half bath. "According to physiological laws, the large vessels of the skin contract after every stimulus of cold and all the more energetically, the stronger the sensation and the colder the water applied has been. After a Kneipp half bath, lasting five to ten seconds only, this spasm of the capillaries persists, after the bather has left the tub." (Winternitz, 1909, 222) After a bath, the capillaries vasodilate, bringing a sensation of warmth.

Warm sensations in the body after experiencing cold water applications are predicated on the golden rule: "Never give a cold or cool bath or pack when the patient is not comfortably warm. Warmth must first be restored by exercise, friction or steam bath." (Judd, 1909, 412-413) C. E. Judd reminds us that "the use of water in curing a disease has made for itself a large place in drugless methods of healing". (Judd, 1909, 411) He also reminds us that water can be "misapplied, often irritate the patient and defeat the very purpose intended." (Judd, 1909, 411) When it comes to Hydrotherapy, it is not enough to just know about compresses or baths, nor can we afford to be careless. We need to have a good understanding of our patients. Judd writes, "Persons of low vitality or poor blood cannot respond any too readily to cold water treatment; hence the treatment should be tempered to suit patient and circumstances." (Judd, 1909, 413) Judd offers us invaluable pearls of how to accomplish triumph using Hydrotherapy in acute diseases.

In 1909, Lust republished a chapter from Kneipp's book, *My Will*, on the subject of douches. Originally, gushes *were* synonymous with Kneipp who originated the use of a simple garden watering can to apply a douche. As time passed, the term, 'gush' was discarded and replaced with douche. Lust includes all of the gushes/douches that are in Kneipp's book such as arm, upper, hip, knee, back, full and lightening douches. It is important to know how and why Kneipp used them. A douche is "given either from a hose or a watering can [and] should spread evenly like a sheet over the [skin]". (Kneipp, 1909, 493) For instance, we learn that a hip douche "regulates the blood in the lower part of the body and has great curative power in cases of piles [hemorrhoids]". (Kneipp, 1909, 493) Although, Kneipp was renowned for his freezing cold water applications, he made every effort to shorten the discomfort. Kneipp writes, "My great rule is to treat the system gently, and this is why I prescribe all the douches of the shortest duration." (Kneipp, 1909, 496) Having experienced Kneipp's douches in European spas, my memory is never with the cold water, but with the exhilaration and sense of warmth after the cold douche.

In 1910, Lust published an article on using the cold bath, wet sheet wrap to treat acute diseases such as "simple cold, measles, typhoid fever or small pox". (Lust, 1910, 85) The cold bath was used to lower a fever, but Lust cautions against prolonged cold baths and excessively cold temperatures. Lust also adds, "Do not forget that we can suppress a fever or inflammation just as easily by cold water or ice bags as by drugs; we never, under any circumstances, use ice bags or ice water, but only water of natural temperature, as it comes from the well or tap." (Lust, 1910, 85) Lust also gives a good description of how to administer a wet sheet wrap and a short bandage.

Following Lust's article on baths and wraps, Robert Biéri, a French Hydrotherapist and a student of the famous Wilhelm Winternitz, attempts to further elaborate on the properties of water. One significant contribution that Biéri makes is that he is including hydropathic terms that were used to denote certain physiological mechanisms. Words, such as revulsion and derivation were common terms used by medical doctors who specialized in Hydrotherapy to describe the movement of blood in response to water. Sadly, these terms were not widely adopted by the early Naturopaths and perhaps, may explain why Hydrotherapy was too easy to discard when the field of nutraceuticals and new modalities showed up on the health scene. For example, Biéri outlines the therapeutic effects using the various hydrotherapies. He notes, "It is requisite before making an appeal to [Hydrotherapy applications] to know to what ailments they should be applied." (Biéri, 1910, 519) When we know the actions of water, we then know for what conditions certain water applications can be best used.

John Leupke, M.D. adds to this discussion of knowing how to use water judiciously commenting, "All cold water procedures must be adapted to the constitution of the individual, his or her age, vitality, surroundings, etc." (Leupke, 1911, 103) Leupke speaks about the value of warm and hot baths to "promote the cutaneous circulation of the blood". (Leupke, 1911, 104) We begin to see a shifting of values among the Hydrotherapists in regards to cold and hot water. Until now, Kneipp's and Priessnitz' beloved cold water treatments had been untouched, unmarred by the notion of hot water.

To witness the gradual undoing of cold water in Hydrotherapy, we can understand Louisa Lust's inclusion of herbal baths as a treatment that Kneipp himself would find useful and very helpful. Louisa used "sage, hay flower, oak bark, pine needles, fenugreek, yarrow, etc.," in hot baths for nervous patients. (Lust, 1911, 231) However, she also prescribed cold wet sheet wraps and also hot wet sheet wraps in order to "loosen up waste matter". (Lust, 1911, 231) Cold wet sheet wraps were always best for reducing fevers. Where there is no deviation from Kneipp is that every hot water treatment ends with a cold water application.

Vinegar, first popularized by Father Kneipp in connection with fevers, was "mixed with cold water, as is done with the vinegar washings, vinegar compressions, clay bandages, etc. of Kneipp." (Habel, 1911, 295) Vinegar applied to the body externally had a cooling effect due to its evaporation and "from the skin, [it] extracts some warmth of the skin and causes by it a local irrational which is the stronger, the quicker the evaporation sets in." (Habel, 1911, 295)

A method to cause sweating in the body was using the heat from freshly mown grass after it is stored in bags. F. Buttgenbach presented this sweating bath and he seemed to be very charmed by its effectiveness. Here are his instructions: "Secure some freshly mown grass from lawns or back yards ... fill it into sacks so it will get quickly self-heated. While the process is going on, make a box about 10 to 12 inches deep and as long and wide as necessary for the perspective person to lie comfortable in." (Buttgenbach, 1912, 522) He continues,

> If the grass is now hot enough to suit you, put a layer, six to eight inches, of it in the box, undress yourself and wash the whole body with water mixed with good cider vinegar (about one-half pint of cold water and one-half teacup of vinegar), then lay down in the box, cover yourself up to the neck with the grass, call somebody else to cover your arms (insulated from the body) tight and good. (Buttgenbach, 1912, 522)

This sweating bath was claimed by Buttgenbach as one of the best ways of getting rid of morbid matter.

Since Kneipp was the man who treated and cured Benedict Lust and Henry Lindlahr, much of the Lust journal focused on Kneipp therapeutics. Vincent Priessnitz died in 1851 and was long gone when Naturopathy was emerging. So, it is a surprise to see Lust write a favourable article depicting Priessnitz' most recognized water application, the abdominal bandage rather than crediting Kneipp directly. In any case, Naturopaths viewed the seat of disease beginning in the abdomen and so the abdominal bandage was most often included in treatment plans. Kneipp applied a compress to the abdomen, whereas Priessnitz wrapped up the abdomen using an inner wet wrap with an outer dry cloth.

Lust provides the instructions for the Priessnitz abdominal bandage. "The internal bandage should be about 7 or 8 inches wide and long enough to reach around the whole abdomen, double on the front, and that means the two ends form a double cover on the stomach part and single on the back." (Lust, 1913, 617)   Much like the wet sheet wrap, the outer dry woolen bandage is wrapped snuggly around the wet cloth.

No book on naturopathic Hydrotherapy would be complete without something about the virtues of wet socks. Wet socks are as naturopathic as you can get. We know that wet socks lower fevers, help with insomnia, warm cold feet, alleviate headaches, and help with foot pains. Lust wrote a list of nine rules for wet socks. One of his rules: "The socks must be kept on much longer than bandages on the abdomen for they do not become warm as quickly as those bandages" (Lust, 1913, 770)

Oh, if only Dr. Carl Schultz words weren't so true!   Schultz writes:

I am sorry to add that many naturopathic physicians have abandoned Hydrotherapy.   Sometimes the physician has not money enough, or thinks he has not money enough, to equip his treatment rooms with the suitable arrangements and appliances. Expensive equipment is not necessary. (Schultz, 1914, 345)

Schultz made this statement in 1914, and by this time in America, the rage of Kneippism and Water Cure was faltering, at least within the naturopathic ranks. Schultz was a scholar and presented three impressive articles on Hydrotherapy.   One is included in this book and the other two can be found in *Principles in Naturopathic Medicine* (Czeranko, 2014), on pages 262-274. I include this particular article by Schultz because he unravels the issue of temperatures used in the various water applications. He presents excerpts from Simon Baruch (1840-1921) who was a modern day Hydrotherapist, keen to resolve the mysteries of water cure by a thorough scientific inquiry. Please do not bypass Schultz' article; it is most impressive and I cannot begin to capture in a few word his contributions to this book.

Occasionally in Lust's publications an article appeared among the advertisements that were at the back end of the magazine. In "Magnesia Sulphate or Epsom Salts Baths", for example, clear directions are given on how to take an Epsom salt bath. The quantity of salt is much more than we typically use today. In an Epsom salt bath, "from three to five pounds of the Epsom salts, according to the capacity of the tub. Let the patient remain in this from ten to twenty minutes, or even thirty minutes sometimes, with the water warm." (Lust, 1916)   Lust continues, "Then rub the body under the water with a coarse sponge. After five or six minutes repeat this rubbing. Take from fifteen to thirty minutes in all for the tub bath." (Lust, 1916)   The Epsom salt bath was exceptional in dissolving uric acid.

Now, onto the famous sitz bath!   There are two articles: one written by Dr. Carl Strueh and the other by Joseph Hoegen, N.D. Dr. Carl Strueh began his career as a medical doctor who wrote dissertations on surgery and gynecology in Munich, German. He moved to Chicago and took up practice. It did not take him long to become disillusioned with medical practice. He began to advertise in Lust's publication almost at the beginning and he would continue to advertise monthly for decades. Although Strueh's articles are succinct, his clinical pearls are worth noting simply because he speaks from clinical experience in one of America's most successful naturopathic practices of his day. One such gem is the following caution: "People afflicted with arteriosclerosis must be cautious about taking cold sitz baths, as a sudden rush of blood to the head may result in apoplexy." (Strueh, 1915, 215) Another concomitant therapy that the early Naturopaths combined with Hydrotherapy was the use of physical exercise. Strueh's tip is worth heeding in a culture that is so sedentary. He used exercise to help induce the reaction needed for a successful water treatment. He writes, "Outdoor exercise should always be taken after a cold or lukewarm sitz bath, otherwise the desired reaction will not take place." (Strueh, 1915, 215)

The second article on the sitz bath by Joseph Hoegen, N.D. provides additional tips. Hoegen in 1916, was selected by Lust to be an editor for a new column, "Hydrotherapy Department" which specialized in the new innovations in water therapies. The column focused less on Kneippian water methods and instead presented a wider range of Hydrotherapy methods. Lust had not only changed the format of his publication by adding numerous new columns to represent the diversity of the emerging naturopathic profession, but he also modified the old name of the magazine, *The Naturopath and Herald of Health* to *Herald of Health and Naturopath*. In the masthead of "Hydrotherapy Department", we learn that Hoegen practices at 334 Alexander Avenue in New York City.

Hoegen considers the sitz bath as one of the essentials in any home that puts a value on health. It is very helpful to read different accounts of the sitz bath to grasp the subtle nuances of a bath that had been so widespread at one time. Hoegen did not condone long durations such as 15 minute or longer cold sitz baths and from his "experience, one to two minutes is sufficient in all cases when the water is cold". (Hoegen, 1916, 468) He "always used a hot foot bath in connection with the cold sitz bath." (Hoegen, 1916, 468) We also learn about when and when not to use a sitz bath. Although water in the sitz bath covered the lower abdomen and pelvis, and it was used for diseases of the lower pelvis, its capacity to act on the whole body and stimulate the cerebral activity and relieve brain congestion were also well noted by Hoegen. (Hoegen, 1916, 468)

Hoegen is an articulate writer and refreshingly doesn't dominate the column with his writings but rather reaches out to some of the most innovative and scholarly Hydrotherapists. He included several articles by Simon Baruch on the subject of the Nauheim bath. Simon Baruch, M.D. (1840-1921) brought a scholarly rigor to the subject of water therapies and published three valuable books that targeted a taciturn medical profession who responded with little support for water. Baruch had served in the Civil War as a medic and used hydrotherapy successfully in the trenches.

Although, Baruch was not a Naturopath, he was an Hydrotherapist through and through. He campaigned for public bath houses in the State of New York and promoted the carbon dioxide baths at Saratoga Springs. We must be grateful for Baruch's disciplined attention to detail and scientific inquiry. If only more Naturopaths could have followed his lead and written articles on Hydrotherapy with the lexicon of their day!

The Nauheim bath is a carbon dioxide bath and the name "Nauheim" is derived from the mineral spring in Germany where it first originated. The use of carbon dioxide in either a wet or dry bath is now world-wide and its benefits well documented. Simon Baruch did much to popularize the carbon dioxide mineral waters of Saratoga Springs in New York State. His other intention was to simulate a carbon dioxide bath in a medical office so that the Nauheim baths were more available to those who did not have access to natural carbonated waters. In his paper, "The Nauheim Bath", Baruch presents his examination of the research of the physiological effects of carbon dioxide upon the heart and respiration. He collaborated with European doctors and would not hesitate to question their errors.

The analogy of being in a bath tub filled with champagne best characterizes a carbon dioxide bath or Nauheim bath. Baruch describes what the carbon dioxide bubbles impart: "The skin shows decided hyperemia wherever it is in contact with the gas bubbles. Decided warmth is felt, together with a sense of comfort and *bien aise*, that is not felt when plain cold water produces a reaction of redness." (Baruch, 1916, 534) Immersed in a Nauheim bath, the sense of comfort that Baruch refers to is vasodilation of capillaries and an overwhelming feeling of warmth. Using cool Nauheim baths, which subjectively feel warmer than the actual temperature, was useful for water applications that required warmer temperatures of water. In this regards, the Nauheim bath was found to be very beneficial for those suffering from congestive heart disease. In any case, Baruch promoted the Nauheim bath which did take off in America as he had planned.

Today, carbon dioxide baths are used in many countries for the treatment of scleroderma, arthritis, diabetes, and heart diseases such as myocardial infarction and yet in America, it has become obscure and found in the esthetic market to reduce cellulite. However, there was a time in

the early 20th century when the Nauheim bath (also called the efferves-
cent bath) was used in the naturopathic medical offices. Some of the
formulations created to simulate the carbonic acid in water consisted of
caustic chemicals and it is no wonder that the Nauheim bath disappeared
in America.

Hoegen's inclusion of Baruch's writings in *Herald of Health and
Naturopath* shows us how progressive Naturopathy became after just
a few years of their existence. With Hoegen, we see more acceptance
of Hydrotherapy that reaches beyond the Kneipp parameters. We learn
immediately what Hoegen thinks about Hydrotherapy. His passion is
effusive and compelling: "If I were to choose between all systems of
drugless healing, having studied nearly all, and knowing what results I can
get, I would select the Water Cure as the most beneficial of all." (Hoegen,
1917, 311) In his article, "Hydrotherapy", he presents a balanced view
of the people who left their mark on Hydrotherapy:

> Within the last century, great and gifted men have taken up the
> Nature Cure method, principally the water cure. These men are
> Priessnitz, Schroth, Graham, Rausse, Kneipp, Kuhne, Just, Rikli,
> and many others. Priessnitz was one of the first to organize the
> use of water into a system, for which he deserves great credit.
> Winternitz, of Vienna, did much in bringing and establishing
> Hydrotherapy on a sound and scientific basis. (Hoegen, 1917, 311)

In this article, one will find a smorgasbord of all the variations and
methods of Hydrotherapy. He provides indications and temperature
ranges for each of the therapies. What is not provided are the details of
procedures. It is clear that by 1917, Hydrotherapy was a given, and did
not require instruction.

In 1917, Benedict Lust translated and published Louis Kuhne's
The New Science of Healing and re-named the book, *Neo-Naturopathy,
The New Science of Healing*. Kuhne had passed away in 1901 and would
not be able to witness how his books impacted Naturopathy in America.
In Lust's Preface, he writes, "In publishing this treatise, my aim is to prove
Naturopathy a logical and exact science; to make this book worthy of
the profession it is devoted to; to make the drugless doctor a bigger and
a better doctor and the patient more appreciative of the merits of natural healing." (Lust, 1917, 4-5) In addition to publishing Kuhne's book,
Lust also included many large excerpts from the book in his magazine.
"My Remedial Agents" was one such article by Kuhne that appeared in
the June issue in 1917 which presented Kuhne's famous steam bath and
friction hip bath.

Kuhne had developed equipment to facilitate the steam or vapor bath which is today obsolete since the advent of plumbing and electricity. Proceeding the cold friction baths, the steam baths helped to promote perspiration and were not recommended for all patients. Kuhne writes, "Weak persons such as seriously ill, more especially nervous patients, should never take steam baths. For such, the most effective cure is attained by the use of friction sitz and hip baths." (Kuhne, 1917, 360)

The friction hip bath differed from the friction sitz bath used by Kuhne by the kind of tub used and the part of the body exposed to water. The friction hip bath was taken in a sitz tub and the water level reached the level of the umbilicus. Kuhne describes this bath: "The water should be at 64° to 68° F/18° to 20° C, and the bather, half sitting and half reclining, should then briskly and without stopping, rub the entire abdomen from the navel downwards and across the body with a coarse moderately wet cloth (jute, coarse linen)." (Kuhne, 1917, 364) The friction sitz bath was not taken in a sitz tub but in a small tub. Kuhne's instruction are as follows:

> In the bath a foot stool, or a wooden seat as made by me, is set. Water is then poured in but only so much, that it rises to a level with the upper edge of the seat, leaving the top dry. The bather then sits down upon the dry seat, dips a coarse linen cloth (jute or a rough towel) into the water and begins gently to wash the genitals and abdomen, always bringing up as much water as possible with the cloth. (Kuhne, 1917, 364)

The patient is not sitting in the tub but rather kept dry on a seat above the level of water.

Kuhne advocated a vegetarian diet and coined the concept that disease began in the digestion. He writes: "If we wish again to raise the vitality of the body, we can only do so by the agency of some means which improves the digestion. The best means known to me are, together with natural diet, are these cooling baths." (Kuhne, 1917, 367)

In the early editions of the Lust magazines, Vincent Priessnitz' lack of recognition could be explained by the fact that no one who lived in the early 20th century would ever have had an opportunity to learn from the master of Water Cure. Since Priessnitz did not leave behind any writings or books that could be studied and implemented. Time would have obliterated this amazing man's work had it not been for the many doctors who came to study his Water Cure.

Not all of the medical fraternity was so eager to learn from Priessnitz.

In Lust's article on Priessnitz, we learn of the intolerance for Priessnitz when his clinic was raided by doctors wanting to know the source of his sorcery. Lust writes what the contemporaries said of Priessnitz:

> "This man has some secret substance, and we mean to find it." They ripped out his tubs, hoping to lay bare the mystery in the linings. They cut up all his sponges, towels, cloths and sheets, but the mystery was not revealed. Priessnitz was forbidden entrance to his sanitarium—the seal of the state was placed on his door. (Lust, 1918, 223-224)

Priessnitz' contributions to Hydrotherapy as practiced a century ago were immense. He devised the compress, the wet sheet wrap, douches, friction, vapor or steam baths, etc., etc. His understanding of diagnosis and establishing treatment protocols were unsurpassed. His words sum up the essence of Hydrotherapy: "Not the cold but the body heat, produced by the reaction to cold water, is the healing factor." (Lust, 1918, 224)

In the closing chapters of this book we witness a decline in articles published in the Lust magazines on Hydrotherapy. This does not bear out in the two remaining books, *Clinical Pearls in Naturopathic Medicine, Volume I & II*, in the Hevert Collection. These two books will highlight the protocols and treatment plans used for various diseases will affirm the value of water in Naturopathy.

In the early years of the Water Cure movement that transcended into Naturopathy, there was a flood of articles on water and especially cold water for the treatment of diseases. Kneipp, the man whom many associated with Hydrotherapy, definitely left behind clinical successes about how he transformed and saved lives. Saving lives was what Kneipp did repetitively with ease and conviction. Another man, Vincent Priessnitz was one such man, an unsung hero, to whom we are forever indebted. The historical figures that got their hands wet with Hydrotherapy were very brave and moral. For many of them faced ridicule, persecution, and prosecution as rewards for their beliefs in the healing power of water as we saw earlier when Priessnitz was challenged by the local doctors.

Cold water as a method of healing became less celebrated. Instead, beginning in 1919, we see a shift towards warmer water temperatures. In "Nature's Cure for Disease" by Lorne Summers, a warm bath is the topic. Summers writes: "The best method to relax the body and soothe the nervous system is by a warm bath taken just before retiring, which will relieve any irritation by assisting in the elimination of fatigue poisons." (Summers, 1919, 343) If we keep reading, we find out that Summers is really just recommending an easy way to have a neutral bath. First, the temperature of water drawn into a bath tub is "105° F/40.6° C; after being in the water a couple of minutes [the doctor] turns on the cold water and cools the bath down to 95° F/35° C. Then the patient remains in the water for about ten to twenty minutes, then dry thoroughly and go to bed." (Summers, 1919, 343) The neutral bath is taken in water that is roughly the same temperature as the body temperature. The water does not feel cold and the water does not feel warm. He adds some benefits for the neutral bath: "Many have found this bath, called the neutral bath, a valuable remedy in the case of insomnia. The neutral bath before retiring is also very valuable in reducing high blood pressure." (Summers, 1919, 343)

In 1920, Summers follows with an article on cold baths indicating that cold water therapies have not completely fizzled away. In response to the germ theory, for example, we learn the importance of the digestive tract as the first line of defense. In this regard, Summers divulges how cold water aids the digestive tract: "The amount of hydrochloric acid produced by the glands of the stomach is increased, as the result of which the appetite and digestion are improved, and the stomach being provided with a better quality of gastric juice, is better prepared to protect itself against injury from intruding microbes." (Summers, 1920, 286) Another way cold water baths aid the fight against germs is by increasing blood circulation. "Experiments made on the body after a cold water bath have shown that the blood distribution has been increased thirty to fifty percent. This means that all tissues will have a better blood supply to carry off waste material and fight any germs that may enter." (Summers, 1920, 286) In the conclusion of his article, he reveals the scavenging forces found in white blood cells, bringing the microscope and microbiology to the naturopathic table.

We return to Priessnitz in the next article written by Robert Biéri, who was a student of Wilhelm Winternitz whom he proudly and fondly calls "the Father of Modern Hydrotherapy". (Biéri, 1921, 224) He continues, "The monumental work which elevated Water Cure once and for all above suspicion, and placed it beyond the scope of charlatanry is the life work of William Winternitz." (Biéri, 1921, 224) Biéri presents a quick snapshot of the history of Hydrotherapy since Priessnitz.

The wet sheet pack is credited to Priessnitz' wisdom and foresight. He would over his short lifetime develop an expertise that still impresses us. The wet sheet pack would be Priessnitz principle water applications when treating hopelessly sick patients from mercury poisoning. Calomel, or mercury chloride, was the golden standard for the Allopaths in the 19th and 20th century and often certain death for the patients who were administered this sinister drug. Those succumbing to calomel would find their way to Gräefenberg and Priessnitz' doorstep. The inestimable wet sheet pack and cold water saved many lives.

William Havard was another who used the wet sheet pack to save lives during the Spanish Flu in 1918. He recognized the merits of the wet sheet: "The method of Priessnitz still holds first rank. It consists of first wrapping the body or a part in wet linen and over this several thicknesses of flannel or woolen blanket." (Havard, 1921, 325) Like Priessnitz, Havard considered the full wet sheet pack for the removal of toxicity. He writes, "The full pack is indicated in all cases where there is a high degree of toxicity or where there is high fever. The higher the fever, the better the patient reacts to the pack." (Havard, 1921, 325)

Havard taught at Henry Lindlahr's school in Chicago and moved to New York City around 1919. Havard wrote several pieces for Lust's publications and each one is coherent and eloquent. I am deeply saddened that Havard did not leave behind any books. They would have become precious classics.

In the article, "Naturopathy in Practice", Havard introduces us to the water applications that he uses to treat acute diseases. He sets the record straight regarding the fever: "Contrary to the popular conception, the treatment in acute disease is not directed to the reduction of fever, or at least should not be. Fever is the indicator of the body's activity." (Havard, 1921, 325) The fever has a purpose and naturally subsides when "all irritating poisons have been oxidized and thrown out from the body". (Havard, 1921, 325) Havard lists and describes the significance of a variety of compresses and wraps in the treatment especially of the fever. Getting different perspectives of how the various water applications were effectively used is exactly what William Havard does.

By the 1920's, the use of cold water by Naturopaths was being challenged by the new kinds of water applications being introduced to Hydrotherapy. The swing from cold to hot and very hot water is exemplified by Benedict Lust's very long piece on the Japanese baths. Lust sets the stage by introducing a few historical highlights and includes some on the Roman baths. "In the year 300 A.D., there were 800 public baths in Rome, besides 14 immense hot baths (*Termae*) in each one of which thousands could bath at the same time." (Lust, 1922, 317) The Japanese hot bath was taken daily by Japanese at temperatures of 50° C/122° F. (Lust, 1922, 319) What a sharp contrast from 60° F/16° C temperatures used in some of the cold water treatments.

Lust, who gained so much from Kneipp, provides his rationale for the change of direction: "I am of the opinion that the hot baths, Roman, Russian and Japanese baths, have one good characteristic quality in common, and that is, that they put the body in a state of an artificial fever, increase the temperature of the blood and thereby dissolve waste matter and force it out through the skin." (Lust, 1922, 319-320) We learn that Lust had been using the Japanese baths for 28 years by this point. This revelation by Lust that he had been using hot water baths since 1894 mystifies me. Lust was so ardently passionate about cold water and Kneipp when he began his publications, *Amerikanischen Kneipp Blätter* and *The Kneipp Water Cure Monthly*. I have no explanation as to why Lust seemed so determined to shift from Kneippian practice. I imagine with the advent of hot water technology in the early 20th century, Lust must have finally realized that fellow Americans were not enamored in the slightest with cold water applications.

Lust redeems himself in part by modifying and lowering the temperatures in the hot Japanese baths to 44° C/111° F and adding cold water to the head. He writes, "This cold shower on the head while in the Japanese bath gives them the real hygienic character! It is this precaution which I deem absolutely necessary when taking a Japanese bath!" (Lust, 1922, 320) In his article, Lust gives a detailed account of how to administer the hot Japanese bath. The prescribed time was one hour and longer [two to four hours] for a curative benefit.

Another new Hydrotherapy application making waves was called the neutral bath. Neutral temperature used in baths was defined as the same temperature of the body [98.6° F/37° C] and was not new in Hydrotherapy. What was new was the length of time spent in a neutral bath. Dr. M. Ferrin writes,

> Lying in a bath tub on soft bed clothes for six hours and knowing that you are actually doing something to promote your health, is no worse than lying in bed for six hours with the consciousness that you are no nearer recovery than when you took your bed, so do not feel sorry for yourself at all, and do not consider that you are wasting time by taking an occasional neutral bath. (Ferrin, 1923, 317)

There were trends in Naturopathy occurring to increase the temperature of the water but also to lengthen the treatment times for Hydrotherapy. The purpose of the long bath times was internal cleansing. "So, in losing the bodily poisons in the neutral bath, you are likely to feel like some great support is gone from you, and so it has, but you do not want your life to be built upon stimulations which come from toxins." (Ferrin, 1923, 318)

Ferrin offers variations to the neutral bath by using some of the old time formulas such as Epsom salts, pine needles or hay flowers. Even the Epsom salt baths were long affairs. "Sometimes even a two-hour bath in warm Epsom salts water works wonders in the removal of surplus carbon from the body." (Ferrin, 1923, 319)

The allure of hot water only intensified with a new bath called, the "blood washing method". The blood washing method was developed by a young man, Christos Parasco, who shared the details with Benedict Lust. This new bath was enthusiastically embraced by Lust who wrote a book on the method, *The Fountain of Youth, Curing by Water* (1923) and taught it at his school and offered the treatment in his clinics.

> The treatment is as follows: put up this special shower head of own invention to a height from 8 to 14 feet and let the hot water fall upon a cork matting, wood crating, air-mattress or just a porcelain or tile floor, where on the body, with extended arms and legs, head and feet, can comfortably spread out or may assume any other position." (Lust, 1923, 524)

Along with the long eight hour shower, patients were given the Arnold Ehret mucusless diet and enemas to enhance further depuration.

Lindlahr also explained how the blood wash works: "The continual dropping of hot water on the body draws the blood to the surface and discharges its impurities through the relaxed and open pores. The morbid excretions are then washed away by the constant flow of hot water". (Lindlahr, 1923, p. 528) In order to make the shower feasible, Lindlahr modified the length of time reducing the shower to two hours.

This shower continued to be one that Naturopaths used. In a conversation with Dr Betty Radelet (1921-1916), an Oregon ND who had practiced for over a half century, she shared with me her own experience of the neglected blood wash. The subject arose when in that conversation I asked her which therapy did she find exceptional among all the therapies she had used over the years in her naturopathic practice? As I heard her story, I caught the gleam in her eye and listened to her firsthand account of the life-changing experience that she had taking and using this unique shower protocol.

In the final article, despite the author's being unknown, is a worthy ending for *Hydrotherapy in Naturopathic Medicine*. "In the course of time, the practical physician has learned to distinguish the limits of water's medical qualities. He has come to the conclusion that while in some cases water offers a radical remedy, in most of the diseases it is useful as an excellent medium to arouse and to assist Nature's curative power." (Unknown author, 1923, 736) In this article, many useful tips are given for the sitz or hip bath. "While the hip baths have the effect to derivate the blood to the splanchnic sphere, the foot baths have the effect to increase the volume of the vascular system in the calves and in the feet." (Unknown author, 1923, 738) Derivation in Hydrotherapy was the process of relieving congestion of a hyperemic part by dilating blood vessels in a remote part of the body by using appropriate hot and cold water applications. Finding mention of derivation in this final article gives one a glimmer of hope for the survival of Hydrotherapy.

Did Hydrotherapy evaporate from Naturopathy? It seems that as the years went by fewer articles about the various Kneipp water applications were printed in the Lust magazines. In their stead, hot or warm water baths and showers took their place.

Reviewing Lust in 1900 on the merits of Kneipp therapy seemed to take a back seat when so many hot water therapies were finding their way into Naturopathy. Lust cited the advantages that Kneipp's system offered as the following:

1) The short duration of all its applications.
2) The application of water upon certain parts of the body only.
3) A natural process of drying after applications.
4) Herbs in form of teas or decoctions for internal or external use.
5) A perfect system of strengthening and hardening the body.
6) A diet based upon Nature's wants. (Lust, 1900, 112)

Using Kneipp as a stepping stone, Lust sprang into action and embraced so many other different healing options and in doing so, effectively replaced Hydrotherapy.

Lust did not hold onto the reins of Hydrotherapy and it only took about 20 years to drain the proverbial bathtub. Sadly, Hydrotherapy would adjust and as we all know today, Constitutional Hydrotherapy would replace all of the miraculous therapies from Priessnitz and Kneipp. In 1923, Otis G. Carroll would refine and consolidate the wet sheet wrap within a tidy 40 minute treatment in a clinical office setting. The previous and traditional wet sheet wrap that could take as long as two and even three hours would be time-prohibitive for a busy naturopathic practice. So, it is no wonder that the time consuming treatments that water therapies entailed were gradually discarded for seemingly more streamlined and efficient modalities.

Alarmingly, in our time many Naturopaths do not turn instinctively to those traditional tools. In a recent conversation with one of our distinguished doctors, for example, I was glad that he reported on his recovery, but took note that antibiotics had been what took the sting out of a bout with pneumonia. It would have been music to my ears to have heard that wet sheet wraps and fasting as primary treatments were considered; however, he resorted as a first measure to antibiotics. While it is good that he recovered, of course, it was not his use of drugs which rattled me most; rather, it was that he praised their virtues without qualification and dismissed traditional therapies as a personal option. Hydrotherapy formed the foundation and starting point in the evolution towards a more comprehensive natural health paradigm. In throwing out the baby with the bathwater, we lost a most precious jewel within our armamentarium.

1897

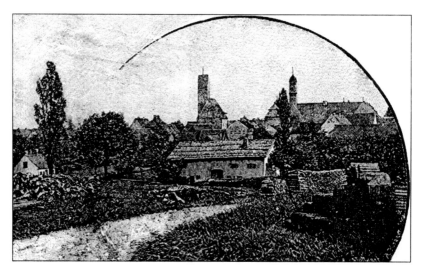

Wörishofen, in 1880, a quiet and remote village to which Father Kneipp was assigned as its priest.

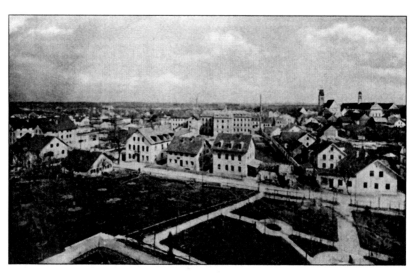

By 1895, Wörishofen had become a bustling city.

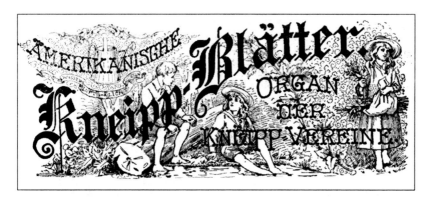

WATER APPLICATIONS*

by Sebastian Kneipp

Amerikanischen Kneipp Blätter, II (15), 186-187. (1897)

GENERAL REMARKS

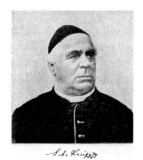

Father Sebastian Kneipp
(1821-1897)

The applications of water used in my establishment and described in this first part are divided into:

Wet Sheets
Baths
Vapor Baths
Gushes
Ablutions
Wet Bandages (packages)
Drinking of Water

The subdivisions of each application are given in Part One of *My Water Cure*. The name and the meaning of the strange sounding practices are explained in their proper place.**

[The aim of water applications is summarized in the following:]

1. to dissolve [the morbid matters]
2. to evacuate the morbid matters
3. to strengthen the organism

In general it may be said that the dissolving is brought about by

---

*This article has been taken from Sebastian Kneipp's *My Water Cure*, "Part 1". —Ed.
**Benedict Lust's introduction to this article is awkward and I have added some text to give context and an explanation. —Ed.

the vapors and the hot baths of medicinal herbs; the evacuation by the
water packages [compresses] and partly by the gushes and wet sheets;
the strengthening by the cold baths, gushes, partly by the ablutions, and
finally by the entire system of hardening.

As every disease originates as previously stated in disorders of the
blood, it is evident that in every case all the respective applications must
be used more or less dissolving, evacuating and strengthening. Further,
not only the suffering part, foot, or hand, or head, as the case may be, is
to be treated, but always the whole body through every part of which the
bad blood is flowing; of course, the diseased part with preference, the rest
of the body only as a fellow-sufferer. It would be partial and wrong to
act otherwise with regard to these two important points. Many instances
in the third part of this book will justify my statement. [See *My Water
Cure*]

Whoever uses water as a remedy, according to my ideas and wishes,
will never think the applications to be for his own whims, i.e. he never
will use an application just because he likes to do so. He will never, like
a fool, take pleasure in being able to "handle, and boast of, and to rave
about many things, about vapors and gushes and packages". To a sensible man, the applications will always be only the means for the purpose,
and if he attain it by the mildest water application, he will be happy.
For his task is only this: to help Nature struggling for health, i.e. for her
own and independent activity, to obtain this activity, to loosen the fetters
of illness, the chains of suffering, and to enable Nature to do the work
herself again, gaily and cheerfully. If this task finished, the treatment
must cease. This remark is important, more important still to observe it.
For there is nothing which so greatly brings the water as healing element
into discredit and bad reputation, as to make applications in an indiscreet
way without measure and reason, as a sharp, strict, rugged procedure.
Those, and only those, I cannot repeat it enough, who consider themselves
to be competent in the system of Water Cures, but frighten every patient
by their endless packages, their vapors almost driving out the blood, etc.,
are causing the greatest harm, which it is very difficult to mend. I do not
call this using the water for healing, but such outrages I call putting water
to shame.

Whoever has a knowledge of the effects of water, and knows how to
use it in its extremely manifold ways, is in possession of a remedy which
cannot be surpassed by any other, whatever its name may be. There is no
remedy more manifold in its effects, or as it were, more elastic than water.
In creation it begins in the invisible globule of air or steam, continues in
the drop, and finally forms the ocean filling up the greater part of the
globe.

This ought to serve as a hint to every water curist to show him that every application of water can be raised from the gentlest to the highest degree, and that in each case it is not the patient who ought to accommodate himself to the package, the vapor, etc., but every application is to be accommodated to the patient.

It is in the selection of the applications to be used that the master hand shows itself. The one who undertakes the cure will carefully examine the patient, but not in a startling way. At first the subordinate sufferings will come under his notice, i.e. those diseases which like toadstools spring up from the interior ground of disease. By them one can, in most cases, easily conclude, where the root of the disease, the principle evil, is to be found. By means of questioning and searching he will find what progress the disease has already made, what mischief it has done; then it must be taken into consideration, whether the patient is old or young, weak or strong, thin or stout, poor of blood, nervous, etc. All these points, and others besides, provide an accurate picture of the disease. It is only then, when this is clear and complete, that he goes to the water apotheca and prescribes according to the principle. The gentler and more sparing—the better and more effective.

A few general remarks may be given here, regarding the whole of the water applications. No application whatever can cause the least harm if it is made according to the directions given.

Most of them are to be made with cold water, either from the spring, well, or river. In all cases where warm water is not expressly prescribed, the word "water" stands for and means cold water. I follow my principle founded on experience. The colder, the better. In wintertime, I mix snow with the water for gushes when they are for healthy people. Do not accuse me of ruggedness; rather, think of the very short duration of my cold water applications. He who has once ventured to make a trial has conquered forever; all his prejudices are entirely removed.

But I am not, nevertheless, inexorable. To beginners in the Water Cure, to weak persons, especially very young or very old ones, to sick people who are afraid of a cold, to such as have not much warmth in their blood, whose blood is poor, or who are nervous, I gladly allow, especially in winter time, a warm room for their baths and gushes (65° F / 18° C) for the beginning, and lukewarm water for every application. Flies are to be attracted not by salt and vinegar, but by honey.

There are special prescriptions for every warm water application respecting the degree of warmth, the time, etc.

Regarding the cold water applications, we must briefly give some hints for regulating the course of action observed before, during and after the application. No one should venture to make any cold application, whatever, when feeling cold, shivering, etc., unless it is expressly allowed in the prescription relating to his case. The applications are to be made as quickly as possible, but without agitation and haste. Also, with dressing and undressing, no delay should be caused by slowness in buttoning or tying up, etc. All this secondary work can be done when the whole body is properly covered. To give an instance: a cold full bath, including undressing, bathing and redressing, should not exceed four to five minutes. It only needs a little practice to accomplish this. If with an application the time "one minute" is given, the shortest time possible is meant; if it is said two to three minutes, the cold application is intended to be of more enduring, but not of longer influence.

After a cold application, the body must never be wiped dry, except the head, and the hands as far as the wrist (the latter in order not to wet the clothes, when dressing). The wet body is at once covered with dry underwear and other articles of clothing. This is to be done quickly, as before remarked, so that the body is not exposed to air. This proceeding will seem strange to many, even to most people, because they will imagine that they are thereby obliged to remain wet all the day long. Let them try it only once before judging, and they will soon experience what this not-wiping is good for. Wiping is rubbing, and, as it cannot be done quite equally over every part of the body and on every spot, it produces disproportionate natural warmth, which is not of much consequence with healthy people, but of very great moment with sick and weak ones. The not-wiping helps to the most regular, most equal and most speedy natural warmth. It is like sprinkling water into the fire; the interior warmth of the body uses the water clinching to the exterior as material for speedily bringing forth greater and more intense warmth. As before said, it all depends upon a trial.

In general it may be said that the dissolving is brought about by the vapors and the hot baths of medicinal herbs; the evacuation by the water packages [compresses] and partly by the gushes and wet sheets; the strengthening by the cold baths, gushes, partly by the ablutions, and finally by the entire system of hardening.

Further, it is not only the suffering part, foot, or hand, or head, as the case may be, is to be treated, but always the whole body through every part of which the bad blood is flowing.

Whoever uses the water as a remedy, according to my ideas and wishes, will never think the applications to be for his own whims, i.e. he never will use an application just because he likes to do so.

Whoever has a knowledge of the effects of water, and knows how to use it in its extremely manifold ways, is in possession of a remedy which cannot be surpassed by any other, whatever its name may be.

This ought to serve as a hint to every water curist to show him that every application of water can be raised from the gentlest to the highest degree, and that in each case it is not the patient who ought to accommodate himself to the package, the vapor, etc., but every application is to be accommodated to the patient.

The gentler and more sparing—the better and more effective.

I follow my principle founded on experience. The colder, the better. In all cases where warm water is not expressly prescribed, the word "water" stands for and means cold water.

Do not accuse me of ruggedness; rather, think of the very short duration of my cold water applications.

No one should venture to make any cold application, whatever, when feeling cold, shivering, etc., unless it is expressly allowed in the prescription relating to his case. Applications are to be made as quickly as possible, but without agitation and haste; also with dressing and undressing no delay should be caused by slowness in buttoning or tying up, etc.

After a cold application the body must never be wiped dry, except the head, and the hands as far as the wrist (the latter in order not to wet the clothes, when dressing).

The not-wiping helps to the most regular, most equal and most speedy natural warmth.

SNOW WALKING*

by Sebastian Kneipp

Amerikanischen Kneipp Blätter, II (21), 279-281. (1897)

FRESH FALLEN SNOW

Walking in newly fallen snow produces even greater effect than that of walking on wet grass or stones. I emphasize "in newly fallen, fresh snow", which forms into a ball or clings to the feet like dust, not in old, stiff, frozen snow, which almost freezes off the feet and is of no use whatever. Moreover, this promenade must never be made in cold, cutting winds, but in spring when the snow is being melted by the sun. I know many people who have walked through such snow water for half an hour, or an hour, even one and a half hours with the best result. The first minutes only caused a little struggle. Later on, they felt no uneasiness or special cold. The regular duration of such a walk in the snow is three to four minutes. I emphatically remark, there must be no stand-still but constant walking.

Sometimes it happens that all too tender toes, which are quite unaccustomed to outer air, cannot bear the snowy cold and get snow-fever, i. e., become dry and hot, burning and painful, and swell. But there is no cause for fear, it is of no consequence if the dry toes are bathed in snow water or rubbed with snow, they will heal directly.

In autumn, the snow walk can be replaced by walking in the grass covered with hoar frost. The feeling of cold is much more painful then, because at that time, at the change of season, the body is still accustomed to the warmth of summer. Even in winter, the snow walk is replaced by walking on stone [walkway], soaked with snow water. The rules for covering the feet and for exercise are the same as in walking on wet grass or stones.**

Generally, the verdict upon this means of hardening is: "Nothing but folly and nonsense," because people are afraid to catching colds, rheumatism, sore throat, catarrh, and every possible complaint. Everything depends on a trial and a little self-conquest. One will soon become convinced how groundless prejudices are and that the dreadful snow walk, instead of causing harm, brings great benefits.

Many years ago, I became acquainted with the wife of a higher officer. This energetic mother set a high value on the hardening of her children.

---

*Benedict Lust first published this chapter on hardening from Sebastian Kneipp's book, *My Water Cure* in a three part series beginning in September 1897. Lust re-published this hardening chapter again in January, 1901. —Ed.

**One of the cardinal rules for Kneipp's water applications was that patients must feel warm before exposing themselves to cold water. Cold feet would not prevent initiating a cold water treatment. —Ed.

Daintiness in eating and drinking were by no means tolerated; complaints about the weather, heat, cold, etc., were always censored. As soon as the first snowfall came, she promised her boys a reward if they ventured to go in the snow barefooted. This she did for many years and her children, in consequence, became strong and vigorous, and all their life long they were grateful for this by no means soft way of education. That mother was fully an expert in her task.

This, then, is the snow walk for healthy people. I will mention two cases to show with what success it can be practiced in many complaints.

A person was suffering for many years from chilblains, which opened, formed ulcers and gave her great pain. According to my advice, she began her snow walks with the first snowfall in autumn, repeated them frequently, and the troublesome tumors ceased to torment her.

Not long ago a girl of seventeen came to me complaining of dreadful toothache. "If you would go through the newly fallen snow for five minutes," I said to her, "your toothache would soon vanish." She followed my advice instantly, went to the garden, and ten minutes afterwards she came back, joyfully exclaiming that her toothache was gone.

The snow walk ought never to take place, unless the whole body be perfectly warm. When feeling cold or shivering, it is necessary to procure normal warmth, by working or exercise. Persons who are suffering from perspiring feet, wounded feet, open or suppurating chilblains, are, of course never allowed to walk in the snow until the feet have first been healed.

WALKING IN WATER

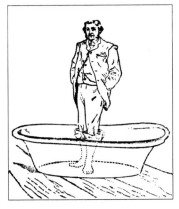

Walking in cold water was one of the best ways of hardening. Kneipp also used water treading for those with insomnia.

As simple as it may appear to walk in water reaching as far as the calf of the leg, yet even this application serves as a means of hardening. Walking in water does the following:

1. influences the whole body, and strengthens the whole system;
2. operates on the kidneys; by this many complaints, originating in the kidneys, the bladder and the bowels, are prevented;
3. operates powerfully on the chest, facilitates breathing; carries gases out of the stomach and;
4. operates especially against headache, congestion, and other sufferings of the head.

This means of hardening can be employed by moving the feet in a bath of cold water, reaching over the ankles. It is more effective for hardening, if one goes into the water up to the shins, and most effective of all, if the water reaches the knees.

As to the duration, one can begin with one minute, then longer, up to five or six minutes. The colder the water, the better. After such a practice, exercise is necessary in winter time in a warm room, in summer in the open air, until the body is completely warm. In winter, snow may be mixed with the water. Weaklings may use warm water in the beginning, then, by and by colder, and lastly, quite cold water.

COLD BATHS FOR EXTREMITIES

For the special hardening of the extremities, arms and legs, the following practice is excellent: to stand in cold water up to the knees or over them, for no longer than one minute; then, after the feet have been covered, to put the arms up to the shoulders in cold water for the same length of time. It is better still to put arms and legs into the water together; in a larger bath, this is easily done. One can just as easily stand in the bath and put the arms and hands in another vessel, standing on a chair. I like to prescribe this practice after diseases, in order to increase the flow of the blood to the extremities.

To those who are suffering from chilblains and cold hands, this dipping in of the arms is of very good service; but one has to be careful, that the hands (not arms) be directly well dried, as they are exposed to the air.

It is essential that before this practice the body should be in normal warmth (not shivering). If the feet are cold up to the ankles (but not the shins), the arms up to the elbows, this need not prevent the application.

KNEE GUSH

As a last means of hardening, I name the knee gush.* It is of special service to the feet, inducing the blood to come to their bloodless veins.

Here I have only to say that the gush on the knees is to be given in a stronger way, if healthy people use it for hardening. This can be done, e. g., by the water jet [shower] coming from a height; by mixing snow and ice with the water in winter time, etc.

This practice can only be undertaken, if the body is warm (not shivering); but cold feet up to the ankles are no impediment. The gush on the knees ought not to be used for more than three or four days, unless it

---

*For directions on how to apply a knee gush, please refer to Benedict Lust's 1900 article on page 113 or Dr. Baumgarten's 1904 article on pages 238–243. —Ed.

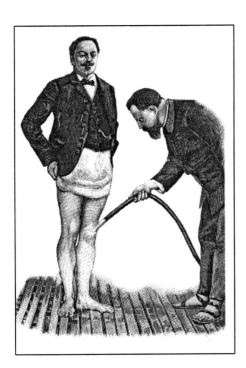

The knee gush was Kneipp's signature water application. Water was originally applied with a simple garden watering can and later a hose was adopted.

is taken in connection with other practices. If undertaken for a longer time, it must be used alternately with the upper gush, or the dipping in of the arms in the morning, the upper gush in the afternoon.

The means of hardening here mentioned may suffice. They can be practiced at every season, and continued in winter and summer. In winter, it would be well to shorten the application itself a little, but to prolong the exercise after it somewhat. For those who are unaccustomed to them, it would be well not to begin with them in winter, more especially those who are suffering from poverty of blood, interior cold, and who are faddled, effeminated, and made sensitive by woolen clothing. I do not say this, as if I were afraid of any harm, but only to prevent people from becoming frightened of such an excellent remedy.

Healthy, as well as weak people, may without hesitation make use of all the applications, both of them observing care and following strictly the directions given. If bad consequences ensue, they are never to be attributed to the applications but always to some greater or lesser imprudence. Even to consumptive people with whom the disease had made considerable progress, I have applied walking in wet grass and stones, snow walking and standing water with great success.

I invite those of my honored readers who perhaps have never yet heard even the name of these things, to give them a small, the very smallest trial before condemning them. If it turns out in my favor, I shall be glad, not for my own sake, but on account of the importance of the matter. Many storms break out in life upon man's health; happy he who has health's roots well fastened, deepened and grounded by hardening.

The regular duration of such a walk in the snow is three to four minutes. I emphatically remark, there must be no standstill but constant walking.

In autumn, the snow walk can be replaced by walking in the grass covered with hoar frost. The feeling of cold is much more painful then, because at that time, at the change of season, the body is still accustomed to the warmth of summer.

The snow walk ought never to take place, unless the whole body be perfectly warm. When feeling cold or shivering, it is necessary to procure normal warmth, by working or exercise.

This means of hardening can be employed by moving the feet in a bath of cold water, reaching over the ankles. It is more effective for hardening, if one goes into the water up to the shins, and most effective of all, if the water reaches the knees.

As to the duration, one can begin with one minute, then longer, up to five or six minutes. The colder the water, the better.

It is essential that before this practice the body should be in normal warmth (not shivering). If the feet are cold up to the ankles (but not the shins), the arms up to the elbows, this need not prevent the application.

In winter, it would be well to shorten the [knee gush] application itself a little, but to prolong the exercise after it somewhat.

I invite those of my honored readers who perhaps have never yet heard even the name of these things, to give them a small, the very smallest trial before condemning them.

FATHER KNEIPP'S SUCCESSORS

by Benedict Lust

Amerikanischen Kneipp Blätter, II (21), 281. (1897)

Three physicians, pupils of the Late Priest Doctor, carry on his world famous cure.
Wörishofen, Bavaria, August 21, 1897. "The King is dead; long live the King!" Poor Father Kneipp is dead, but Wörishofen lives. The many guests here often speak of the kind hearted old priest who spent his life amid these hills for the sake of relieving the ills that flesh is heir to.

Wörishofen now exists as a cure resort of some pretension. It has entered into competition with the outside world, and I think, seems destined to be reckoned among the permanent health resorts of Europe.

Wörishofen has three men who claim to know the Kneipp cure and affirm that they can cure with it many of the ills which man is heir to. Of course, no one would think for a moment

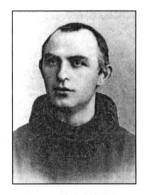

Father Bonifaz Reile

Superior of the Brotherhood of Mercy in Wörishofen and the successor to Father Kneipp.

that they will have the success that Father Kneipp had, nor have they his extraordinary knowledge in the different applications of water and herbs to cure disease. Nevertheless, I think that it can be truthfully said that they know the Kneipp cure thoroughly, and will have great success.

Among these three men first comes Dr. Albert Baumgarten. Dr. Baumgarten is a Prussian from the Rhine district. He is quick, energetic, and has the perseverance of the Prussian. For six years, he studied and practiced the cure under the eye of Father Kneipp. He is a firm believer in it. His knowledge of German, French and English, together with his knowledge of the cure, brings him a large number of patients. After the doctor, the Prior, or Rector of the Brothers of St. John, who number thirty, has charge of the large Kurhaus in Wörishofen. Prior Reile is his name.

Six or eight years ago, Father Kneipp determined to perpetuate his cure in Wörishofen by means of some religious order which would reside and always remain in Wörishofen. The Order of the Brothers of St. John, who have many hospitals in Europe, accepted the offer to continue the cure. Father Kneipp built a very large Kurhaus, gave it to the brothers, and the general of the society placed the Brothers of the Kurhaus under a young and brilliant Brother, well versed in herbs, who henceforth, was called Prior Reile.

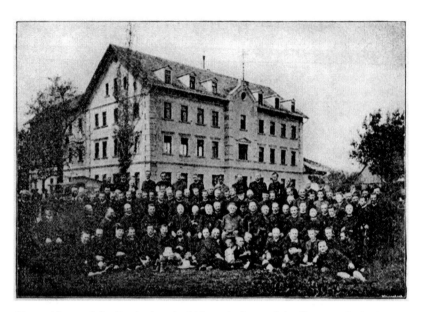

The residents of the Brotherhood of Mercy in front of the first new Sanitarium at Wörishofen.

The Prior was given the duty to heal all people who applied to Father Kneipp by letter. The Prior often received 200 letters a day. He gathered around him a group of clerks to take charge of the large correspondence. The Prior has been healing in the Kurhaus and curing by correspondence during the six years that Dr. Baumgarten has been practicing the cure in the village.

The business of the Prior became so great that it was necessary for him to have the aid of a physician to help him diagnose the cases brought to him. Dr. Mahr, a clever Bavarian doctor, of an established reputation, was brought from Munich. Dr. Mahr also learned the cure from Father Kneipp; so that today, Wörishofen has three men with more than ordinary talent who have learned the cure from its inventor, and practiced it for many years under his directions.

At present each of them has its own clientele, and their respective patients are more than satisfied. Two thousand five hundred "Kur-guests" are here from all countries, together with a large gathering of the highest nobility of Europe.

Wörishofen has three men who claim to know the Kneipp cure and affirm that they can cure with it many of the ills which man is heir to. Of course, no one would think for a moment that they will have the success that Father Kneipp had, nor have they his extraordinary knowledge in the different applications of water and herbs to cure disease.

Dr. Baumgarten is a Prussian from the Rhine district. He is quick, energetic, and has the perseverance of the Prussian. For six years, he studied and practiced the cure under the eye of Father Kneipp.

After the doctor, the Prior, or Rector of the Brothers of St. John, who number thirty, has charge of the large Kurhaus in Wörishofen. Prior Reile is his name.

Six or eight years ago, Father Kneipp determined to perpetuate his cure in Wörishofen by means of some religious order which would reside and always remain in Wörishofen.

Dr. Mahr also learned the cure from Father Kneipp; so that today, Wörishofen has three men with more than ordinary talent who have learned the cure from its inventor, and practiced it for many years under his directions.

WET SHEETS

by The Late Mgr. Sebastian Kneipp

Amerikanischen Kneipp Blätter, II (23), 310-311. (1897)

COVERING WITH WET SHEETS

A large, coarse piece of linen* is folded 3, 4, 6, 8, or 10 times length-wise, wise and long enough to cover the whole body, beginning at the neck. The sheet ought not to end on both sides as if cut off, but hang down a little on the right and left of the body. The so prepared sheet is dipped in cold water (in winter, warm water may be used) well wrung out and then put on the patient lying in bed in the way described above. A woolen blanket or a piece of linen doubled two or three times, is laid upon it, in order to close the wet covering tightly and to thoroughly prevent the entering of the air. The whole is covered with a feather quilt. As a rule, I wrap a rather large piece of woolen material round the neck to prevent the air entering from above. Care must be taken that the covering up is well done, otherwise the patient would easily take cold.

The wet sheet is applied from forty-five minutes to an hour. If longer duration is prescribed, in order to operate by cold, the sheet having been warm, must be wetted again in cold water.** As soon as the prescribed time has expired, the wet sheets are taken away; the patient dresses himself and takes some exercise, or remains in bed for a short time.

This application operates especially on the expelling of gases detained in stomach and bowels.

This practice, like the following ones, demands that the body be warm.

LYING ON WET SHEETS

To the covering with wet sheets corresponds the lying on wet sheets, which, in case both applications are used alternately, must be applied first. The following remarks are to be made regarding it.

As this application is also to be made in bed, a piece of linen, and over it a woolen blanket, are laid upon the mattress, to prevent it from getting wet. Then the same piece of coarse linen, as used for the preceding application (doubled 3 or 4 times), dipped in water and wrung out, is placed

---

*Kneipp used coarse linen that was known as "Kneipp linen mesh" for his compresses. The coarse linen was not new nor stiff which would not adhere to the body and cause unnecessary exposure to air. —Ed.

**The differences between Kneipp and Priessnitz in their water applications shows up in subtle ways. Priessnitz encouraged warming of the body during a treatment using more blankets to wrap the patient in and did not change the warm compress by getting it cold again. Kneipp changed the warmed compress by washing it again in cold water. —Ed.

lengthwise upon the blanket, so that it reaches from the end of the neck to the end of the [spine], i. e., the whole length of the back. The patient lies down on his back, wraps himself up in the extended blanket from both sides, in order to prevent the air from coming in, and then covers himself with a blanket and feather [covering or duvet]. This lying on wet sheets is also to be applied for three quarters of an hour; if longer, the wetting of sheets with cold water must be repeated, because its effect, like that of the covering with wet sheets, is produced only by cold. The same rules as given above are to be followed.

This application is especially effective for strengthening the back bone and the spinal marrow, for pain in the back and for lumbago. I know many cases in which lumbago was entirely removed by two applications of wet sheets made on the same day.

Also against congestions, in the heat of fever, this lying on wet sheets is of very good effect. In which individual cases it is to be used, and how often it is to be repeated, is said in the part of this book, [My Water Cure] where the diseases are spoken of.

Covering With And Lying On Wet Sheets

The two applications can be taken one after the other or both together. The sheet for lying on is prepared as given in the previous example; that for covering likewise prepared, is laid near the bedside. The patient lies down undressed on the one wet sheet and covers himself with the other. The final covering with blanket and feather covering [duvet] is easily done. If there is another person attending, it is well to tuck in both blanket and feather duvet on both sides, to prevent the entering of the cold air. It is important that the blanket, lying under the wet sheets broad-wise, be large enough to wrap up both the wet sheets like a bandage.

The duration of this application ought not to be less than three-quarters of an hour, and not more than an hour.

It is of very great service against great heat [fever], gases, congestions, hypochondriasis, and other sufferings.

Compress On The Abdomen

The patient lies in bed. A piece of linen, folded four to six times, dipped in water, and thoroughly wrung out, is laid upon the abdomen (from the stomach downwards) and covered with the shirt and finally carefully with blanket and feather duvet.

The application may be made of three-quarters of an hour to two hours; in the latter case, it must be renewed after an hour, i.e. wetted anew. This application is of good service against indigestion, cramps, also where the blood is to be led away from the chest and heart.

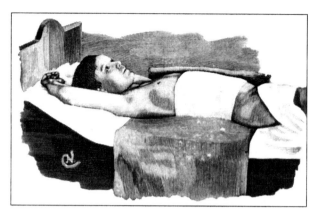

An abdominal compress.

For wetting the linen, vinegar is very often used instead of water, also decoctions of hay blossoms, shavegrass, oat straw, etc. In order to save the vinegar, a twofold piece of linen doubled 2 or 4 times, which is dipped only in water. The covering is done as stated before.

The so prepared sheet is dipped in cold water (in winter, warm water may be used) well wrung out and then put on the patient lying in bed in the way described above. A woolen blanket or a piece of linen doubled two or three times, is laid upon it, in order to close the wet covering tightly and to thoroughly prevent the entering of the air. The whole is covered with a feather quilt.

The wet sheet is applied from forty-five minutes to an hour. If longer duration is prescribed, in order to operate by cold, the sheet having been warm, must be wetted again in cold water.

As this application is also to be made in bed, a piece of linen, and over it a woolen blanket, are laid upon the mattress, to prevent it from getting wet.

This lying on wet sheets is also to be applied for three-quarters of an hour; if longer, the wetting of sheets with cold water must be repeated, because its effect, like that of the covering with wet sheets, is produced only by cold.

The patient lies in bed. A piece of linen, folded four to six times, dipped in water, and thoroughly wrung out, is laid upon the abdomen (from the stomach downwards) and covered with the shirt and finally carefully with blanket and feather duvet.

1898

ICE AND BLEEDING

FOOT BATHS

THE WARM FULL BATH
Sebastian Kneipp

KNEIPP CURE INSTITUTES IN AMERICA
A. N. Tally, M.D.

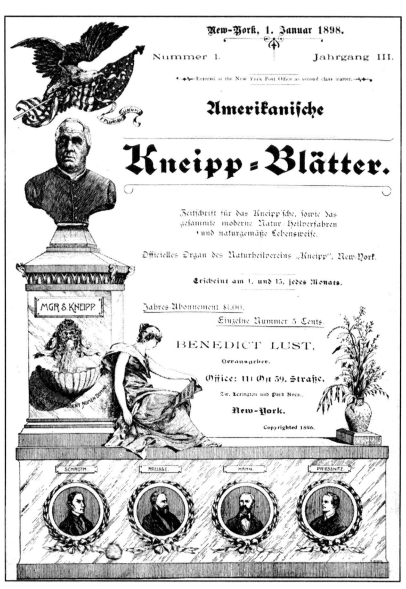

This ornate cover appeared on the *Amerikanische Kneipp Blätter* issues published in 1898. At bottom, left to right, are: Johann Schroth (1798-1856), Johann Heinrich Rausse (1805-1848), Johann Sigmund Hahn (1664-1742) and Vincent Priessnitz (1799-1851).

ICE AND BLEEDING*

by Sebastian Kneipp

Amerikanischen Kneipp-Blätter, III (14), 126-127. (1898)

I have been asked many times what principles I follow with regard to coverings with ice, bleeding, etc. These I will briefly state.

Whoever wishes to reconcile himself with an enemy, and for this purpose offers him his hand with knitted brows, will find greater difficulty in succeeding than if he met him with a bright face and a joyful heart. It is something similar to this with ice and water. I have always considered the application of ice, especially on the nobler parts of the body, (head, eyes, ears, etc.) to be among the most rugged and violent remedies ever used. They do not help or encourage Nature to recommence its work; they force it with violence to do so, and that must revenge itself. Ice cloths and ice bags, or whatever the names of those things may be, are entirely excluded from my [water cure methods]. Only imagine these enormous counteractions: inside the body a burning heat, outside a mountain of ice, and between them a suffering member, the organ of tender flesh and blood, worked on by both. I have always waited with great anxiety for the result of such work, and in most cases my anxiety was justified.

I know a gentleman who was ordered to have ice laid upon one of his feet day and night, for a whole year long, without any interruption. It would surely take nothing less than a miracle to prevent this mountain of ice from taking away not only all heat, but also the indispensable natural warmth! Nothing was to be seen of the healing of the foot.

But, someone will reply, in many cases it has really done good. Yes, for it may be that the disease could not withstand the means of compulsion. However, what were the consequences? Innumerable persons have come to me who had partly lost their eyesight, become more or less deaf, others with rheumatism of every kind, especially in the head, or with great sensibility of the head, etc. What was the cause of all this? "Yes, there, and then," I was answered, "the tiresome ice bag did it. I have been burdened with this complaint for so many years." Certainly, most of them will be burdened with it to their last breath.

I repeat again that I oppose absolutely any application of ice and I assert, on the contrary, that water applied in the right way is able to soften and to extinguish any heat, even the most violent, in whatever part or organ of the body it may be raging. If a fire can no longer be put out

---

*Benedict Lust, in the early years, as a young and aspiring publisher would draw from his mentor, Sebastian Kneipp's works to obtain content for his magazine. This article on "Water Applications" was published again in the June issue, 1901. —Ed.

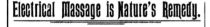
by water, ice will do just as little for it; that is easily understood by every-
one.

I said just now that a regular application of water will bring help.
I do not mean that for instance with an inflammation in the head, it would
be advisable to use as many packages as there were ice bags formerly used;
100 ice bags and packages will not stop the blood rushing to the inflamed
spot and thereby increasing the heat. I must try to lead the blood away, to

distribute it to the different other parts, for example, I must make applications on the whole body, besides those on the suffering part. I shall, for example, attack the enemy in the head, first of all at the patient's feet, and then gradually proceed up the whole body.

Nevertheless, the ice is of good service to my Water Cure by indirect use. In summer, it cools the water when it is getting lukewarm.

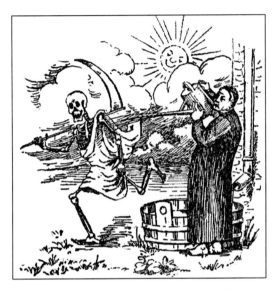

The Kneipp Water Cure Terrorizes Death.

What is my opinion with regard to bleeding, leeches and all the different kinds of blood extractions? Well, I will state it plainly. Fifty, forty, thirty years ago there was seldom a woman who was not bled two, three or four times a year; the half holidays and, of course, the most favorable days were faithfully chosen for this purpose in the beginning of the year and marked in the calendar with red or blue strokes. The country physicians, the surgeons and barbers, themselves, called their own work in this way, a real butchery. Institutions and convents, too, had their appointed time for bleeding and the strictly regulated diet above all. Congratulations were made to one another after having endured the bloody toils, which may have been no small ones sometimes. A priest of that time assured me that he had undergone this bleeding for 32 years, the process being repeated four times every year, and each time he lost 8 ounces of blood, making in all $8 \times 4 \times 32 = 1024$ ounces.

Besides this bleeding, leeches were used, and scarifying and other processes practiced. Young and old, high and low, men and women, were all well provided for.

How times are changing! For a long time these doings were looked upon as the only and absolutely necessary means of being and remaining healthy! And what is thought of them now-a-days? We smile at and ridicule this false opinion of the old, this false natural science, to imagine that any man should have too much blood! About two years ago, a foreign physician, who was also an active literary man, and who was following a new school told me that he had never in his life seen leeches.

Many physicians attribute the poverty of blood in the present days, to the former misuse of bleeding. They may be right; however, this is not the only cause of it.

But to the subject! My conviction is this: in the human body everything corresponds so wonderfully, the particle to the part, and every part to the whole, that one cannot help calling the organism of the body an incomparable work of art, the idea of which could only originate in the creative mind of God, and the execution of which was only possible to the creative power of God. The same order, the same measure, the same harmony exists between the raising and consumption of the ingredients necessary to the support of the body, provided man himself, reasonable and independent as he is, cooperates with the will of God by rightly using what is given to him, provided he does not overturn the order by misusing it, and so bringing dissonances into the harmony. As this is the state of the case, I cannot imagine how the formation of blood alone, this most important of all processes in the human body, should go on without order, without number and measure, unarranged and immoderately.

Every child, so I imagine, receives as an inheritance from its mother, together with the life, a quantity of material for the formation of blood, call it what you will, which is, as it were, the essence without which no blood can be prepared. If this essence is exhausted, the formation of blood, and with it life itself, ceases. Fading away, decaying, I do not call living. By every loss of blood, whether it be caused by a fall, an accident, or by bleeding, leeches, or scarifying, a particle or part of this stock of blood, of this essence of life, is lost and in the same measure the body's life is shortened. Every extraction of blood means nothing less than a shortening of life; for life lives in the blood.

The objection to this will be: nothing is more quickly accomplished than the formation of blood; losing blood and gaining blood is almost one and the same thing.

Yes, the formation of blood takes place with an incredibly wonderful speed; I quite agree with this argument. But excuse me, if I give another one based on experience; it will interest my readers who are engaged in farming, and they will be obliged to confirm it. If a farmer wishes to fatten cattle quickly, he draws a good quantity of blood from them, and after having done so, he feeds them well. In a short time plenty of fresh blood is formed, and the cattle progress and fatten. After three or four weeks, the bleeding is repeated; then good and nourishing food, as well as many strengthening potions, are given. The progress is excellent and even with old cattle, as much and as nice blood will be found when they are killed as with young cattle. But let us look more closely at this blood. The blood produced artificially is only watery, weak blood without vitality. The cattle have no longer any strength or power of endurance, and if not soon killed, will get dropsy.

Should it be otherwise with man? Having lived more than 75 years and gained some experience and knowledge of human life, I know that precisely the immoderate bleeding of our ancestors has influenced the capacities, talents and duration of life of their offspring. The gentleman mentioned in the beginning of our treatise, who had lost so many ounces of blood, died of dropsy in the best years of manhood. And if a man (I state facts only) had been bled 150, another 200 times, and had thereby become unspeakably weak and ill, must not the following generation be sickly and frail, inclined to cramps and other sufferings?

I willingly acknowledge that there can be cases, but only exceptional ones, where an immediate danger is removed by bleeding, other quickly operating remedies not being at hand.

Otherwise, I ask every reasonable, impartial person: "Which is preferable, to have the thread of life extorted from you piece by piece, or to have the blood distributed by proper water applications in such a way that even the most full-blooded has not a too great quantity of blood?" How and by which application this distributing is to be done, I have discussed several times in the proper place.

It is generally said that in cases of impending strokes, bleeding is the only means of escape. I remember, just now, a case in which a stroke had taken place; the first physician quickly bled the patient; the second one, however, declared that precisely in consequence of this bleeding the patient would die, which indeed was verified. It is not fullness or profusion of blood which generally leads to a stroke, as people erroneously think, but poverty of blood. "He died of a stroke" generally means that the blood having been consumed, life was consumed also. The oil ceased its flowing and nourishing; therefore the glimmering wick was extinguished. Of what useful service the water is immediately after strokes can be seen in the third part of the book, [My Water Cure]. I will only state here that my predecessor in the office of curate had a stroke three times, and after the third time, the physician declared that he could not live any longer. The water has not only saved his life for the moment, but has preserved him to his congregation for several years.

[Ice applications] do not help or encourage Nature to recommence its work: they force it with violence to do so, and that must revenge itself. Ice cloths and ice bags, or whatever the names of those things may be, are entirely excluded from my [water cure methods].

I have always considered the application of ice, especially on the nobler parts of the body, (head, eyes, ears, etc.) to be among the most rugged and violent remedies ever used.

I repeat again that I oppose absolutely any application of ice, and I assert, on the contrary, that water applied in the right way is able to soften and to extinguish any heat, even the most violent, in whatever part or organ of the body it may raging.

Every extraction of blood means nothing less than a shortening of life; for life lives in the blood.

I must try to lead the blood away, to distribute it to the different other parts, for example, I must make applications on the whole body, besides those on the suffering part.

By every loss of blood, whether it be caused by a fall, an accident, or by bleeding, leeches, or scarifying, a particle or part of this stock of blood, of this essence of life, is lost, and in the same measure the body's life is shortened.

Foot Baths*

by Sebastian Kneipp

Amerikanischen Kneipp-Blätter, III (15), 137. (1898)

The foot bath can be taken warm or cold.

The Cold Foot Bath

The cold foot bath consists in standing in the cold water as far as the calves of the legs or higher, for 1 to 3 minutes.

In diseases, the cold foot bath serves principally for leading the blood drawn from the head and chest; but it is generally taken in connection with other applications, sometimes in cases in which a full or half bath cannot be endured by the patient for different reasons.

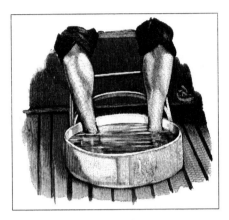

Foot Bath

When taken by healthy people, it aims at giving freshness, and strength; it is especially advisable for country people in summer time, if after a hard and fatiguing day's work, they are unable to sleep at night. This bath takes away weariness, and brings rest and good sleep.

The Warm Foot Bath

The warm foot bath can be taken different ways: salt, hay flower, oat straw and malt foot baths.

Salt Foot Bath

A handful of salt and twice as much wood ashes are mixed in warm water 88° to 90° F/31° to 32° C. Then the foot bath is taken for about 12 or 15 minutes. Sometimes, but always by special order, I give such a foot bath with a temperature as high as 100° F/38° C; but then a cold foot bath of half a minute's duration must always follow.

The foot baths are very useful in all cases where vigorous and cold remedies cannot be used on account of weakness, fragility, want of vital

---

*Benedict Lust republished this article on "Foot Baths" twice more, in the July issue in 1901 and again in September, 1902. —Ed.

warmth, etc.; as little or no reaction takes place, i.e., the cold water cannot produce sufficient warmth for want of blood. These foot baths are suitable for weak, nervous people, for those who have poor blood, for very young, and very old people, mostly for women, and are effective against all disturbances in the circulation of the blood, against congestions, complaints of head or neck, cramps, etc. I do not recommend them to people who suffer from perspiring feet.

Our country people like these cold foot baths, and their effect is acknowledged by the general use of them.

HAY FLOWER FOOT BATH

A sanitary foot bath is that made from hay flowers. Take about three to five handful of hay flowers,* pour boiling water upon them, cover the vessel, and let the whole mixture cool to the warmth of 88° to 90° F/31° to 32° C, the most comfortable temperature for a foot bath. It is of no consequence, whether the hay flowers remain in the foot bath, or whether the decoction only is used. Poorer people use the whole to save time and trouble.

These foot baths operate by dissolving, evacuating, and strengthening; they are of good service for diseased feet, especially sweating feet, open wounds, contusions of every kind (whether arising from a blow, a fall, etc., or bleeding or black and blue with blood), for tumors, gout in the feet, gristle on the toes or putridity between them, for whitlows and hurts caused by too narrow shoes, etc. In general, it may be said that these foot baths are of excellent service for all feet the [fluids] of which are more morbid and more inclined to putridity, than safe and sound.

A gentleman suffering to a great extent from gout in his feet, was freed from pain in an hour by one of these foot baths, together with a foot package, dipped in the decoction.

OAT STRAW FOOT BATH

The foot bath with oat straw is closely connected with the preceding one. The oat straw is boiled for half an hour in a kettle, and a foot bath of 88° to 90° F/31° to 32° C is prepared with the decoction, which is to be taken for 30 to 40 minutes.

According to my experience these foot baths are unsurpassed as regards the dissolving of every possible [callous] of the feet. They are useful against gristle, knots, etc.; against the results of gout, articular disease, podagral [gout of the feet], corns, nails grown in and putrid, and against blisters caused by walking. Even sore and suppurating feet, or

---

*Sebastian Kneipp: "What I call hay flowers are all the remains [found at the bottom of a hay stack] such as stalk, leaves, blossoms and seeds, even hay itself."

toes wounded by too sharp foot sweat, can be treated with these foot baths.

A gentleman had cut his corn, and the toe became inflamed. An ugly ulcer seemed to threaten with blood poisoning. The foot was healed in four days by taking daily three foot baths with oat straw, and applying packages, dipped in the decoction, reaching to above the ankles.

A patient was in danger of having all his toes rotted off; they were swollen and dark blue color. He, too, got frightened about blood poisoning but the foot baths and foot packages cured him in a short time.

In many cases, I prescribe these foot baths to be taken like the full warm baths (see respective passage on "The Warm Full Bath" in Kneipp's book, *My Water Cure*), changing three times, and concluding with the cold bath.*

A constant exception to this rule, however, is made with regard to the warm foot bath of 88° to 90° F/31° to 32° C with admixture of ashes and salt, (mentioned under salt foot bath). The object of this is, to draw the blood more powerfully downwards, and there to distribute it. But if after this warm foot bath a person were to apply a cold bath or ablution to end with, he would thereby drive the blood, which had been strongly led down to the feet, back again. It would by no means flow again so plentifully to the feet as it had done by means of the warm water with ashes and salt. The first desired effect would in this manner be, at least partly, destroyed, and the aim frustrated. Therefore, the warm foot bath with ashes and salt is never to be followed by a cold one.

Malt Grain Foot Bath

I wish to mention here a special kind of foot baths which are more of a solid than a fluid nature. If there is a possibility of using them, do not reject them! I have used them often, very often, with great success. Take malt grains, when still warm, and put them into a foot bath. The feet penetrate easily into them and soon feel comfortable in the salutary warmth. This bath can last from 15 to 30 minutes. Those who are suffering from rheumatism, gout, and such like, will soon find out its sanitary power.

There is one remark to be made concerning all the foot baths. For persons affected with varices, the foot bath ought never to reach higher than the beginning of the calf, and never exceed the temperature of 88° F/31° C.

Foot baths with warm water only, without anything being mixed with it, I never take or prescribe.

[The hay flower] foot bath operates by dissolving, evacuating and

---

*The reference made to "changing three times" refers to alternating the warm foot bath with a cold foot bath three times. More time is spent in the warm water and the cold water is for one minute generally.

strengthening; they are of good service for diseased feet, especially sweating feet, open wounds, contusions of every kind (whether arising from a blow, a fall, etc., or bleeding or black and blue with blood), for tumors, gout in the feet, gristle on the toes or putridity between them, for whitlows and hurts, caused by too narrow shoes, etc.

In diseases, the cold foot bath serves principally for leading the blood drawn from the head and chest; but it is generally taken in connection with other applications, sometimes in cases in which a full or half bath cannot be endured by the patient for different reasons.

A handful of salt and twice as much wood ashes are mixed in warm water 88° to 90° F/31° to 32° C. Then the foot bath is taken for about 12 or 15 minutes.

Take about three to five handful of hay flowers, pour boiling water upon them, cover the vessel, and let the whole mixture cool to the warmth of 88° to 90° F/31° to 32° C, the most comfortable temperature for a foot bath.

These foot baths operate by dissolving, evacuating, and strengthening; they are of good service for diseased feet, especially sweating feet, open wounds, contusions of every kind (whether arising from a blow, a fall, etc., or bleeding or black and blue with blood), for tumors, gout in the feet, gristle on the toes or putridity between them, for whitlows and hurts, caused by too narrow shoes, etc.

According to my experience [oat straw] foot baths are unsurpassed as regards the dissolving of every possible [callous] of the feet.

Therefore, the warm foot bath with ashes and salt is never to be followed by a cold one.

For persons affected with varices, the foot bath ought never to reach higher than the beginning of the calf, and never exceed the temperature of 88° F/31° C.

The Warm Full Bath

by Sebastian Kneipp

Amerikanischen Kneipp Blätter, III (20), 193-194. (1898)

The warm full bath like the cold one is useful both for the healthy and the sick. The manner of taking it is two-fold.

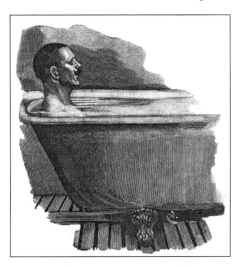

The one bath (a) is sufficiently filled with warm water to cover the whole body, and in this bath the person remains for 25 to 30 minutes. At the end of that time, the other bath (b) filled with cold water, is quickly entered, the person dipping in up to the head, but not with the head. If no second bath is there, the whole body is washed as quickly as possible with cold water. This cold bath, or cold washing, must be finished in one minute. The clothes are then put on, quickly, without drying, and exercise taken for at least half an hour, either in the room or in the open air, until one feels quite dry and warm. Country people may immediately return to their work. The water for this first bath must have a temperature of 90° to 95° F / 32° to 35° C, for aged persons 95° to 100° F/ 35° to 38° C. It is advisable to measure carefully and accurately with a thermometer, which is easily obtained. But it is not sufficient to put the thermometer into the warm water, and take it out again at once; it must remain in the water for a while. Those who prepare a bath should do it earnestly, being aware of their responsibility. Indifference and carelessness are nowhere less pardonable than in such important services of charity.

The second way to take this bath is the following. The bath is filled as mentioned before, but the water has the temperature of 100° to 112° F /38° to 44° C. With these baths 112° F/44° C should never be exceeded, but also no lower temperature taken than 95° F/35° C; on the average I advise and prepare them myself with 102° to 106° F/39° to 41° C.

Those who take this bath go into the warm water not once, but three times, and also into the cold water three times. This is the so-called warm full bath with three-fold change. The whole bath takes precisely 33 minutes; the different changing is done as follows:

> 10 minutes in the warm bath,
> 1 minute in the cold bath,
> 10 minutes in the warm bath,
> 1 minute in the cold bath,
> 10 minutes in the warm bath,
> 1 minute in the cold bath.

Without exception the [warm full bath with three-fold change] must always be concluded by the cold bath. Healthy, strong people sit down in the cold water bath, and dip in slowly up to the head. Sensitive persons sit down and quickly wash chest and back* without dipping under. A whole ablution answers the same purpose for those who are too much afraid of the cold bath. The head is never wetted; if it has become wet, it must be dried. Likewise, after the last cold bath, no other part of the body is to be dried except the hands, and these in order not to wet the clothes when redressing. For the rest, especially as regards the necessary exercise after the bath, the same rules are to be observed as regarding the first baths.

I owe a few remarks here. Warm baths alone, i.e. without subsequent cold baths or ablutions, are never prescribed by me. The higher degree of warmth, especially if it lasts and operates for a longer time, does not strengthen, but it weakens and relaxes the whole organism; it does not harden, but makes the skin still more sensitive to the cold; it does not protect, but it endangers. The warm water opens the pores, and lets the cold air in, the consequences of which are to be seen even in the following hours. The cold baths or cold ablutions following the warm ones act as a remedy to the latter (I do not allow any application of warm water without the following cold one,) the fresh water strengthens, by lowering the higher temperature of the body; it refreshes by washing off, as it were, the superfluous heat; it protects by closing the pores, and making the skin more firm. The same prejudice against the sudden cold following the warmth meets us again here. It is precisely on account of the cold bath following that the warm one can and must be given at a higher temperature than is usual, or than I myself would agree to generally. The body is filled with so much warmth, armed as it were, that it is able to stand the shock of the penetrating cold.

---

*The patients throw as much water over their shoulders as sufficient to wash the back.
—*Sebastian Kneipp.*

Those who are too much afraid of the cold bath at first, may begin with a whole ablution; they will thereby get courage. It depends entirely upon the first trial. Those who have once tried it will never take a warm bath again without the following cold one, if only on account of the comfort it gives. To many who at first trembled with fear, but later on became used to the strange changing and liked it, I was obliged to dictate strict limits to prevent the excess of good from turning to evil.

The prickling and crawling sensation on the skin, which is strongly felt upon going back to the warm bath, after the cold one, especially on the feet, need not frighten anyone; later on it will seem like an agreeable rubbing.

For these two kinds of full baths there is no necessity of preparations, e.g. to bring the body to the right temperature.

Here, as for all the warm baths, I never, or at least very seldom, use warm water alone; decoctions of different herbs are always mixed with them.

THE WARM FULL BATH FOR THE HEALTHY

If I order warm full baths for healthy persons, i.e. comparatively healthy, (healthy, but weak persons,) I do so only in cases where such weakened people cannot make up their minds to take cold baths, and solely for the purpose of preparing and ripening them by this warm full bath, with the cold one following, for the fresh cold bath.

My principles and my practice with reference to this are as follows. I seldom, or almost never, order warm baths for quite healthy and strong natures, whose fresh, rosy complexion sparkles, as it were, with warmth and vital fire. Nor do they desire them either, for they long for the cold water like a fish. I recommend them for younger people who are weak, poor of blood, and nervous, especially those who are inclined to cramps, rheumatism and such like complaints; and before all others to the mothers of families, who are worn out so early by every possible hardship. Such a bath with 95° F/35° C and subsequent cold ablution, taken for 25 to 30 minutes, every month, would be sufficient for them. For those who are inclined to articular diseases, gout, podagra [gout of the feet]; two such baths a month would be better than one. Younger persons should try the cold full bath in summer time.

To aged and weak people I recommend at least one warm full bath every month of 95° to 100° F/35° to 38° C taken for 25 minutes and concluding with a cold ablution, for cleanliness of the skin, for refreshment and for strengthening. They will feel quite renewed after such bath on account of the greater perspiration activity of the skin and more vivid circulation of the blood.

This cold bath, or cold washing, must be finished in one minute. The clothes are then put on, quickly, without drying, and exercise taken for at least half an hour, either in the room or in the open air, until one feels quite dry and warm.

Without exception the [warm full bath with three-fold change] must always be concluded by the cold bath.

Warm baths alone, i.e. without subsequent cold baths or ablutions, are never prescribed by me.

The cold baths or cold ablutions following the warm ones, act as a remedy to the latter (I do not allow any application of warm water without the following cold one,) the fresh water strengthens, by lowering the higher temperature of the body; it refreshes by washing off, as it were, the superfluous heat; it protects by closing the pores, and making the skin more firm.

I seldom, or almost never, order warm baths for quite healthy and strong natures, whose fresh, rosy complexion sparkles, as it were, with warmth and vital fire.

Kneipp Cure Institutes In America

by A. N. Tally, Jr. M.D.

Amerikanischen Kneipp Blätter, III (22 & 23), 227-228. (1898)

The absolutely convincing results of Hydrotherapy are lucidly evidenced not alone by an ever increasing favoritism and preference among the laity, but especially by the far more demonstrative fact that the practice is rapidly invading and conquering the ranks and file of the intelligent body of men compromising the medical profession. Should this be very surprising? Not at all. For if we but open our eyes and scan the threatening horizon of untold woe and misery of this great world of ours and notice the steady and ever onward march of suffering and the thousands of chronic invalids in the very face and at the threshold of legion of so-called remedies, we cannot help to think that something must be vitally wrong, and we cannot condemn people when they are losing confidence in existing remedial agencies and we are compelled to welcome the delight the intellectual rays that are dawning and pervading with their brightest illuminatory influence all classes of society. *Back to nature* are the enchanting words that were hurled like a terrific thunderbolt against the artificial but perverted ideas menacing a sad and erring mass of humanity by the greatest philanthropist the present century produced. Back to nature. Yes, back to nature a proper mode of living, mentally, morally and physically, and a rational usage of water, were the magnetic doctrine which seemed to electrify the entire world and was re-echoed from one end of the globe to the other. The man who thus dared to assail the prevailing but erroneous and aged ideas, that had wandered far from their home, to return beneath the motherly roof of a kind Nature's care, and to whom is due the lion's share of the monumental edifice and popularization of modern Hydrotherapy, was no more or less that simple and humble clergymen and physician at Wörishofen, Father Kneipp, who has since been called to this eternal home to accept the long earned reward he so eminently deserved.

Monsignor Kneipp was a great man in every sense of the word and one of those intellectual and clear seeing giants who are so rare in our times. By means of his keen analytical faculties, grafted upon individual observations and an enormous experience, he soon became convinced of the superiority and efficacy of Water Cure, and hence inaugurated a new era in the annals of the healing art by establishing a system of his own, which was rapidly gained renown in all civilized portions of the globe and is universally known as the Kneipp Method of Water Cure. The powerful and all conquering spirit which dominated this apostle of charity, who sacrificed himself relentlessly at the shrine of humanity, the unequalled results which have crowned his laborious task among suffering humankind is best attested by the thousands of sufferers who annually came to Wörishofen, which, through the brilliant achievements of Father Kneipp, became the largest hydrotherapeutic sanitarium of the world. The best proof however, of the efficiency of his method is demonstrated by the fact that numerous sanitariums were soon in demand and erected both in Europe and in America, where the Kneipp system of Water Cure is practiced, by means of which hundreds have been restored to health. Many have improved and all have learned to appreciate the salutary influence of water if applied rationally and in suitable cases.

People having been actual observers of these facts and thoroughly imbued and convinced of the unexcelled and immense advantages to be derived by suffering humanity from the inauguration of a method of such simple, uncomplicated, yet thoroughly effective nature, have erected sanitariums on the Kneipp system at different parts in this country.

First, we mention the St. Francis' Sanitarium at Denville, which was opened May 15th, 1895. During the short period of its existence, it has formed an interstate reputation and today enjoys an ever increasing and desirable patronage. Denville is situated in Morris County, New Jersey, thirty miles west of New York City, on the Delaware, Lackawanna & Western Railroad.

Denville is a highly healthful resort and well fitted by Nature for a sanitarium. The air is pure and bracing. The grounds of the sanitarium comprise over two hundred acres situated on the heights of Denville, on both sides of the beautiful Rockaway River. The place abounds in sunny meadows and shady forests. The property comprises a beautiful lake in the woods.

Here, removed from the bustle and turmoil incident to large cities, the sufferer finds an alleviating balm for his spiritual and physical ills in the unsurpassed bounty of Nature, which goes a great ways towards restoration of his health, particularly if such hygienic surroundings are supplemented by careful nursing and special attention as each individual case may demand.

PATIENTS ADMITTED AND DISEASES THAT HAVE BEEN SUCCESSFULLY TREATED BY THIS METHOD

Above all, this treatment is to be recommended to such persons as are enfeebled by overstrain resulting from severe intellectual application, and to people who are confined, day by day, the entire year in their workshops or [work place[, breathing the impure atmosphere of their surroundings, thereby acquiring early a material disposition for various diseases. Incalculable would be the benefit for our overworked generation, were they to devote two or three weeks each year to such a treatment, instead of going to the luxurious summer resorts where usually the last fraction of health force is sacrificed incidental to the dissipation and excitement demanded by the tyranny of society. If they would undergo the invigorating action of water for two to three weeks each year in a sanitarium of pleasant location and quiet environments, they would relieve their organism of the foul contaminating material with which it is charged, harden themselves so that they could easily withstand the continual onslaught of disease and return to their business with renewed vigor and cheerfulness.

Persons with acute affections, i.e. if their ailments are not of a contagious nature, for in the latter instance the welfare of their fellow patients would be endangered.

Diseases of the respiratory organs, catarrhal bronchitis, asthma, spitting of blood, primary stages of consumption, catarrhal affections of the pharynx and larynx, etc.

Diseases of the heart, palpitations, debility, and general functional derangements of that organ.

Kidneys and bladder diseases, Bright's disease, chronic inflammation of kidneys or bladder, hematuria, etc.

Acute and chronic infections of muscles and joints, rheumatism, gout, inflammatory conditions of joints i.e. if such are not of malignant nature, hip joint disease, etc.

Diseases of the nervous system, chorea or St. Vitus dance, sciatica, neurasthenia, nervousness, neuralgia, headache, hysteria, insomnia, melancholia, etc.

Chlorosis and anemia or disorders resulting from a faulty formation or circulation of the blood.

Paralyses, particularly of the paralysis of spinal origin frequently found in children.

Eruptive diseases in general.

Scrophulous conditions, inherited or acquired, particularly the latter where through faulty digestion and assimilation of food, the healthy and robust development of the organism is impossible.

Stomach and bowel affections, dyspepsia, diarrhea, constipation, etc.

Diseases peculiar to women.

Obesity or undue accumulation of fat in the body.

Back to nature *are the enchanting words that were hurled like a terrific thunderbolt against the artificial but perverted ideas menacing a sad and erring mass of humanity by the greatest philanthropist the present century produced. Back to nature.*

By means of his keen analytical faculties, grafted upon individual observations and an enormous experience, he soon became convinced of the superiority and efficacy of Water Cure, and hence inaugurated a new era in the annals of the healing art by establishing a system of his own, which was rapidly gained renown in all civilized portions of the globe and is universally known as the Kneipp Method of Water Cure.

Incalculable would be the benefit for our overworked generation, were they to devote two or three weeks each year to such a treatment, instead of going to the luxurious summer resorts where usually the last fraction of health force is sacrificed incidental to the dissipation and excitement demanded by the tyranny of society.

1899

MOUNTAIN AIR RESORT "BELLEVUE" BUTLER, NEW JERSEY
LOUISA STROEBELE

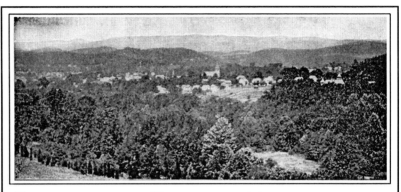
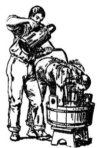
Louisa Stroebele purchased 60 acres of land near the village of Butler, New Jersey, in the late 19th century. Here, she built a very successful health retreat called the Bellevue and hired Benedict Lust as her resident Hydropathist.

Mountain Air Resort "Bellevue," Butler, New Jersey

by Louisa Stroebele

Amerikanischen Kneipp Blätter, IV (3), 141. (1899)

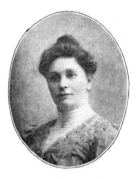

Louisa Stroebele
[1864-1925]

Most romantically situated on the top of a hill, about ten minutes' walk from the depot, "Bellevue" comprises thirty acres of woodland, laid out with shady walks along a picturesque brook of clear water, known as Trout Brook, and with its beauty-spots in the shape of quiet nooks, sheltered from the sun, its numerous springs along the hillside, its grand view into the Ramapo Mountains, is an ideal summer resort for lovers of Nature.

The view from the celebrated "Kick Out" Mountain, one mile from Bellevue, is beyond description, and at once reminds the spectator of the Alps in Switzerland. It is only of late that this northern part of New Jersey, with its mountain ranges and its attractive sceneries, has become the favorite spot of the people of New York and neighboring cities as a mountain air resort, being recommended for its pure, bracing, and invigorating air by numerous prominent physicians of New York City.

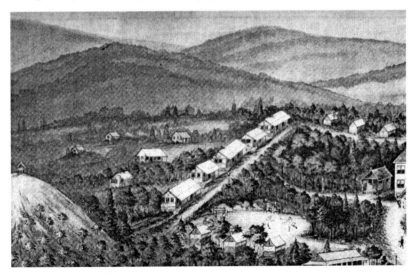

This ad published in 1917 indicates that the Butler Yungborn was open all year round, and used only drugless methods.

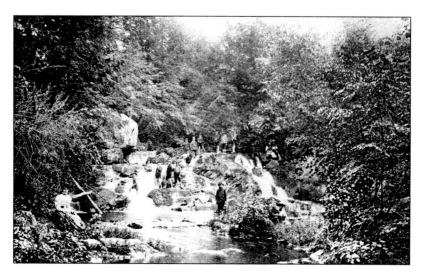

The Butler Yungborn was renowned for its beautiful vistas and had two brooks traversing the property.

The mountains are from 1,100 to 1,400 feet high. A number of lakes, as Greenwood Lake, Echo Lake, Pompton Lake, and others are within reach for a day's outing, and may be approached either by private conveyance or by railroad.

Many who formerly spent the summer months in the Catskill Mountains give now the reference to these regions, finding the air here as pure as there, with the advantage of being here nearer to their homes and to the seashore. Butler being only thirty miles from New York City, parties wishing to spend a day for a change in the latter place can leave Butler by a morning train and return in the evening, the fare for a trip both ways being only $1.00 by using the so-called ten trip tickets.

BELLEVUE also offers the advantage of having an open air swimming bath on its own grounds, besides the Turkish-Russian baths in the building, and the air and sun baths in tents especially arranged for the purpose. Here removed from the bustle and turmoil incident to large cities, one finds an alleviating balm spiritually and physically in the unsurpassed bounty of Nature, which goes a great ways towards recuperation of health, particularly if, as is the case at BELLEVUE, such hygienic surroundings are supplemented by a common-sense diet, cooking being done in such a manner that food is not only prepared to please the taste, but upon scientific principles, which insures the best results nutritionally. Aside from carefully selected food such as cereals, meats, fish and fowl, and vegetables in large variety, the table is abundantly supplied with rich milk and fresh butter, also with fruits at all seasons.

Butler is a station on the New York, Susquehanna & Western

Railroad. The Railroad Company is constantly improving its train service, there being at present fourteen trains to and from New York on week days, and four on Sundays. It has also been stated that the Electric Railroad Company having now a line from Hoboken to Singac (only six miles from Butler) will before long continue the line through Pompton Plains to Butler and Greenwood Lake.

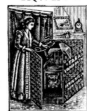

Expenses at the BELLEVUE are $15.00 per week, baths included, invariable to be paid in advance. Children under twelve, half price. Parties desiring carriage on their arrival, for which there will be a reasonable charge, should give notice beforehand. For circulars and other detailed information address:

Miss L. Stroebele, Bellevue, Butler, New Jersey
Or to the New York City Office: 111 E. 59th St., New York City

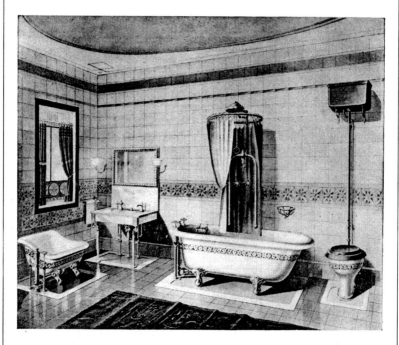
State of the art bathroom in the late 19th century

1900

The Pfarrer Sebastian Kneipp Medicine Company on Astor Street was one of the first in America to promote Kneipp products. In 1896, Benedict Lust launched his own publication, *Amerikanischen Kneipp Blätter,* which would promote the work of Father Kneipp and also provide an excellent way to advertize Kneipp products at his store in New York City.

The Kneipp Gushes Or Pours

by Benedict Lust

The Kneipp Water Cure Monthly, I (1), 6-7. (1900)

While the public in general is under the impression that walking in the grass is the principal means of healing in the Kneipp cure, there is a little more to understand, a little more to know for the practitioner of the Kneipp Water Cure than simply the how and when to take a walk in the grass.

Kneipp's gushes in connection with a well-regulated diet form a very important factor in the Kneipp cure. The cold water gushes are the means of producing heat and invigorating the whole system. Not everyone knows how these gushes have to be applied. The application of the Kneipp gush is an art which must be learned, the nature and effect of which must be studied to be sure of beneficial results. Experience is as necessary as understanding but experience will be the best teacher.

All patients are not equally strong; therefore, it is the duty of the Kneipp practitioner to study the strength of the system of the patient and regulate according to it the length and strength of the gushes. With some people's reaction, the flushing of the skin sets in very quickly, with others it takes more time, but this reaction has to come in every case.

The Kneipp gushes are: head gush, face gush, ear gush, breast gush, arm gush, upper gush, hip or thigh gush, knee gush, back gush, full gush and the lightning gush.

The Head Gush

The water gush or pour is directed against the head, not against a single spot but the whole head. The water pour must be moved in a circle five or six times.

The Face Gush

Begin on the chin; then go up to the left eye over the forehead, down to the right eye and back to the spot where the gush was started. This is done five or six times. The patient stoops forward so that the water has a good flow.

For head and face gush the patient remains clothed.

The Ear Gush

For this gush the [position] of the patient is a bent one, so that the water can run off. The gush is directed round the ear four or five times.

THE BREAST GUSH

This gush is started on the arm from the hand up to the shoulder and across the breast and back again for about one or two minutes.

THE ARM GUSH

Start with the gush at the right hand and go up to the shoulder and remain there for a little while. Repeat the same with the left arm. The gush lasts from one to two minutes.

THE UPPER GUSH

This gush is a difficult one and requires some practice on part of the attendant. Start the gush at the right hand, go upwards to the shoulder, then move the gush down the back to a spot near the centre of it. Rest here for a little while so that the water covers the back well. The chest is not gushed and it must be carefully avoided to let the stream of water fall directly upon the spine. The gush lasts from one to two minutes. When treating weak people it will be advisable not to rest in the spot mentioned but to cross over the left side of the patient's back, to move up to the left shoulder and down the left arm. Then seek a spot on left or right side from whence the water may flow over the back.

THE HIP OR THIGH GUSH*

Start at heel of the right foot, move the gush up the centre of the calf, rest here for a little while, so that the water washes the whole thigh, move up slowly to the waist and go back to the starting point. The same is done with the left foot. This has to be repeated three or four times with each foot. Then the patient has to turn round and the same process is repeated in the front, starting at the right foot. The more equally the gush is applied the greater the benefit. It has to last from one to three minutes.

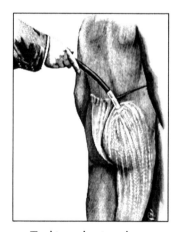

The hip gush using a hose.

------

*Benedict Lust published an article in the April issue in 1908 on the thigh gush and here is what he writes: "Kidney troubles, hemorrhoids, stomach troubles, congestions, asthma and any excitements are especially cured by thigh gushes. Father Kneipp did not treat children to these gushes, but plunged their whole bodies into water; and old people he treated leniently by applying cold water at 68° F / 20° C." (Lust, 1908, 112) —Ed.

The Knee Gush

The knee gush is started in the manner as the hip gush but only carried up as far as the middle of the calf. From this point let the water flow so that the whole calf is covered. Then do the same with the left foot and repeat the process four or five times. Have the patient turn round and start at the toes of the right foot, go up to a point a little above the knee and keep the gush directed to that spot for some time. Do the same with the left foot. The gush has to last from one to two minutes.

The Back Gush*

This gush is started at the heel of the right foot, carried up to the waist and back again. Then start at the left foot, go up with the gush to the waist, cross over to the other side of the waist and up to the right shoulder, go again back with the gush to the right waist, over to the left side and up to the left shoulder. The front part of the body is not gushed. The gush has to last from one to two minutes.

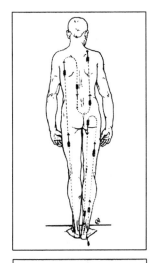

---

*Benedict Lust adds the following advice for the back gush: "During this gush the flush touches a large field of nerves; that is the vertebral column with its articulations. After this application some have pains in the sacral region; others lose their breath; others again have cramps in the muscular apparatus of the back. If the asthmatic complaints increase, the gushing has to be stopped and the breast to be washed with cold water.

People who have a weak spinal cord, rheumatism or gout will be cured by these gushes; people with weak lungs can only take them if they are not nervous; also paralyzed ones will be benefited by them. ... If the back gushes cannot be followed by a thorough reaction, they will be more of detrimental than of beneficial effect. The reaction will be brought on by stooping, stretching of the body and raising the scapula. If the patient has no natural warmth, he ought not to take back gushes." (Lust, 1908, 112)   —Ed.

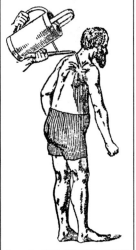

The back gush using a watering can.

The Full Gush

This gush is started in the same way as the back gush, but from the left shoulder the gush has to be carried up to the neck. If the patient a strong person, one may at once start on the chest in the front, and let the water spread over the abdomen and thighs, but with weak people one will do better to go slow and start at the toes of the right foot, go up to the thighs and back again. Start at the toes of the left foot, move the gush up to the thighs, go over to the right side and up to the right breast. Then move back again to the left side of the abdomen, go up to the breast and from there to the centre of the breast.

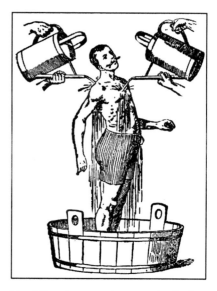

The full gush covers the entire body, first on one side and then on the other.

The Lightning Gush

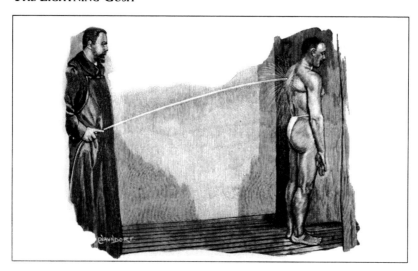

The lightning gush uses pressurized water.

This gush finished the Kneipp system of gush treatments. The lightning gush is very complicated; it covers every inch of the body, front and back. A practitioner of great experience and skill only will be able to apply this gush in the way it ought to be applied. It is impossible to understand the theory of the application of this gush without having seen how it is done, without receiving detailed instructions. The *whipping* forms an essential part of it and follows the complicated maneuvers with the jet or full stream of water. It consists of quick movements of the jet and produces an effect like the one which would be attained by whipping the body, front and back, with a whip made of water. The whole lightning gush lasts from five to eight minutes.

These gushes produce effects not known heretofore. Kneipp's system or the Kneipp cure as it is known, potentially heals all diseases in any way curable, for these various applications of water tend to remove the roots of the disease. The whole system of gushes will dissolve morbid matter in the blood, evacuate what is dissolved, make the cleansed blood circulate rightly, and harden and strengthen the enfeebled organism.

A man who is accustomed to these treatments, a man who went through the lightning gush treatment, does not need to worry that a change in temperature will affect his system. He will be a different man altogether. It makes the old feel young again, and the young strong, healthy and happy.

The application of the Kneipp gush is an art which must be learned, the nature and effect of which must be studied to be sure of beneficial results. Experience is as necessary as understanding, but experience will be the best teacher.

With some people's reaction, the flushing of the skin sets in very quickly, with others it takes more time, but this reaction has to come in every case.

The lightning gush is very complicated, it covers every inch of the body, front and back. A practitioner of great experience and skill only will be able to apply this gush in the way it ought to be applied.

The whole system of gushes will dissolve morbid matter in the blood, evacuate what is dissolved, make the cleansed blood circulate rightly, and harden and strengthen the enfeebled organism.

HYDROPATHIC MEDICAL ADVISER

by Ludwig Staden, Hygienic Physician (Naturarzt)
The Kneipp Water Cure Monthly, I (1), 14. (1900)

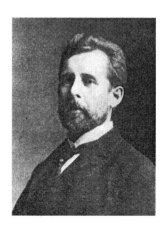

Ludwig Staden

Mr. G. M., Scranton, Pennsylvania—
ASTHMA

Most cases of asthma have their real origin in dysemia of the blood, which causes more or less accumulations of morbid matter in the muscular fibres of the five branches of the wind pipe. General treatment consists in hardening the entire system through cold sponge bath every morning directly after rising; thereafter, a good energetic rubbing of the whole body or to bed again for 10 to 15 minutes in order to rewarm the body. Three or four times weekly a bed steam bath from one to one and a half hours, with one hot water bottle enveloped in a wet towel applied to the feet and one to the calves and thighs of both legs. Thereafter, the first time, a knee douche; the second time, an upper douche; the third time, a back douche according to Kneipp,

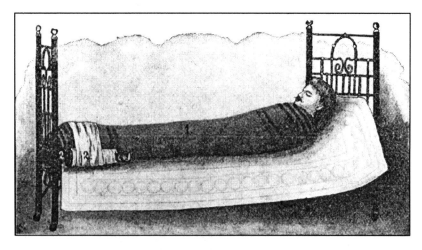

The steam bath in bed resembles a wet sheet wrap with the addition of hot water bottles placed alongside the wet sheet before wrapping the patient in a woolen blanket. The size of the compress can be an abdominal, three-quarter, or full wet sheet.

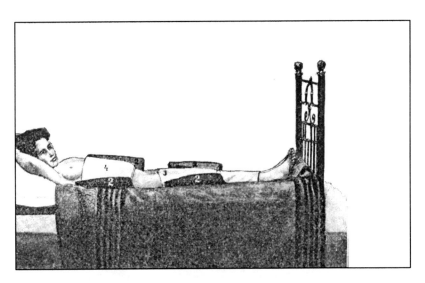

The hot water bottles are lying next to the patient's body in the bed steam bath.

and for the rest of the body a cool sponge bath. Three times a week before going to bed an alternate foot bath, put the feet in water 100° to 105° F / 38° to 40.6° C about one foot high for five minutes; then directly in cold water about 60° F / 16° C for a half minute and repeat this twice. If constipated a lukewarm injection 90° F / 32° C daily or every other day. In case of a bit of asthma, which often occurs during the night, put thick hot compresses on the chest and hold the feet and hands for five minutes in hot water and immediately afterwards in cool water for a half minute. This may be repeated four to six times. The hot compresses have to be renewed when getting cold. A vegetarian, non-stimulating diet is of great benefit, especially fruits, berries, fruit juices, milk, whole wheat bread, all kinds of vegetables and cereals, also tea of ribwort. Avoid strictly beer, wine, brandy, etc., coffee, tea, beef tea, meat, soup, etc., and smoking. Sleep by the open window and be in fresh air as much as possible. Deep and slow breathing through the nostrils is a special exercise outdoors.

S. R., Stamford, Connecticut—Sick Headache

Overloading the stomach, constipation, and errors in diet are the principle causes. Do not eat except when you feel really hungry; give up meat and all stimulants and try a non-irritating diet, plenty of fruits. During an attack, take a tea with a spoon of lemon juice every 15 minutes and lay down, also a warm sitz bath 95° F / 35° C for 20-25 minutes and cool sponge bath thereafter. Further, an injection of warm water 95° F / 35° C, one to one and a half quarts, followed directly after evacuation by a cold

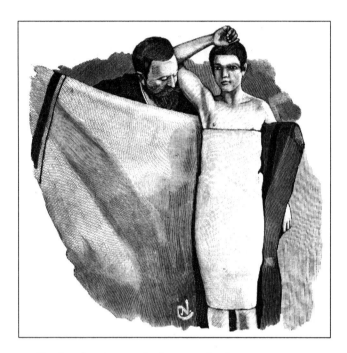

The short bandage or also known as the three-quarter wrap.

enema of about a half wine glass full of water which has to remain in the rectum. A three-quarter pack or short wrap according to Kneipp once or twice a week will be very beneficial. Needless to say: plenty of fresh air.

Ludwig Staden, Hygienic Physician (Naturarzt)
346 Schermerhorn Street
Brooklyn, New York

The Spanish Mantle, Half Bath And Foot Vapor Bath

by Benedict Lust

The Kneipp Water Cure Monthly, I (3), 36-38. (1900)

This strange appellation is not of Kneipp's invention. Other Hydropathists rendered the treatment with great and good results and Kneipp, too, found it of great service in certain cases; therefore, he had no reason to change its name.

The Spanish mantle is a whole application in itself like the full bath or the short packing, because its effects extend to the whole organism. Nevertheless, it should only be used alternately with other water applications in cases of serious and dangerous illness.

Here is a description of the Spanish mantle:

A sort of a long shirt is made of coarse linen; this shirt should be open in front and must reach down to the toes, it should resemble a very wide, long night gown, open in the front. This mantle is dipped into cold water, wrung out and put on like an ordinary night shirt, one part folded will cover the other in front. Those who are afraid of cold water, weak or aged people or those of poor blood may dip the mantle into hot water. The bed must be prepared beforehand. Woolen blankets are spread over it in such a way that the patient may lie down on them. He is then closely wrapped in the blankets. The putting on of the wet mantle and the wrapping up in the woolen blankets must be done as quickly as possible. This is very important for the exposure to the fresh air must be limited to as little time as possible.

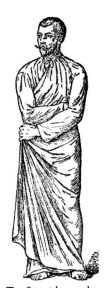

The Spanish mantle

Once, a patient who was suffering from all sorts of ailments came to Kneipp. A faintness of the heart caused him great trouble and congestions and hemorrhoids tormented him. Kneipp applied the Spanish mantle once or twice a week for some time and soon, all the above mentioned complaints, as well as many others, which ailed the patient were gone. He himself said, he felt as when his pains and ailments were blown away. Since that time, the gentleman in question uses the Spanish mantle as a sort of universal remedy. He puts it on when he goes to bed and takes it off when awakening during the night or in the morning. To make the help of others unnecessary, he has a second Spanish mantle made of wool which he puts over the wet linen one.

As a rule, this application should not last longer than from one to two hours at the most. The duration of it depends upon the strength of the patient, especially upon his corpulence. For a weak farm laborer, one hour or one hour and a half may be sufficient, while a fat brewer, for instance, will need the application for at least two hours.

The strong and beneficial operation of the Spanish mantle is easily proven. Simply inspect the water in which the mantle after the application is washed. By the way, it must be washed after every treatment. You will be astonished and think it almost incredible, dear reader, the amount of dirt extracted from the body. Father Kneipp experienced cases in which the white linen of the mantle seemed to be dyed yellow. No washing but only bleaching in the sun could remove the yellow and give back to the linen its white color.

All the chief pores of the whole body are opened by the Spanish mantle in a very mild way; the dirt and phlegm are excreted. It is easy to understand how beneficial the effect must be upon the temperature of the body and upon the general health of the patient.

For general catarrhs, mucous, fever, gout, smallpox, typhus, etc., etc., there is no better remedy as the Spanish mantle, as Father Kneipp has found out. In cases of gout, gravel, etc., the Spanish mantle may be dipped into a decoction of hay flowers, oat straw or pine sprigs. As a rule, the effect of the application will be greater when the mantle is dipped into a decoction of such herbs as may possess healing qualities for the ailment to be cured.

THE HALF BATH

There are cases for which the full bath offers too much and the foot bath too little effect. Therefore, Kneipp used in such cases what he called the half bath. He applied this bath in three different ways:

1. The patient stands in the water so that it reaches above the calves or above the knees.

2. The patient kneels in the water so that the whole of the thighs is covered.

3. Patients sit in the water so that it reaches to about the navel. This third application is the original Kneipp half bath.*

Of course, only cold water is used. As a means of hardening these applications are excellent. Healthy people who want to become stronger

---

*Benedict Lust credits Kneipp with discovering the Half Bath, but in fact, Priessnitz deserves this honour. —Ed.

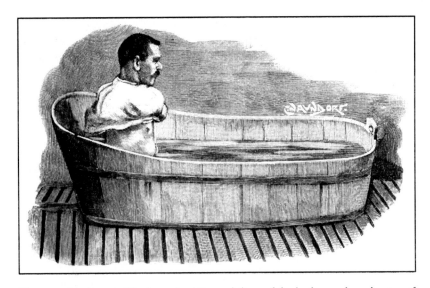

The water level in a half bath reached the umbilicus of the bather and used water of different temperatures. Kneipp and Priessnitz were ardently fond of cold water in a half bath.

can do nothing better than take a half bath once in a while, weak people, as well as, convalescents will be greatly benefited and soon get entirely well and strong.

In diseases they should be taken when especially and expressly prescribed; experiments ought not to be made with them, for in some cases they may do harm.

Other applications should always follow the half bath which should never last longer than from a half a minute to three minutes.

Kneipp used the standing and kneeling applications (No. 1 and No. 2,) upon patients in thorough decline and always with great success. With these applications he commenced his Water Cure. There are many people who in the beginning cannot bear the pressure of the water in a full bath. The reason is either their great weakness or wretchedness, consequently a discrete, moderate and considerate application of cold water is necessary. Sometimes this must be done for weeks, until such patients get strong enough to be able to endure more.

As a second means of hardening, a dipping in of the arms up to the shoulders is connected with the half bath [Nos. 1 and 2, standing and kneeling].

To healthy people the real half bath cannot be recommended too highly. The disorders and diseases of the lower part of the body are by this bath suffocated in the germ or removed where they are already settled. Upon the bowels the effect of the half bath is very great. They are preserved and their strength increases. Many people wear a bandage as a protection against cold, etc. Does such a bandage really protect? No, it weakens, not considering other effects even worse than the one mentioned.

Piles, wind colic, hypochondria and hysteria will soon greatly diminish after a regular use of the half bath.

Healthy people should wash the upper part of their bodies with cold water in the morning and in the afternoon or evening take a half bath.

Before concluding the article, we cite some instances of successful cures by means of the half bath.

Typhus had weakened a young man so that he was quite unable to work. He started the treatment with the kneeling in the water every second or third day, first only for one minute and later on for two or three minutes. This mode of treatment was kept up for some time and soon the patient was as well and strong as before his sickness.

Another patient was suffering from violent congestions. The upper part of the body was washed one day and the next day the kneeling in the water followed. This mode of treatment was kept up for a certain time and soon the congestions ceased.

For pains in the stomach caused by retained wind, this same treatment will be of great benefit. A special effect of the half bath is the evacuation of such gases which are so troublesome after diseases.

THE VAPOR FOOT BATH

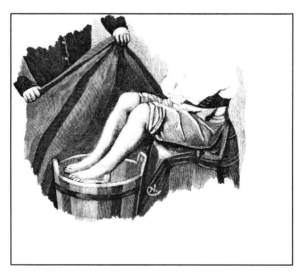

The foot vapor bath

In our last month's issue, we spoke about the vapor head bath. This time we will throw some light upon the vapor foot bath and its merits. The application of this bath is rendered as follows:

A rather wide and thick blanket is placed lengthwise on a chair upon which the patient sits down with bare feet and legs. A wooden foot bath, a little more than half filled with boiling water is put before him. On the upper edge of the bath at the handles two small pieces of wood are fastened, on which the patient can easily put his feet. Great care must be taken, however, about secure fastening, in order to prevent the danger of their giving way and scalding the patient's feet. As soon as the patient is in the position, the thick blanket is put around his feet and the tub in such a way as to entirely prevent the steam from escaping.

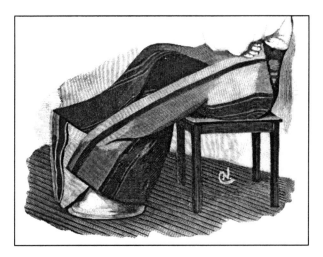

A woolen blanket wrapped around the legs retains the steam during a foot vapor bath.

Kneipp used a light, boiling decoction of hay flowers or put the hay flowers themselves into the boiling water.

The effect as well as duration of this application can be increased by putting a hot brick into the water every five or ten minutes.* This must be done carefully; there must be no splashing as otherwise the splashing may scald the feet of the patient. The greater the effect intended shall be, the longer the bath has to last. In cases of sweating feet, for instance, only the

---

*With the advent of modern appliances, such as an electric water kettle, the use of bricks is obsolete. —Ed.

soles of the feet are to be brought into perspiration, again in other cases it is necessary to bring into perspiration the whole legs, the thighs included, sometimes the abdomen and sometimes the whole body.

Kneipp treated many cases by this simple application after which the patient was bathed in sweat as when covered by half a dozen blankets. As a rule, the application should last in cases where there is only a mild form of treatment wanted no longer than from 15 to 20 minutes, but to produce the highest effects of a real vapor bath it will be necessary to renew the hot brick every 5 or 10 minutes and have the bath last for 25 or 30 minutes.

The vapor bath must always be followed by a cooling application which has to extend over all parts which perspired. If only feet and legs have been sweating, wash the same with a wet towel; strong people may take a knee gush. If the thighs and abdomen have been perspiring, a half bath has to follow the vapor foot bath. Should the perspiration extend all over the body, a half bath in connection with the washing of the upper part of the body will answer the purpose of cooling or a full bath may be taken. (See Kneipp, *My Water Cure*)

The benefit of the application of the vapor foot bath will be great for all the manifold sufferings of the feet, as there are for instance, badly smelling perspiration, swollen feet, in many cases caused by accumulations of juices and blood, and cold feet to which the blood cannot find its way. The vapor foot bath will also be of great service for whitlows, nails grown in, blood poisoning set in consequence of badly cut out corns, torn out nail roots, etc., etc. A quickly applied vapor foot bath will do good work in all such cases.

Against headaches originating in the congestion of blood in the head, an increased application of the vapor foot bath will work wonders.

Slight vapor foot baths have been of good service to those who need a general warming up of the body before a cold water application can be made. This vapor foot bath should not be applied oftener than once or twice a week, three times in one week only in special cases. The vapor foot bath is most undoubtedly far superior to any sweating bath applied in the old style.*

---

*Lust is alluding to the "blanket sweating bath" employed by Vincent Priessnitz. These baths could last as long as four hours and patients would perspire copious amounts.
—Ed.

Nevertheless, [the Spanish mantle] should only be used alternately with other water applications in cases of serious and dangerous illness.

This mantle is dipped into cold water, wrung out and put on like an ordinary night shirt, one part folded will cover the other in front.

The bed must be prepared beforehand. Woolen blankets are spread over it in such a way that the patient may lie down on them. He is then closely wrapped in the blankets.

As a rule, this application should not last longer than from one to two hours at the most. The duration of it depends upon the strength of the patient, especially upon his corpulence.

All the chief pores of the whole body are opened by the Spanish mantle in a very mild way; the dirt and phlegm are excreted.

For general catarrhs, mucous, fever, gout, smallpox, typhus, etc., etc., there is no better remedy as the Spanish mantle, as Father Kneipp has found out. In cases of gout, gravel etc., etc., the Spanish mantle may be dipped into a decoction of hay flowers, oat straw or pine sprigs.

Patients sit in the water so that it reaches to about the navel. This third application is the original Kneipp half bath.

Kneipp used the standing and kneeling applications (No. 1 and No. 2) upon patients in thorough decline and always with great success. With these applications he commenced his Water Cure.

Kneipp used a light, boiling decoction of hay flowers or put the hay flowers themselves into the boiling water.

The vapor bath must always be followed by a cooling application which has to extend over all parts which perspired. If only feet and legs have been sweating, wash the same with a wet towel; strong people may take a knee gush.

Against headaches originating in the congestion of blood in the head, an increased application of the vapor foot bath will work wonders.

NATURAL HEALING IN AMERICA, PART I

by Benedict Lust

The Kneipp Water Cure Monthly, I (4), 55-56. (1900)

KNEIPP AND OTHER SOCIETIES FOR THE ADVANCEMENT OF NATURAL HEALING

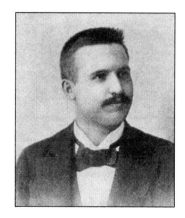

Benedict Lust [1872-1945]

According to an old saying, it is the habit of Germans to form some society or other as soon as there are three of them together.

We don't know, if it is really as bad as that, but we are sure that should there be two followers of Kneipp among the above mentioned three, these two would found a Kneipp society with the object to make a Kneippian of the third.

This is not intended to be a joke, for there is hardly one follower of our great master who is not fully convinced of the blessings the Kneipp system affords to the healthy as well as to the suffering and who would not be ready and willing to prove to this fellow beings that the Kneipp cure is one of the best roads to health and happiness.

Wherever there meet a few Kneippians, a society is soon founded. Meetings are held to which outsiders are invited. These are taught that there is a little more in the Kneipp system than walking in the grass. By and by sick people suffering from chronic or acute diseases come to these meetings and listen to the speakers. Soon they take confidence in the matter and try the new system of healing. A cured patient who was formerly treated in vain by physicians has always been the best advertisement for such societies and after the first successful treatment plenty of new members are soon [won] over to our cause.

Nothing is more successful than success and we may justly claim that the methods of Kneipp are a great success in this country and with the well-earned success have made a progress which nobody dreamt of a few years ago.

In many principal cities there are larger or smaller Kneipp societies. But the believers in the other systems are just as much in earnest and work just as hard. The systems may differ but their object is the same; that is, the improvement of the health of humanity and the diminution of the burden of sickness.

NEW YORK

In New York there are five societies devoted to this noble cause.

THE KNEIPP SOCIETY

This society holds its meetings every first and third Tuesday in the month in McGaffrey's Lodge Rooms, 139 East 59th Street.

Members have to pay 50 cents initiation fee and a monthly fee of 25 cents. All those who want to get information on all matters pertaining to any system of natural healing are welcome and may learn all they want to know free of charge. Specialists of great experiences and knowledge are always present. Their lectures make the meetings very interesting.

The President of this society is Benedict Lust, the editor of this monthly, who has devoted many years to the earnest study of natural healing and was treated and cured of serious lung trouble by the late Reverend Sebastian Kneipp in Wörishofen. His own treatment and effected cure turned his mind and energies to natural healing. He worked hard to get the knowledge necessary. This being accomplished, he decided to devote his life to suffering humanity.

NATUREHEILKUNDE

At 79 East 4th Street, in Hoppe's Hall, Natureheilkunde meets. The society, a German word which means, translated into the English language, 'science of natural healing'. This society treats all systems alike; taking the best of every one of them according to cases and circumstances. The President of this Society is Mr. Fr. Dittmar.

THE PRIESSNITZ SOCIETY

The Priessnitz Society meets at 206 East 86th Street. Besides the other systems of healing, the Priessnitz Society devotes its energies partly to the advancement of the system of Priessnitz, as its name indicates, a definition of which our readers will find in the January 1900 issue of *The Kneipp Water Cure Monthly*.

MORRISANIA

The Society of Natural Healing of Morrisania meets monthly in Count Zacharzowski's Hall, NW corner of 152nd Street and Courtland Avenue. This society of Morrisania is devoted to the science of natural healing in general.

DOLGEVILLE

We are informed, a new society of natural healing was formed some time ago. Mr. William Jahn is President and Mr. Chas. Fallier, Secretary.

NEW JERSEY

In the neighborhood of New York, in the State of New Jersey, there are societies for the advancement of natural healing in Newark, Paterson, and Camden.

NEWARK

In Newark, there are two such societies. Both are prosperous and are doing their best in the interest of their noble cause. Professor Charles Lauterwasser, 252 Littleton Avenue, is the President of one. This gentleman is a hydropathic physician and natural scientist of 20 years' experience in Europe and America and one of the best authorities on natural healing.

CENTRAL KNEIPP SOCIETY

This society was founded by George Rauch, a hydropathist, who has studied under the late Rev. Sebastian Kneipp in Wörishofen. G. Rauch is the President of this Society which meets in 80 Hamburg Place, Newark, New Jersey.

PATERSON

There is The Paterson Society for Natural Healing, which meets in Brummer's Hall, 28 Cross Street. This society has a very large membership.

CAMDEN

The Camden Society of Natural Healing holds it meetings in Liberty Hall, Camden. The secretary of this society, Mr. J. Knauer, 1031 Kaighns Avenue, who is doing all in his power to advance our cause. Great interest is shown by the members and the membership list is growing constantly.

From Camden right across the Delaware River is situated Philadelphia, which counts one society of natural healing.

PENNSYLVANIA

PHILADELPHIA

The Philadelphia Society of Natural Healing was founded in 1891 and meets in the Society Hall, corner of 2nd and Huntington Streets. A large membership list and good attendance of the meetings show that there is great interest for our cause in Philadelphia. Mr. V. Huster, 2957 North 22nd Street, is the secretary of the Society.

In Pennsylvania are also societies of natural healing in Monaco and Allegheny.

Massachusetts

Three societies are in Massachusetts. Boston may justly be proud of having one of the largest societies of natural healing in this country.

The Boston Society Of Natural Healing

This society holds its meetings in the Boylston Abt Club Hall. The officers are Dr. M. C. Groppner, President; Mrs. Emma Schmidt, Vice-President; Miss Katzer, Secretary; Mrs. Auguste Miller, Financial Secretary; Mrs. M. Kormann, Librarian; Trustees: Ferdinand Schlichting and Mrs. Anna Donath; Treasurer, Mrs. R. Starke.

Lawrence Society Of Natural Healing

The officers of this society are Dr. Louis Eidam, President; Charles Oehlschlaegel, Vice-President; Ernst Ammon, Recording Secretary; Louis Eidam, Correspondence Secretary; William Burger, Treasurer; Mrs. Emma Schaefer, Librarian; Trustee, Louis Nitzhle.

The Adams Society

The Adams Society meets at 17 Willow Street. Mr. Paul Tuerke is the President and Mr. William Krause the Secretary and Treasurer.

Connecticut

In Connecticut are two societies devoted to natural healing. One is in Rockville and the other in New Britain.

Rockville

Mr. W. Suesslerich is the President and Mr. H. Giesdorf the Secretary, Dr. R. Sarrazin, Hydropathic Physician in charge. The meetings take place in Chink's Hall on Village Street.

New Hampshire

There is one society, in Manchester. Mr. Ed. Hornig is the President of it; Emzil Zussy, Vice-President; H. Roedelsberger, Corresponding Secretary; August Hanke, Recording Secretary; R. Erlmann, Treasurer; Mrs. Therese Simon, Cashier; Librarians: Gottfried Lein and Frank Gleitzmann.

Rhode Island

Rhode Island has two societies, one is Providence and one in Menton.

MISSOURI

ST. LOUIS, MISSOURI, KNEIPP INSTITUTE

There is also one society of which Dr. Siebert, 2317 S. 12th St., is the President; E. Ressler, Vice-President; Mart. Funk, Secretary, and E. Bennecke, Treasurer.   This society contemplates the foundation of a Kneipp Institute for which purpose wealthy friends of the Kneipp cure have subscribed large amounts.

ILLINOIS

CHICAGO

Also counts one prosperous society of which Dr. E. Gleitsmann, 634 N. Hoyne Ave., is the President.

KNEIPP AS AUTHOR

by Benedict Lust

The Kneipp Water Cure Monthly, I (5), 67. (1900)

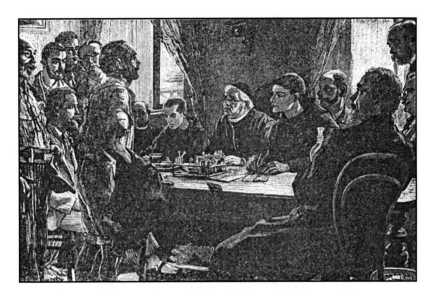

Sebastian Kneipp with his clerical assistants consulting patients. Notice the number of medical doctors in the background observing the consultation.

Before Kneipp ever thought of writing his works on his Water Cure, he wrote and published several books on agricultural topics. These have been published in four and five editions, certainly a proof that whatever Sebastian Kneipp did, he did it well. But who would know Sebastian Kneipp had he not written *My Water Cure*? A few German beekeepers and farmers perhaps, while today his name is known by nearly every human being and his works are read by all who take an interest in the welfare of humanity. Written in plain every day language, they are understood by everybody, a ray of light and a gospel of hope for suffering humanity. Would Kneipp have chosen the language of science which is supposed to delight the so-called educated people of today, people whose tongues may be trained to cover their ignorance by well-sounding phrases, meaningless and valueless though, would he ever have become the "Father Kneipp" he was and the benefactor of mankind he still and always will be! We doubt very much. The few educated would have read his books, shrug their shoulders and bought the same pills and drugs, they always bought. Kneipp wrote for the poor, common, every day people. They not only understood him, but followed his advice. The success the Kneipp cure had with the poor opened the eyes of the rich and the educated.

Kneipp Literature.

The Kneipp Cure, American edition of
"My Water Cure", paper cover,......... 60
Bound in cloth,.....................$1.10

My Water Cure, tested for more than
35 years and published for the cure of diseases and the preservation of health by
Seb. Kneipp, parish priest of Wörishofen
(Bavaria). Translated from the 36th German edition. With 100 illustrations and
a portrait of the author, 389 pages. Bound
in cloth,.............................. 1.65

Thus shall thou live. Hints and advises for healthy and sick people, suggesting a plain, rational mode of living and a
natural method of curing by Seb. Kneipp.
Bound in cloth,...................... 1.65

My Will. A legacy to the healthy and the
sick, by S. Kneipp. With 29 photographs
taken from life, and numerous illustrations, and a portrait of the author. Bound
in cloth............................. 1 65

The Care of Children in Sickness and
Health, by Mgr. Kneipp. Contains instructions how to bring up children and
how to cure diseases they are subject to.
Fine edition, cloth,................... 1.35

Ma cure d'eau ou hygiène et medication
pour la guérison des maladies et la conser-
vation de la santé par Séb. Kneipp. Avec
de nombreuses figures dans le texte. Price
bound,.............................. 1.30

Comment il faut vivre, advertisse-
ments et conseils s'addressant aux malades
et aux gens bien portants pour vivre d'
après une hygiène simple et raisonnable
et une thérapeutique conforme à la nature
par Séb. Kneipp. Cinquième édition.
Avec un supplement: Manier de pratiquer
les applications d'eau à Wörishofen sous
le contrôle de M. l'abbé Kneipp. Price,
bound,.............................. 1.30

Mon Testament. Conseils aux malades
et aux gens bien portants par Mgr. Séb.
Kneipp. Price,...................... 1.25

This latest work of Mgr. Kneipp should be
in the hands of all who wish to try his treatment, as it explains thoroughly all forms and
the latest modifications of the different baths,
gushes, etc., and contains a number of excellent
illustrations, adding greatly to its value.

On receipt of price postpaid.

Benedict Lust made available to his clients all of Kneipp's books in his Kneipp Store
located at 111 E. 59th St., New York City (1896-1902).

Without the benefits the poor derived from the Water Cure, no rich man or woman would ever thought of making use of it. Did not the learned and highly educated doctors tell them that the Water Cure was the same kind of a humbug as the rest of such cures and that Father Kneipp may be or may have been a good man, but that he was mistaken? They ought to know it, for did they not study their profession! How could Kneipp know when he had never had made a study of the treatment of diseases? In the opinion of these learned doctors, Kneipp was a dreamer while all other Hydropathists were humbuggers. Who can describe the astonishment of the learned and educated doctors when they heard that the poor and rich not only understood Kneipp's plain language but were able to treat themselves? What was more, in many cases, the learned and highly educated doctors were able to cure themselves of ailments which these learned gentlemen had previously treated in vain.

Kneipp's *My Water Cure* was translated into fourteen languages and was sold in every country. It was published for the first time in 1886 and since then has had 73 issues.

In 1889 Kneipp published his second work under the title *Thus shallst thou live*. While *My Water Cure* shows how one should use water as a healing factor, the second work shows to suffering humanity the right mode of living. This second work of Kneipp was translated into nine languages and published in 24 issues inside of seven years and a half.

A handbook for the well and the sick with a little herb atlas followed, while in 1890, the first issue of his celebrated book *The Care of Children* was published. This little book cannot be recommended too highly to parents who will find in it advice for all sorts of children's ailments as well as rules for children's diet, etc., etc.

In 1891 Kneipp published his *Advisor of the Sick and Well*, which was printed in 40,000 copies. This book contains nothing new and is nothing but a condensation of *My Water Cure* and *Thus Shallst Thou Live*. A work intended for the poor who could not afford to spend much.

In 1894 follows *My Will* and in 1896, *Codicil to My Will*. Both works are supplementing his other books which in connection with his lectures complete the list of Kneipp's works.

The European editions of the *Kneipp-Blätter* and *Kneipp-Almanach* contain many valuable items written by Kneipp and will be read for years and years to come by all who are interested in natural healing. Kneipp's *Atlas of Herbs* and medical plants will assist every follower of our great master who has his own apotheca. This Atlas gives true pictures and descriptions of all plants which are useful according to Kneipp and which one may gather in forest or field after studying this little book.

Written in plain every day language, they are understood by everybody, a ray of light and a gospel of hope for suffering humanity.

Kneipp wrote for the poor, common, every day people. They not only understood him but followed his advice.

Who can describe the astonishment of the learned and educated doctors when they heard that the poor and rich not only understood Kneipp's plain language but were able to treat themselves? What was more, in many cases, the learned and highly educated doctors could do, they were able to cure themselves of ailments which these learned gentlemen had previously treated in vain.

Kneipp's My Water Cure *was translated into fourteen languages and was sold in every country. It was published for the first time in 1886 and since then has had 73 issues.*

NATURAL HEALING IN AMERICA, PART II

by Benedict Lust

The Kneipp Water Cure Monthly, I (5), 79. (1900)

SANITARIA AND HYDROPATHISTS

In my first item I spoke about the Kneipp and other societies for the advancement of natural healing in America. Before such societies existed it was a difficult task for the Kneipp Physician or Hydropathist to gain followers and patients. Many hours were spent by the first advocates of natural healing in convincing the suffering of the honesty of these efforts. Many hours were spent in showing to these poor sufferers that there was only one road to health and happiness, only one road but a road which was built on a foundation laid by Nature. Nothing is more successful than success. The first successful cures convinced the healed as well as many of their friends, so that today the army of believers in natural healing is very large and growing every day.

Today there are many sanitaria and Hydropathists all over the country. Of course it is impossible for us to mention everyone, but those we are mentioning can be relied upon as ladies and gentlemen of great knowledge and ability gained by years of study and practical experience. The science of natural healing cannot be gained from books, experience is the best and only teacher of it.

In New York there are quite a number of Kneipp Physicians and Hydropathists.

NEW YORK KNEIPPIANUM

The New York Kneippianum was found by Miss Elise Amend, who is an accredited graduate of Wörishofen, the high school of Kneippism and the Kneipp Water Cure. The authorities in Wörishofen are very strict and whoever is accredited by them may be relied upon as an expert on all matters pertaining to Kneipp's Water Cure.

Miss Amend's sanitarium is situated in a very healthy neighborhood of New York, at the corner of 124th Street, opposite Mount Morris Park, 1931 Madison Ave. A skillful physician is in attendance who examines all patients. Miss Amend has been very successful and has cured many patients which were pronounced incurable by their physicians. The herb steam bath is a specialty of Miss Amend who has also cured many cases of excessive stoutness.

BADEKUR

The sanitarium, the Badekur at 21 East 83rd Street, stands under the direction of the well-known and celebrated hydropathist John H. Scheel, an American of great knowledge and experience who has studied all systems of natural healing. His motto is: "Study everything, keep the best and use it in the interest of suffering humanity." For years, Mr. Scheel has made a special study of the ailments and conditions of delicate young people and children. Today, this gentleman can claim to possess a system of healing for all such cases which will produce a cure in a very short time. His sanitarium is one of the best equipped and cannot be recommended too highly to parents who want to secure a long healthy life for their weak children as well as to all those who suffer from any disease.

PROFESSOR F. W. RITTMEIER

Professor F. W. Rittmeier, who has studied medicine in Europe, is counted among the best representatives and practitioners of natural healing. In his sanitarium at 115 East 82nd Street,* he gives individual treatment for all chronic ailments according to Kneipp's, Priessnitz' and Kuhne's systems. The Professor also makes a specialty of massage treatment and Swedish gymnastics.

BROOKLYN

In Brooklyn are two sanitaria which have been credited with many successful cures.

THE LIGHT AND WATER CURE INSTITUTE

At 346 Schermerhorn Street, Brooklyn, of Naturarzt Ludwig Staden and Carola Staden is a modern institute of natural healing in the fullest sense of the word. Mr. and Mrs. Staden are both highly educated and have gained knowledge by years of earnest study and by years of practical experience and success. Carola Staden is a graduate of Lindner's Hygienic Institute, Dresden, Germany.

---

*The address cited by Benedict Lust does not correspond to the address in the advertisement placed by Rittmeier on the facing page. —Ed.

Treatment of all chronic diseases by means of a perfect method of Natural Healing is practiced. Professor Staden's light baths are wonderfully effective, while Carola Staden has saved the lives of many a woman and mother by means of her Thure-Brandt massage treatments.

W. F. H. KRUEGER

W. F. H. Krueger is a young hydropathist who has a bright future before himself. Quite a number of successful cures have been effected by him. Professor Krueger's office is at 200 Maujer St., Brooklyn.

NEWARK, NEW JERSEY

In Newark, New Jersey, also are two sanataria of natural healing.

FIRST KNEIPP AND NATURE CURE SANATORIUM

The first and oldest one, established in 1891, is the first Kneipp and Nature Cure Sanatorium.

Charles Lauterwasser, the proprietor and director of this institution of natural healing, has 20 years experience devoted to the study of Nature Cure in all its branches. Knowledge gained by experience is good knowledge and can be relied upon. Thousands of successful cures are the best proofs that Charles Lauterwasser possesses such knowledge. His sanatorium is at 252 Littleton Avenue, Newark, New Jersey.

RAUCH'S KNEIPP SANITARIUM

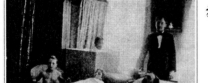

The other sanatorium in Newark is Rauch's Kneipp Sanitorium, 66–68 Barbara Street, Newark. Professor Rauch follows the rules of the Kneipp system strictly and gained his experience in Wörishofen. Professor Rauch is a young man of good ability.

SANATORIUM BELLEVUE

Our list of sanitaria in and around New York would not be complete if we would not mention the Sanatorium Bellevue in Butler, New Jersey. Situated in the midst of beautiful forests and hills at the slopes of the Ramapo Mountains, it is an ideal place for Nature Cure. A place where in the pure air the sick get well and the well feel stronger and happier. Sanatorium "Bellevue" is the place for quiet and rest and offers every comfort of a well-equipped home. The sick will be treated according to the rules of the Kneipp system in connection with light, air, and sun baths. Miss L. Stroebele is the proprietress of this sanatorium.

THE NEW ORLEANS KNEIPP WATER CURE

As stated above there are quite a number of sanitaria throughout the country. The South possesses one of the best in New Orleans: corner of Flood and Levee. This Water Cure institute is open all year and has healed thousands of suffering human beings.

LETTER TO THE EDITOR

by Richard Metcalfe

The Kneipp Water Cure Monthly, I (10), 186. (1900)

September 3rd, 1900.

Mr. Benedict Lust,
Editor, *The Kneipp Water Cure Monthly.*

Dear Sir!
I am much obliged to you for the Water
Cure journals received with your letter.
I beg to enclose £1 for one years' subscription
for four copies to be sent to me monthly.

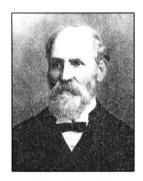

Richard Metcalfe,
a Hydrotherapist from
London, England.

As requested, I herewith send you a list of
the Hydro's in England, though I doubt very
much as to whether they will be of much help
to you.

Many of our hydropathic establishments
are so in name only, being merely a kind of rendezvous for pleasure seek-
ers. Hydropathy in England during the 20 years has degenerated, which
is due in a measure to the desirability of the directors of the various com-
panies to make the establishments a financial success, regardless of the
medical part. The medical faculties have drawn daggers against any inno-
vation on their presences, and so long as this state of things exists, I am
afraid there will be very little headway made in England. On the continent of Europe, amongst the medical men, they are more open to accept
any new remedies that are calculated to benefit the human race and add
to their medical remedies.

Individually, I am a firm believer in the Water Cure, as practiced by
Priessnitz and Father Kneipp, and will do everything I can possibly to render you any assistance so far as England is concerned. Judging from my
personal experience of over 40 years in the largest city in the world, I am
sure you will credit me with some knowledge of the ways and means of
approaching the people, and I venture to make the following observations
regarding your Journal.

First, I should be careful in not making the Journal too much of Father
Kneipp's Water Cure; admit articles of every description bearing upon
hygienic remedial measures. I have visited Gräefenberg (the birth place
of the Water Cure) twice during the last five years, and was astonished to
find that there had been no advance since the death of Priessnitz and the
annual number of invalids had considerably diminished.

The geographical position as a health resort, is as good now as it was a hundred years ago, and the accessibility to Gräefenberg by rail or by road is unique. The only possible cause for the reduction is due to the proprietors not adding new hygienic remedies to their hydropathic appliances like other parts of Austria and Germany, where better medical results are gained in much less time.

Secondly, of course as time rolls on, certain improvements are continually taking place in every system under the sun; for instance, the introduction of the Roman bath for the people, both as a medical and sanitary agent.

Thirdly, electricity and massage during the last 20 years have proved very important agents, and are advocated very extensively by the medical faculty.

Fourthly, diet and exercise is another matter that is occupying the attention of the faculty, including clothing.

Fifthly, the craze on the air cure which I have advocated for the last 40 years, and which is just now attracting the attention of the medical faculty, and also the public. By inserting these subjects, I feel sure you will have a better chance of procuring subscribers in England and in fact all over the world. There is a great opening for a Journal which advocates all hygienic things that relate to life health and disease.

Lastly, (which I may say is of vital importance) that you should try and get some good firm as agents in London, who would in their catalogue bring your Journal before the English people. I send you by the same post a copy of the life of Priessnitz, and two or three treatises by myself, from which you can make any extracts you please.

Wishing you God speed in your undertaking,
I am Yours very faithfully,

Richard Metcalfe
Metcalfe"s London Hydrotherapy Ltd.
Richmond Hill, Surrey

Individually, I am a firm believer in the Water Cure, as practiced by Priessnitz and Father Kneipp, and will do everything I can possibly to render you any assistance so far as England is concerned.

First, I should be careful in not making the Journal too much of Father Kneipp's Water Cure; admit articles of every description bearing upon hygienic remedial measures.

PROFESSOR REINHOLD PRAISES THE COLD WATER CURE

by August F. Reinhold

The Kneipp Water Cure Monthly, I (11), 206. (1900)

For thousands of years physicians pretended to minister to the ills of mankind. Not one of their vast numbers ever thought of the possibility of curing chronic ailments. It was reserved for an illiterate German peasant, Vincent Priessnitz, in the beginning of the present [19th] century to demonstrate the curability of all diseases by plain water.

He attained the most phenomenal success, and not only prominent people, but numbers of doctors from all over the globe flocked to him. These doctors, after studying his method and seeing the wonderful effects of plain water, returned—enthusiastic converts—to their native places, renouncing drugs, establishing institutes for Water Cure everywhere and propounding the method of Priessnitz in many a voluminous work.

That in water we possess the long-sought-for panacea, or cure-all, can easily be demonstrated. Hydropathists hold that all diseases are caused by impurities in the body. In many acute cases, the body possesses vitality enough to throw out this matter in the form of pimples and ulcers; but in chronic diseases, our vitality is too low to operate spontaneously.

CAUSES OF DISEASE

The special ailments are produced by the particular place where the sick matter happens to be deposited. If it attack the eye, it causes blindness; if the ear, it leads to deafness; if the limbs be preferred by it, we get rheumatism, gout or paralysis, etc., but in every instance, sickness is caused by the presence of matter which does not belong in our body.

Now, if all the different kinds of diseases have only one common cause, namely, deposits of matter, it is obvious that the diverse forms under which sickness appears must be curable by any single method which is capable of removing this unnatural encumbrance—and it has been found that ordinary water answers this purpose admirably.

This sick matter is introduced into our body by a perverse way of living, and by our many excesses and vices. It is astonishing to what extent people sin against the simplest rules. Some like indigestible food; others overload their stomachs, others are fond of spices; some again take their meals excessively hot or cold; others swallow them without mastication, forgetting that the teeth are placed in their mouths for masticating, and that their stomachs are destitute of grinding implements.

Any substance insufficiently digested is not assimilated and remains foreign to our system. This foreign matter is the cause of every sickness. A large amount of matter is brought into our body in the form of drugs.

In order to effect a rapid and permanent cure, two things are necessary, viz.; we must avoid introducing injurious substances into our body, and secondly, we must purge our body of what is already deposited. This latter end is easily effected by Water Cure. I recommend for your study these books on water as a curative agent: *The True Healing Art*, by Russell Thacher Trall; *My Water Cure*, by Sebastian Kneipp, and *New Science of Healing*, by Louis Kuhne, and *The Natural Healing System*, by Friedrich Eduard Bilz.

OPPONENTS OF HYDROTHERAPY

About thirty years ago the Water Cure movement waned, not because it had been weighed and found wanting, but because not every physician could start an institute. Then again, it is much easier to write out a prescription which takes but a minute, instead of giving a treatment, that may last from one to three hours. Last, but not least, under water treatment people are cured too quickly and lastingly, and they are taught how to avoid future relapses, so that by a general adoption of this method the physicians would cut their own throats.

These considerations not only explain why the water treatment was allowed to sink into oblivion, it also explains why its revival is due to non-medical men, such as Father Kneipp and Louis Kuhne. Even today the medical doctors selfishly try to suppress this method of cure by sneering at it and calling it a humbug.

All the Hydropathists for the last century have made it their study to devise milder and milder processes, until today it is a regular child's play and a veritable treat for everyone.

The Water Cure also obviates operations, and many a life is saved by it that otherwise would have fallen a sacrifice to the knife.

As we, horror-struck, contemplate the outrages perpetrated during the dark Middle Ages against dissenters and witches, I doubt that in the years to come, people will fail to understand how we could authorize a class of men—the medical doctors—to undermine our health with thousands of deathly drugs and to hack, slash and saw us all to pieces.

It is not a shame that even today medical doctors, with all their pretended lore, their colleges and universities, their libraries and professors with high-sounding titles, and the great esteem in which they are held and hold themselves; that in spite of all their countless remedies and innumerable costly instruments, and their thousands of Latin and Greek terms by which they dazzle the ignorant crowd as well as themselves, I say, is it not a shame that they are unable to effect any of the cures which were readily achieved by the peasant Priessnitz some sixty years ago?

Language has no expressions strong enough to denounce the crimes committed by the doctors against their fellowmen. Or is it no crime if they know of better methods and decline to adopt them? As the past shows, medical men would willingly deliver the Water Cure to eternal forgetfulness. Hence, it becomes the sacred duty of every one to enlighten himself on this subject and to arouse public sentiment so as to abolish by law all dispensing of poisons.

—*N. Y. World*

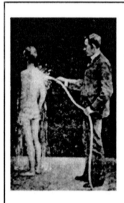

REINHOLD'S INSTITUTE

FOR

WATER CURE,

Rev. KNEIPP'S METHOD.

60 LEXINGTON AVENUE

NEW YORK.

APPLY FOR CIRCULAR.

Reinhold's Nature Cure Sanitarium

and Physical Culture Home

has removed to **LITTLE ROCK, ARK.,** the "City of Roses". in the "Sunny South". Treatment a veritable treat. In Aug. 1901, we publicly proposed that a committee select test cases of any disease, we to treat them free of charge, subject to a **forfeiture of $1000**. We cure all, usually deemed incurable. Room, board and treatment, per week $17, per 4 weeks $58. Circular free.   12m.

Professor Reinhold was one of the early supporters of Benedict Lust's efforts to consolidate natural healing in America. He placed monthly advertisements in Lust's publications in 1897 to promote first Water Cure clinic in New York City near Park Avenue. Three years later, he placed a notice to announce his move to Little Rock, Arkansas.

Not one of their vast numbers ever thought of the possibility of curing chronic ailments. It was reserved for an illiterate German peasant, Vincent Priessnitz, in the beginning of the present century to demonstrate the curability of all diseases by plain water.

These doctors, after studying his method and seeing the wonderful effects of plain water, returned—enthusiastic converts—to their native places, renouncing drugs, establishing institutes for water cure everywhere and propounding the method of Priessnitz in many a voluminous work.

In many acute cases, the body possesses vitality enough to throw out this matter in the form of pimples and ulcers; but in chronic diseases, our vitality is too low to operate spontaneously.

In order to effect a rapid and permanent cure, two things are necessary, viz.; we must avoid introducing injurious substances into our body, and secondly, we must purge our body of what is already deposited.

About thirty years ago the Water Cure movement waned, not because it had been weighed and found wanting, but because not every physician could start an institute. Then again, it is much easier to write out a prescription which takes but a minute, instead of giving a treatment, that may last from one to three hours.

As we, horror-struck, contemplate the outrages perpetrated during the dark Middle Ages against dissenters and witches, I doubt that in the years to come people will fail to understand how we could authorize a class of men—the medical doctors—to undermine our health with thousands of deathly drugs, and to hack, slash and saw us all to pieces

1901

Benedict Lust 's school's location and name changed often during its tenure. This advertisement for the Naturopathic College appeared in the 1901 June issue of *The Kneipp Water Cure Monthly*, a year before launching *The Naturopath and Herald of Health*.

The Butler Yungborn would eventually become a second campus site for those studying Naturopathy with Benedict Lust in the early 20th century.

Naturopathic Adviser*

by Ludwig Staden, Naturarzt
The Kneipp Water Cure Monthly, II (6), 170. (1901)

U nder this column FREE advice according to the rules of the Natural
Method of Healing will be given to all subscribers of *The Kneipp
Water Cure Monthly.*

C. P. D., Los Angeles, California

You are suffering from sciatica.
Every day a chair steam bath. Put a
kettle with boiling water under a cane
chair, sit on it and cover yourself from
the hips to the feet with a blanket so that
no steam can escape. As soon as you
are in mild perspiration, take a half bath
or sitz bath, 75° F /24° C, ten minutes,
combined with a sponge bath of the
whole body. Before going to bed a foot
steam bath or alternate foot bath, five
minutes, 100° F/38° C, one-half minute
cold water, three times repeated. Every
morning cold sponge bath of the whole
body, three times weekly, combined with
thigh gush. Make good use of going to

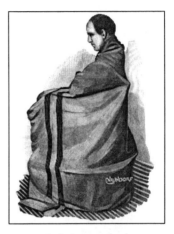

A chair steam bath

the sea shore; lay in the sun on the hot sand until very warm all over the
body, then take a short ocean bath. Avoid meat and alcohol. Live on a
vegetarian diet, especially plenty of fruits of all kinds, almonds, etc. Every
day the juice of three to five oranges mixed with the juice of two or three
lemons. If constipated, use injections [enema].

W. H. B. & Co., Stockport, Illinois

Question 1. Should or should not soap be used in taking the morning sponge bath?

Answer:

Soap should never be used except for special cleaning purposes;
it deprives the skin of its oily nature.

---

*Ludwig Staden had a similar monthly column in *The Kneipp Water Cure Monthly* in
1900 called, "Hydropathic Medical Advisor". —*Ed.*

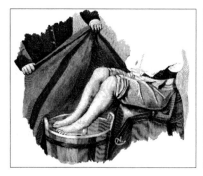 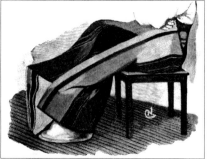

The feet of patients would rest on a board placed on top of the hot water tub in the foot steam bath and then the legs are securely wrapped in a blanket.

Question 2. Do you advise the drinking of hot water for cleansing stomach and bowels?

Answer:

All the applications and treatments in Naturopathy have to be given according to the individual condition of the patient. What is beneficial for one may not be for another. This is the reason why some are in favor of it, some against it. Certainly you may try it.

Question 3. Are you able to give a fixed rule for (a) just what overeating is and (b) what is proper and improper food?

Answer:

(a) Your own nature alone can give you a rule how far you have to go in eating. If you live on a raw food diet, you will find the limit easy; if you live on cooked food, especially on a meat diet, it will be more or less difficult, because the spices and irritating influences of such a diet will induce man to eat more than he needs. They also cause an artificial thirst. See article "Who is Right" July, 1900.*

(b) Naturopathy recommends as proper food a non-irritating, non-stimulating fruit and vegetable diet. Read the famous book *Fruit and Bread* by Schlickeisen.

Question 4. After going to bed in cold or cool weather my feet are nearly always cold. How should this be prevented?

Answer:

Chronic cold feet are a symptom of false circulation of the blood, which is the cause of many chronic ailments. Every evening before

---

*In *The Kneipp Water Cure Monthly,* Staden refers to a letter he received from Rev. Albert Stroebele, Louisa Lust's brother, inquiring about whether or not a person should eat breakfast. He cites Dr. Dewey's book, *No Breakfast Plan,* in which the author suggests skipping breakfast and eating two meals a day allows people to work more efficiently. —*Ed.*

going to bed an alternate foot bath, three times weekly upper gush and three times knee or thigh gush, walking barefooted; during the night wet abdominal bandage. Lukewarm enema if constipated. If everybody would ask in the way as you did, we could answer in the way as you suggest.

MAB. H., BOSTON, MASSACHUSETTS

Consequences of appendicitis. In order to avoid another attack, your husband should use a hygienic diet, as often described here. Instead of three boiled eggs every morning, let him have grape nut, with lukewarm milk or Irish oats with milk, strawberries, baked apples, stewed prunes, oranges or any fruits he should like, with rolls one day old. For the second meal: rice, macaroni or a few potatoes, with any vegetable, especially spinach, sprouts, carrots, peas, string beans, asparagus, etc. Vegetables must be steamed and flavored with a little whole wheat flour, tomatoes, parsley, celery, onions, etc. Some vegetables you may cook in water, like asparagus, oyster plants, but use the water for soup, which gives a fine taste like chicken broth. Soups must always be thick. Use very little salt, no other spices. Now and then he may eat some chicken, turkey, lamb, mutton, or fish, with vegetables. With every dinner, plenty of lettuce or water cress, prepared with lemon juice and olive oil. One cup of malt coffee before meals. No drinking during meals or directly afterward. Every morning cool half bath two to three minutes, combined with sponge bath, every night a wet abdominal bandage; in case of pain on the region of the appendix, a thick extra compress of clay salve. (Potter's clay mixed with water prepared to a thick salve.) If circumstances permit it, sun baths, especially on the abdomen. In constipation, enemas of chamomile tea.

MRS. J. C. D., LEBANON, ILLINOIS

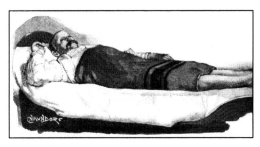

The three-quarter pack was convenient for a patient to apply by themselves.

For the child troubled with enlarged tonsils, apply a wet neck bandage every night and every other night an abdominal bandage; twice weekly a bed steam bath, after rising in the morning a cold sponge bath, especially of the neck and chest. Allow the child to walk barefooted, also a sun bath now and then. The best treatment for ordinary colds in small children is a three-quarter pack or bed steam bath, three-quarters to one hour with lukewarm half bath to follow about ten minutes, or a warm hay blossom bath, 98° F / 37° C, five to eight minutes, with a three-quarter pack or dry pack to follow three-quarters to one hour, then cool sponge bath of the whole body. Enemas of peppermint tea. Very simple diet, no meat or beef, tea, coffee, etc. Lukewarm milk, soup with rolls or bread, farina, milk, rice, oatmeal, hominy, etc., stewed fruits, baked apples, Dr. Lahmann's cocoa.

In case of too profuse menses, apply a four-folded compress dipped in vinegar and water on the abdomen and renew as soon as it gets warm, two hours, then two hours rest and repeat. On the fourth or fifth day, an oak bark sitz bath, 90° F / 32° C, for twenty minutes. The oak bark has to soak in water twelve hours, then cook it forty or fifty minutes. (Six ounces to one bath.) Cool enema every day about one pint. Between the menses every other day one cool sitz bath, 70° to 65° F / 21° to 18° C, for three to five minutes. During the night abdominal bandage. Moderate riding of bicycle.

H. A. H., FALL RIVER

Hayfever. This is a catarrh of the bronchial tubes, the nose and eyes, and attacks mostly people who eat and drink too richly and too much. A very simple vegetarian diet is the first *conditio sine qua non*. Avoid alcohol in any form, strong coffee, tea, spices. Begin right away with bed steam bath every other day, one hour duration with cool half or sitz bath ten minutes to follow. Instead of a bed steam bath you can take a sun bath which is more powerful. Every morning cold sponge bath with alternating thigh gush and upper gush. Gargle several times daily with lemon water. Every morning and afternoon breathing exercises in fresh air for about five minutes; inhale slowly through the nostrils, retain the breath in the lungs for a few seconds and exhale slowly through the nostrils. In constipation, daily enema with lukewarm peppermint tea. Sleep with open windows. During an attack, also alternate foot bath.

J. F. H., CHICOPEE FALLS, MASSACHUSETTS

You are run down and you cannot digest any food. Live on a very simple food diet, do not eat much at a time, but oftener. Breakfast: one cup of Dr. Lahmann's Cocoa, or lukewarm milk, with toasted bread, a few strawberries or an orange or baked apples or raw tomatoes and lettuce. Dinner: Rice with raw tomatoes or baked apples or lettuce or stewed prunes, peaches, etc. Fruits of all kinds with whole wheat bread. Supper: Lukewarm milk or black malt coffee with whole wheat bread. The juice of one lemon mixed with one raw egg, fruits and berries. Avoid sugar, meat, spices, vinegar, coffee, tea, alcohol; use very little salt. Before going to bed, one cup of the following mixed teas: aloe powder, crushed juniper

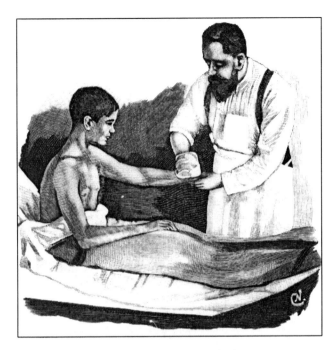

Every morning, a sponge bath

berries, gentian and fennel; ¼ of a teaspoon to one cup, you may add a little pure honey.

Every morning, sponge bath, two times weekly bed steam bath with extra compress on the stomach. One and a quarter hours hereafter, sitz bath 80° to 85°F / 26.7 to 29° C for 15 minutes. Four times weekly, clay compress on the stomach (potter's clay mixed with water) one and a half to two and a half hours, can also be used every night combined with wet abdominal bandage. Sun bath for ten to twenty minutes; later thirty to forty minutes every other day if they can be taken. There is no physical treatment in the world that has more healing power than a sun bath if taken properly. Enemas if constipated.

Ludwig Staden
346 Schermerhorn Street
Brooklyn, New York

To Whom It May Concern

Patients who desire advice by mail have to send $2 in advance for first letter, $1 for any additional service. Otherwise no answer in future.

THE KNEIPP CURE

by Friedrich Eduard Bilz

The Kneipp Water Cure Monthly, II (8), 211-213. (1901)

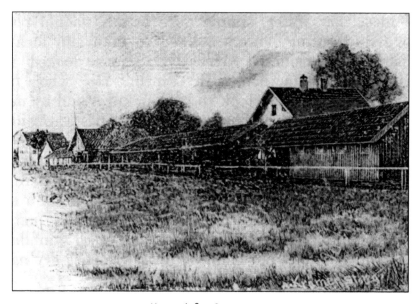

Kneipp's first Sanitaurium

W ho was Kneipp, the man who made his name so famous in recent years by his curative methods? Kneipp was a Roman Catholic priest in Wörishofen, in Bavaria. He was born at Stefansried, Bavaria, on the 17th of May, 1824, the son of a poor weaver. As a boy, he displayed great natural intelligence, and was possessed with a yearning desire to study for holy orders; but his parents had not the means of giving him the necessary opportunities, and he was obliged to follow his father's trade. In the introduction to his work, *My Water Cure*, he describes his career in the following words:

> I was twenty-one years of age when I left home with my travelling permit in my pocket. The document described me as a weaver's apprentice; but on the tables of my heart had been graven, from the days of my childhood, a very different description. With pain unutterable, and a yearning desire for the fulfillment of my ideal, I had looked forward for long, long years to that departure. So I began my journey, hurrying from place to place, and seeking—not, as my friends hoped I should, to ply the weaver's shuttle, but—for someone who would be willing to help me to study. The Reverend Chaplain Merkle interested himself in me, gave me private instruc-

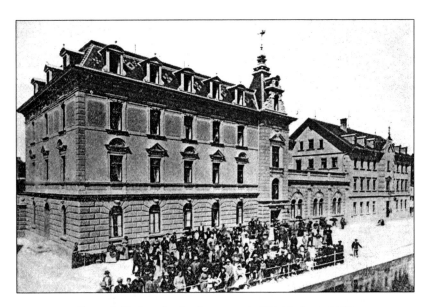

Kneipp's "Kurhaus" or healing center in Wörishofen in 1895

tion for two years in succession, and prepared me with such an unwearied zeal for my examination that, at the end of the second year, I was received into a Gymnasium (High School). The work was not light and to all appearance was destined to be fruitless. After five years of the greatest privations and efforts, I was broken in body and mind. My father fetched me away from the town, and the words of the landlord of the inn, at which we rested, are still ringing in my ears, "Weaver," said he to my father, "you are bringing your student home for the last time." The landlord was not alone in his opinion; it was shared by others. An army doctor of high repute at that time, who was also distinguished for his great benevolence and large hearted kindness to poor patients, had visited me ninety times in the last year of that period of five years, so earnestly had he wished to be of use to me. However, the progress of my illness had triumphed over his professional knowledge and his self-sacrificing humanity. I myself had given up hope and looked forward with resignation to my end.

Chance placed in my hands a modest little volume. On opening it, I found that it dealt with Hydropathy. I read its pages again and again; they contained what seemed incredible. The thought flashed upon me that at the eleventh hour I had found out my own condition. I read further; it was right; it agreed and harmonized with my own experience; it suited me to a hair. What joy! What comfort! New hope electrified the drooping body, and the yet more drooping spirit. The little volume was at first the straw to which I clung as a drowning man; it became in a short time the staff supporting the invalid. Today, it is the lifeboat which was sent to me by a merciful Providence in the nick of time, in the hour of extreme peril.

The little book, which treats of the healing power of cold water, from the pen of a physician, Dr. Sigmund Hahn. I tried the cure for three months; then for another three months. Though unconscious of any decided improvement, I felt none the worse. This gave me courage. The winter of the year 1849 arrived, when I was once more in Dillingen. Two or three times a week I repaired a secluded spot on the bank of the Danube, and took a plunge in the river. If I walked quickly to my bathing place, I walked home still more quickly to my warm room. These cold dips did me no harm, and on the other hand, as it seemed to me, not much good. In the following year I was in the Georgianum, in Munich, where I found a poor student in worse case than I was myself. The physician of the establishment declined to give him the necessary certificate of health to entitle him to the benefits of Institution, because—so ran the medical report—he would not live long. I now had a beloved colleague. I initiated him into the mysteries of my little book, and we two vied with each other in proving and practicing its prescriptions. After a short time my friend obtained his desired certificate from the doctor; and he is still alive and well. I myself gained strength more and more; became a priest; and have followed my sacred vocation for thirty-six years. Friends flatter me by saying that they wonder now, when I am nearly fifty years older, at the power of my voice, and are astonished at my bodily strength. Water remained to me a tried and faithful friend. Who can blame me for proving myself a fast friend to it?

The above is, in fact, a compendium of history of the life of Father Kneipp, and at the same time, the history of the origin of the "Kneipp Water Cure". As Kneipp himself says in his work, he does not in any degree claim to be the originator of a special method of cure. His method, critically considered, is only a branch of the modern combined Hygienic Treatment; he relies, according to his work, above quoted, chiefly on the cold Water Cure as practiced in his day by Vincenz Priessnitz, in Gräefenberg, in Austrian Silesia.* But to Kneipp belongs, undoubtedly, the merit

---

* To put the Kneipp and Priessnitz chronology into perspective, it is important to note that Kneipp is trying Hydrotherpay in 1848, and three years later in 1851, Priessnitz' death is mourned by the world. —Ed.

of having directed the attention of mankind anew to the remedy which had almost passed into oblivion—that remedy being water.

The expression, "The Kneipp Cure," refers to the curative system carried out by Father Kneipp at Wörishofen, in Bavaria. From the Natural Method of Healing which, as is known, employs only the natural healing factors, air, water, diet, etc., Father Kneipp so far deviated, in his practice, as to prescribe the use internally of decoctions or infusions or such herbs and plants as appeared to him to have a therapeutic value, as well as of warm or steam baths charged with the ingredients of plants.

These trifling deviations from the Natural Method of Healing, pure and simple, have been sometimes criticized with undue severity by the disciples of that drug denying method; but they do not in the least detract from the practical success of Kneipp's system. His patients are to be found in every rank and calling, from the princely landholder to his humblest subject. The very reverend gentlemen, a priestly personage of a stalwart and vigorous type, attracted the favorable notice of the invalid public by his gentle and sympathetic manner when giving advice, and by the pains which he bestowed on the treatment of his patients, rich and poor alike. To those circumstances the flourishing progress of the method of healing may in no small degree be attributed.

Kneipp's theory is that the cause of all disease lies in the blood— either from the fact of the blood being vitiated by the presence in it of morbid matter can be expelled by water. For the purposes of his cure he employs water in the form of wraps, compresses, packs, steaming, washings, and affusions. He holds that cold water is more effective than warm, and he ascribes to the other applications a subordinate importance only. The specialty of Kneipp's method is the shortness of the time during which the applications are continued—cold and short being the rule, especially for affusions. He says, however, in his work, that not every patient can bear that rule of treatment; and in case of such inability, he adopts our modified practice. Kneipp has many markedly successful cures to show as the results of treatment carried out under his experience and watchful eye. The great attractive power of Wörishofen was due in the first place to Kneipp's personality, but in a great measure also to the Roman Catholic priesthood and their press. Physicians journeyed in great numbers to that town to study Kneipp's treatment on the spot. Kneipp hydropathic establishments sprang up like mushrooms out of the earth; yet Kneipp himself said that many and many a practitioner assumed the Kneipp title for himself and his establishment; and few among them all were fit to hold it.

KNEIPP'S DIAGNOSIS

As Father Kneipp never examined a patient by auscultation or percussion, and yet achieved such remarkable results in the cure of disease, it is worthwhile to enquire how he arrived at his diagnosis, and arranged his plans to treatment.

1) His first look at the patient, which, owing to the number of sufferers whom he had to look at, was a very keen one—generally enabled him to form an opinion of the case. If the individuals were pale and thin, he concluded that their blood was poor and of bad quality, and that they lacked natural warmth. His first object then was to stimulate their appetite and circulation, which he accomplished for the most part by partial washings or affusions; local applications and packs, being in such cases appropriate. If the lack of the natural warmth was very marked, cold applications were preceded by warm ones, such as steaming of that part of the body which was immediately afterward to receive a cold affusion. As a consequence of the improved appetite and circulation which followed that treatment, the supply of blood and natural warmth were increased, and the whole system was roused to greater action.

2) In the case of corpulent persons, his attention was directed to augmenting the excretions; an object which must be pursued with caution if the heart of the patient is affected, as is frequently the case in corpulency in a greater or less degree. Although, the physician rejects water entirely in cases of heart complaint, Kneipp was of a wholly opposite opinion. He said to himself,

A well-ordered circulation is beneficial to the sufferer from heart complaint, and that can only be attained by the proper employment of water. By knee, thigh and back affusions, for instance, the blood is drawn downwards from the weak heart, which is thereby relieved. At the same time the warmth of the blood is better distributed, and the natural strength of the patient is increased, so that it becomes possible to proceed to upper, or even full affusions.

Out of every hundred persons ninety are nervous.* There must, therefore, be gradations of treatment in every case. With most patients, the mild applications come first; a beginning being made with the feet;

---

*The word "nervous" was used before the term, "neurasthenia" would replace it. Neurasthenia encompassed a host of symptoms that included fatigue, nervous exhaustion, palpitations, and pains. —Ed.

walking barefooted in the house, or on the grass when the sun shines. In that way, the circulation of the blood in the feet is enlivened, and it is then possible to proceed with the stronger applications. When nervous pains and spasms call for relief, warm applications are prescribed.

In some diseases, pain may actually be caused by the first stages of the cure; but there are signs of returning health. For it is not to be expected that a circulation which has been irregular for years can be brought into good order without a slight revolution, of which such pains are the best proof. In this way slight attacks of cough, or pain in the back, increase or cessation of the regular functions, may occur at the beginning of the cure. All such symptoms are, as a rule, so many proofs that the patient will certainly recover. Indeed, if they are altogether absent in chronic cases, the course of the cure is generally unsatisfactory, from the want in the patient of the reactive force required for the healing process. It is to be regretted that some invalids allow themselves to be frightened by these symptoms into changing their method of treatment for some other which removes them still farther from the desired goal of recovery. Upon such and similar natural and reasonable grounds Kneipp based his plans of treatment.

Sad to say, it was not permitted to the great Samaritan of Wörishofen to continue his work as long as—in the interests of the spread of his doctrine of the Natural Method of Healing, and of suffering humanity— could have been desired. A malignant malady, an insidious formation on the bladder, carried off the hale and vigorous old man in the course of six months. He died on the 17th of June, 1897, deeply mourned by the many thousands whom he had succored, as well as by all the friends and followers of the natural healing art.

Honor to his memory!

FUNDAMENTAL RULES OF THE KNEIPP CURE

The following are fundamental rules and maxims, which should be borne in mind in the application of the Kneipp affusions, baths, etc.:

The shorter the application the better its effect.

The colder the water, the shorter must be the time of its employment; and the greater the reaction will be. Weak patients must, nevertheless, begin with water of a moderate temperature; at first 66° F/19° C, cooler after a time, down to 59° and 55° F/15° and 13° C, and at last quite cold. The body must be as warm as possible before the application of cold water. If there is a lack of natural warmth, the first applications must be warm.

There should be no drying of the body by artificial means after the use of water; but the clothes should be put on quickly, and in order to help bring on a reaction, exercise should be taken, rapid at first and slower by degrees. If there is no reaction, or if the patient is very weak, the warmth of bed should be sought.

Hardening the body is the best means of preserving the general health, and of protection against attacks of disease.

SPASMS IN THE ABDOMEN

Hay seed (remnants of hay and grass) steeped in hot water, used for warm compresses and packs in combination with other resources of the natural method of healing, are a powerful and reliable means of relief. For abdominal complaints, which are caused through obstruction of the kidneys by mucous, lime blossom tea furnishes an excellent remedy. Decoction of peppermint or water mint, taken in warm milk, soothes pain. Rue tea, or rue (*Ruta graveolens, L.*) soaked in spirit, twice daily or twelve drops on sugar, or the same quantity of it in olive oil, answers the same purpose. The last mixture must stand in a warm place for some length of time.

VIOLENT SPASMS IN THE ABDOMEN

These yield to chamomile tea. Such spasms are frequently nothing but the result of an accumulation of gases, and are accompanied by vomiting and cold hands and feet. In such cases, an infusion of peppermint, water mint, aniseed, or fennel—or a mixture of them all—will be of great service. Besides taking chamomile tea, the patient should, on the first day of attack, wash three times with warm water and vinegar; on the second day, twice, and afterward only once a day. Thus, equable warmth and normal circulation of the blood will be reestablished.

—*The Natural Healing Method,* Friedrich E. Bilz

THE BILZ BOOK

A Golden Guide to Health, Strength, Happiness and Old Age

A COUNSELLOR TO THE SICK—A GUIDE TO THE HEALTHY

25 Gold Medals and Diplomas.   Translated into 18 different languages. Enormous sale of nearly 3,000,000 copies
These are the strongest arguments in Favor of the Bilz Book

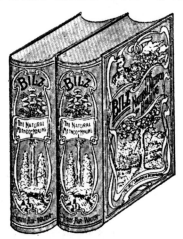

HEALTH IS WEALTH

The BILZ BOOK is the greatest Encyclopædia, which shows you the only correct and reasonable way of treating all Diseases at *Home without Medicine,* and teaches in the clearest possible manner how you can *protect yourself* and your family *against Disease.* If you are thoroughly healthy, you are able to work and earn money whereby to maintain and keep yourself, your wife and children in Happiness and Comfort, but if you—the Breadwinner—become ill, *your Family is then in danger* of starving and becoming ill also.

Sorrow, disease, distress, pain and grief then reign in your Family, instead of Happiness, Joy and Health, and the danger for the Family becomes more serious, when the Breadwinner's illness gets worse and worse, and his state at the end hopeless.

You can ward off this misery and terror from you and your Family if you live in accordance with the rules of the great BILZ DOCTOR BOOK.

NATURE, THE GREAT HEALER
All diseases may be cured by natural self treatment
The Famous B I L Z B O O K
Exhaustively and exclusively describes the wonderful methods developed and inaugurated by the celebrated F. E. BILZ of the famous Bilz Sanatorium

What the Bilz Book Teaches

The Bilz Book scarcely needs an introduction to the American public, for its fame in many lands has caused it to be widely spoken of here.

The Bilz Book teaches no complicated doctrine —no intricate formula—it simply consists of a wise, thoughtful and lucid expression of the Natural Method of Healing, so successfully practised for so many years by the eminent F. E. BILZ.

The adherents of this method of healing number millions—high and low, rich and poor. It is efficacious for all—economical for all. It teaches you how to utilize God's good gifts for your preservation and health. *The Ingredients are free*—the advantages open to all.

The Bilz Book is a wonderful compilation of over 2,000 pages. It describes minutely the best method of cure for every disease and ailment of humanity. *The Bilz Book is the Doctor in the Home.* You simply turn to its pages, and then, as thousands of others have done, you cure yourself.

The greatest tribute to this treatment lies in the fact that many eminent medical men treat their patients according to its methods. *With the aid of the Bilz Book you can treat yourself.*

Friedrich Bilz' *The New Method of Healing* (1898) was a two volume encyclopedia offering a foundation for Water Cure practitioners.

Kneipp's theory is that the cause of all disease lies in the blood—from the fact of the blood being vitiated by the presence in it of morbid matter that can be expelled by water.

The specialty of Kneipp's method is the shortness of the time during which the applications are continued—cold and short being the rule, especially for affusions.

The great attractive power of Wörishofen was due in the first place to Kneipp's personality, but in a great measure also to the Roman Catholic priesthood and their press. Physicians journeyed in great numbers to that town to study Kneipp's treatment on the spot.

As Father Kneipp never examined a patient by auscultation or percussion, and yet achieved such remarkable results in the cure of disease, it is worthwhile to enquire how he arrived at his diagnosis, and arranged his plans to treatment.

His first object then was to stimulate their appetite and circulation, which he accomplished for the most part by partial washings or affusions; local applications and packs, being in such cases appropriate.

In the case of corpulent persons, his attention was directed to augmenting the excretions; an object which must be pursued with caution if the heart of the patient is affected, as is frequently the case in corpulency in a greater or less degree.

In some diseases, pain may actually be caused by the first stages of the cure; but there are signs of returning health, for it is not to be expected that a circulation which has been irregular for years can be brought into good order without a slight revolution, of which such pains are the best proof.

The colder the water, the shorter must be the time of its employment; and the greater will the reaction be.

The body must be as warm as possible before the application of cold water. If there is a lack of natural warmth, the first applications must be warm.

Hardening the body is the best means of preserving the general health, and of protection against attacks of disease.

Vincent Priessnitz

by Richard Metcalfe

The Kneipp Water Cure Monthly, II (8), 218-220. (1901)

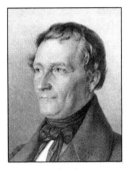

Vincent Priessnitz
[1799-1851]

Water applications have been used and appreciated throughout the ages. Vincent Priessnitz, who earned the title "Father of Hydropathy", was neither the discoverer of nor the first to use water as a remedial agent in disease.

That discovery was probably coeval with the appearance of man in his present condition. When we see that some of the lower animals possess an instinctive knowledge that water is good for them when wounded, and in certain conditions of sickness—or they have been seen to seek that element which they are suffering—we should be derogating from man's dignity and superior intellectual endowments if we denied to him a similar instinct and equal observing powers.

Histories that carry us back to remote ages show that the practice of water ablution, both for sanitary and religious purposes, existed amongst most ancient peoples.

Among the Jews, bathing was enjoyed by a code of specific regulations, which served to secure personal cleanliness and to convey the idea of moral purity. The association of water with the cure of disease is illustrated by Elisha's command to Naaman the Syrian to wash seven times in Jordan and by that of the Savior to the blind man to go and wash in the pool of Bethesda. Among the Egyptians, Greeks and Romans, baths were in common use. Most of us have heard of the Greek *gymnasia* and the Roman *thermae*, in which the plunge or affusion was largely employed as an invigorator of the body.

Mahomet enjoined the use of the bath, and wherever his followers were, it was in daily use. In almost all countries, hot or cold, civilized or savage, some form of bathing has been and is practiced. Its utility for purposes of health, cleanliness and comfort is practically acknowledged everywhere.

The fathers of the healing art, whose names have become familiar to us, were well aware of the therapeutic virtues of water. Pythagoras (B. C. 530) and, somewhat later, Hippocrates (B. C. 460) used water with friction and rubbing, in spasms and disease of the joints, and watery applications in a great variety of diseases, particularly pneumonia, gout and rheumatism. The successors of these sages, up to the time of Galen (A. D. 131-200), valued water in the treatment of disease. Galen himself gave water the highest place in his list of remedies. "Cold water," he says, "quickens the action of the bowels, provided there be no constriction from spasms, when warm is to be used. Cold drinks stop hemorrhages and sometimes bring back heat; cold drinks are good in continued and redundant humors by stool, or by vomiting, or by sweat." He recommends tepid and warm water drinking, with hot baths followed by tepid or cold in cases of biliousness, spasms, fever of the stomach, hiccup, cholera morbus, obstinate ophthalmia and plethora.

Not much is recorded of the use of water in disease after Galen's time until the Arabian physicians Rhazes (923) and Avicenna (1030) are found advocating the use of cold water in fevers, measles, smallpox, vomiting, nausea and diarrhea. About this time, the Arabs were prosecuting their researches in chemistry and pharmacy. Many new drugs were introduced and water was ignored, and judging from the results of the Arabian treatment of disease, this was not to the advantage of the patients.

Here and there, in the medical history of Europe, there occurs the name of a doctor who recommends water-drinking, washing, bathing, or swimming to preserve health and cure disease. But there is nothing of special importance until the beginning of the eighteenth century (1702), when our countrymen, Sir John Floyer and Dr. Baynard, published their book, *History of Cold Bathing, both Ancient and Modern*, the first part of which contains interesting letters by Floyer, written between the years 1696 and 1702. In Italian, at Naples (1723), appears Lanzani's, *Right Methods of Using Cold Water in Fevers and Other Maladies, Internal and External.*

Niccolo Lanzani mostly confines his advocacy of water to his employment internally in fevers of all kinds, for which he holds water drinking to be the best remedy.

About the same time appeared another interesting book by a distinguished clergyman, John Hancocke, D. D., Rector of St. Margaret's, Lothbury, London, Prebendary of Canterbury, entitled, *Febrifugum Magnum, or Common Water the Best Cure for Fevers and probably for the Plague* (1722), in which he gives many instances of the curative effects of water, use in case of fever, violent colds, etc., unassisted by any kinds of medicine. These publications, with the actual practice of the authors, again drew attention to water as a remedial agent. Floyer and Baynard employed water freely and with the success in chronic diseases, such as rheumatism, gout, paralysis, indigestion, general debility and nervous affections. Externally, they administered the plunge bath, and they gave copious doses of water internally.

About this time several pamphlets about water treatment appeared. Among them was the following:

The Curiosities of Common Water; or The Advantages Thereof in

Preventing and Curing Many Distempers, etc. by John Smith. (London 1723).

Thomas Taylor, the "Water Poet," is responsible for a pamphlet with the following title: *Kick for kick, and Cuff for cuff,* a refutation of a bombastic, scurrilous postscript, written by one who calls himself Gabriel John. Others still will have it Daniel Dafoe, which he calls reflections on my Hudibrastick reply to his Flagellum or dry answer to Dr. Hancocke's liquid book, etc. With two remarkable instances of cures by common water, one of a malignant fever and no less than seven in one family of the pestilence." Published in London, 1793.

In German, there appeared a book, *On the Power and Effect of Cold Water* (1758) [first edition published 1737], by Johann Sigmund Hahn, who lived in the neighborhood of Gräefenberg, and whose father, Dr. S. Hahn, was a worshipper of cold water. This Hahn, though he used other remedies, employed water so extensively in curing diseases that he may be considered a sort of Hydropathist. He recommends cold water in chronic diseases particularly; also washing in smallpox and eruptions of the skin, falling baths [douches] in inflammation of the brain, douches in maimings, cold injections in diarrhea, injections into the nostrils for colds, and into the ears for deafness, and foot baths in chronic injuries. Hahn's work had, in 1754, passed through four editions. It did not, however, succeed in winning over the faculty to the cause of the Water Cure; and as for the public of Germany, though they liked to drink water, they did not care to have it applied externally.

V. Perez, a Spanish physician, sought to cure most diseases by the use of water, and he published at Madrid in 1753 a small book entitled, *El Promotor de la Salud de los Hombres, sin dispendio el menor de sus caudales; admirable methodo de curar todo mal con brevedad, securidad, y à placer. Dissertacion histórico, critic, medico, prática, en que se establece el aqua por remedio universal de las dolencias.*

Somewhat later, in England, Fredrick Hoffman published his ideas (London, 1761) with a somewhat similar title: *An Essay on the Nature and Properties of Water,* showing its prodigious use; and proving it to be a universal medicine, both for preventing and curing the diseases to which the human body is subject."

About 1777, an English doctor, Wright, was led to try the Water Cure. Dr. Wright, having caught fever from a sailor, undressed, threw a cloak about him, and went on deck, where, doffing his cloak, he had three pails of water thrown over his head. Repeating the process as often as the feverish heat returned, he quite recovered. Afterwards, he treated fevers successfully in Edinburgh by the cold affusion, and published a report of his proceedings in the *London Medical Journal* (1786). By the same method, Dr. Currie of Liverpool (1750-1805) treated with great suc-

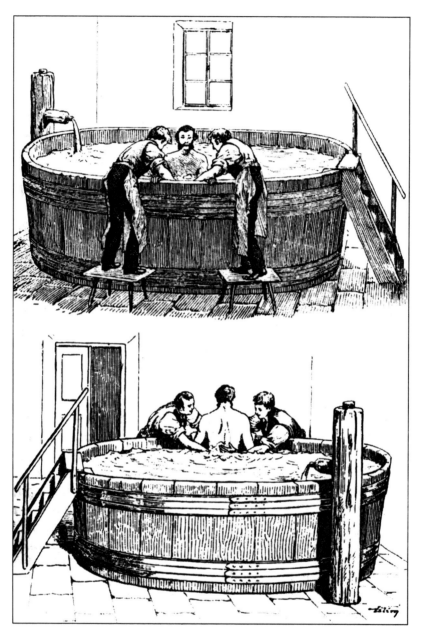

The size of Priessnitz' bath tubs at Gräefenberg were between 20 to 30 feet wide. Priessnitz did not condone using water warmer than 74° F/23° C in his cold water baths.

cess a contagious fever which was prevalent in that town, and in 1797 made public his views and experiences with a list of cures effected by his measures. Though he by no means anticipated the discoveries of the founder of Hydropathy, his reports on the effects of water in fevers and other diseases are considered to possess much practical value.

Dr. Currie found imitators both in England and on the continent, to whose names and achievements it would be tedious to refer. But in connection with the therapeutic use of water it would be unpardonable to omit mention of the name of the great German physician, Hufeland, who may be regarded as an apostle of bathing. After Hufeland, and before Priessnitz, by far the greatest water doctor was Professor Oertel, of Ansbach, whose numerous writings on the subject became popular. Oertel's motto, "Drink water in abundance, the more the better; for it prevents and cures all evils," found a large measure of acceptance with the people of the Continent. Water societies were formed in Germany, and water was extensively used dietically and medicinally, with as was supposed, admirable effect. Still, there was no system and what was done was done very much at random.

It remained for one greater and more far-sighted to grasp at once the whole secret of water treatment, and to develop and systematize it in one short lifetime. That man was Vincent Priessnitz.

The fathers of the healing art, whose names have become familiar to us, were well aware of the therapeutic virtues of water. Pythagoras (B. C. 530 and, somewhat later, Hippocrates (B. C. 460) used water with friction and rubbing, in spasms and disease of the joints, and watery applications in a great variety of diseases, particularly pneumonia, gout and rheumatism.

In German, there appeared a book, On the Power and Effect of Cold Water *(1758), by Johann Sigmund Hahn, who lived in the neighborhood of Gräefenberg, and whose father, Dr. S. Hahn, was a worshipper of cold water.*

It remained for one greater and more far-sighted to grasp at once the whole secret of water treatment, and to develop and systematize it in one short lifetime. That man was Vincent Priessnitz.

FOMENTATIONS

by Benedict Lust

The Kneipp Water Cure Monthly, II (9), 241. (1901)

A fomentation is a simple and effective method of applying moist heat to any part of the body by means of flannel wrung out of boiling water, milk, or any medicated hot fluid. It possesses advantages in many cases, and is to be preferred to poultices, as it is lighter and cleaner, and can be frequently repeated without much trouble. In extensive inflammations, especially of the abdomen, in erysipelas, and to allay spasms in deep-seated parts, as in cases of renal and biliary calculi, repeated milk fomentations are always to be preferred. When moist heat is prescribed for inflammatory diseases of the joints, or as a mild derivative* in rheumatic fever, to relieve the articular pain, milk fomentations will be found serviceable. Much depends on the way in which the fomentation is prepared. It ought to be applied as hot as the skin can bear, and although moist, the hot liquid should be thoroughly squeezed out of the flannel applied to the skin. A large piece of course flannel folded is employed for the purpose. After being soaked in the boiling liquid, it should be enveloped in a coarse towel. The hot liquid may be wrung out of the flannel by simply twisting the ends of the towel several times round the fomenting cloth. Have two pieces of flannel and a pail of hot water in which to wash out each cloth before applying it a second time. After the operation, wash out the flannels well and hang them in the fresh air (and sunshine if possible) until again required. To protect the hands use a wringer made by fixing a wooden rod to each end of the towel. To retain the heat, it is advisable to apply a dry flannel or towel over the wet one. If it is desired to produce a soothing effect add half pint of Kneipp's Curative Herb Tea to two quarts of boiling liquor, or a few drops of turpentine if the object be to induce slight counter-irritation. The milk must be sweet and good, also thoroughly boiled. Almost every form of disease will be much relieved and more speedily cured if mild fomentations are applied. Carefully sponge the fomented part with cool water, and use gentle massage after.

---

*Derivation is a Hydrotherapy term referring to the drawing of blood from one part of the body by increasing blood to another part. Derivation reduces congestion by moving blood to a distal area. —*Ed.*

A fomentation is a simple and effective method of applying moist heat to any part of the body by means of flannel wrung out of boiling water, milk, or any medicated hot fluid.

In extensive inflammations, especially of the abdomen, in erysipelas, and to allay spasms in deep-seated parts, as in cases of renal and biliary calculi, repeated milk fomentations are always to be preferred.

It ought to be applied as hot as the skin can bear, and although moist, the hot liquid should be thoroughly squeezed out of the flannel applied to the skin.

To retain the heat, it is advisable to apply a dry flannel or towel over the wet one.

BATHS AND THE WATER CURE

by Benedict Lust

The Kneipp Water Cure Monthly, II (9), 241. (1901)

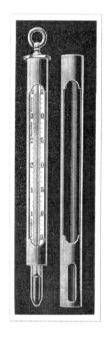

B aths are of various kinds, and are distinguished according to the substances of which they are composed, such as air, earth, sand, vapor, or water. According to their temperature as cold, tepid, or hot, and applied as affusion, compress, douche, drop, electro, eye fomentations, fountain, full pack, half pack, hot air, or Turkish baths, injections, plunge, rain, shower, sitz, sponge, sun, towel, vapor, or Russian [steam bath], wind, etc., according as they are general or partial, natural or artificial. Bathing, besides serving the great ends of bodily cleanliness and comfort, is very important in the preservation or restoration of health. Never bathe within less than three or four hours after a meal, or when exhausted. Cold baths are harmful when the powers of the body are too languid to bring on a reaction, but beneficial in cases of nervousness or general debility. They should always be taken with caution. Many errors are committed by staying in a cold bath too long. Never take any food immediately after bathing. Always sponge the body all over with cold water after taking a hot bath, as it tones up the nerves and leaves the skin in good condition. The most delicate and feeble person may take a cold bath with benefit and pleasure if they begin with a hot one. The temperature of a cold bath may be from 33° to 70° F / 0.5° to 21° C; a tepid bath from 80° to 96° F / 27° to 36° C; a hot bath from 100° to 112° F / 38° to 44° C. Some people can bear the temperature raised to 116° F / 47° C.

It is a great fallacy for elderly people or for any one suffering with heart trouble, anemia, colds, fevers, etc., to imagine that a good, hot bath, to be followed by a quick rub over with cold water and dry towels, will do harm. It is not so by any means. How can the bath be dangerous when it relieves the system by the elimination of impurities through the skin? Note the surprising quantity of scurf that can be got off by occasional baths and light friction. Excessive use of the hot bath in any form is bad, as it tends to make the skin dry, harsh, and scaly, by diluting the secretions of the sebaceous glands, the oil of which is intended by Nature to keep the skin smooth, glossy, and soft.

I have not sufficient space to give a full detailed account of the various processes of Hydropathy. The works of Father Kneipp, Dr. Trall, and other writers should be carefully read by those who wish to know more about it.

Cold baths are harmful when the powers of the body are too languid to bring on a reaction, but beneficial in cases of nervousness or general debility.

Never take any food immediately after bathing.

Always sponge the body all over with cold water after taking a hot bath, as it tones up the nerves and leaves the skin in good condition.

The most delicate and feeble person may take a cold bath with benefit and pleasure if they begin with a hot one.

The temperature of a cold bath may be from 33° to 70° F/0.5° to 21° C; a tepid bath from 80° to 96° F/27° to 36° C; a hot bath from 100° to 112° F/38° to 44° C. Some people can bear the temperature raised to 116° F/47° C.

Excessive use of the hot bath in any form is bad, as it tends to make the skin dry, harsh, and scaly, by diluting the secretions of the sebaceous glands, the oil of which is intended by Nature to keep the skin smooth, glossy, and soft.

BAD HEALTH

by Friedrich Eduard Bilz

The Kneipp Water Cure Monthly, II (11), 287-291. (1901)

TREATMENT FOR EVERY ILLNESS, ALTHOUGH THE NAME BE UNKNOWN

The uninitiated cannot always know the nature of a disease; and not only these, but in many cases even physicians are ignorant of it, for their diagnosis (distinguishing the character of a disease by its symptoms) is most deceptive, and it is often that medical men who err in this respect that have acquired a great name as authorities—I must tell the reader that the name of the disease is of no consequence whatever. When a person is ill, his whole body suffers; and the whole body in the first place always comes under treatment.

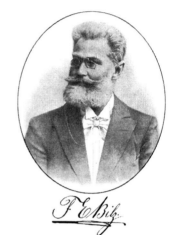

Friedrich Eduard Bilz (1842-1922) was a devout follower of Kneipp.

The best thing, suitable for every patient, is always the universal remedy, the steam bath in bed.* He should never wait till the disease has quite broken out and till he knows what disease it is, but the great point is to nip it in the bud, to take preventative measures at its very first appearance.

For the application of a steam bath in bed, the following rule is to be observed:

In acute attacks of illness, attended with fever, the patient is kept in the steam bath for from half an hour to one hour, but above all, only as long as he feels comfortable, and until the fever has again obtained the upper hand. It should be followed either by a lukewarm bath (88° F / 31° C), or by wet rubbing of the whole body in tepid water (73° F / 23° C). It may be repeated as often as required.

An extra compress is applied to the inflamed and painful parts of the body during a pack, which may frequently be substituted here for the steambath in bed.

In chronic (protracted) diseases, however, the duration of the

---

*The steam bath in bed resembles a wet sheet wrap with the inclusion of hot water bottles placed within the pack. Directions for a steam bath in bed is given by Ludwig Staden on page 116. —Ed.

steam bath in bed is usually one hour to one and a half hours, and even longer, and from two to four of them are given weekly. An extra compress may also be applied in this case to the affected part. A bath or rubbing with the wet towel of the whole body should follow the pack as above described. I must not omit to mention here that the patient must be taken out of the pack the moment he feels uncomfortable in it, a point to be strictly observed in all diseases, whether acute or chronic.

In acute cases (when there is a fever), the linen sheet should not be wrung so dry as in chronic cases.

Besides the steam bath in bed, the abdominal compress (which may also justly be designated a universal remedy) can be applied. In cases when the conditions of illness assume a feverish character, a somewhat thicker linen sheet is used, dipped in tepid water (73° to 77° F /23° to 25° C), wrung out less thoroughly than usual, and put round the body. It is changed as soon as it gets hot or irksome. In chronic diseases, on the other hand, a sheet less thick is employed, wrung out well and applied (if in the day time) from two to four hours in bed; if in the evening, it may be left on all night. Be it again expressly mentioned that in every disease the air must be fresh, in or out of doors (sleep with the window open). In most cases the diet must be non-stimulating; above all, the bowels kept open, if necessary by all means of enema, which should also be applied for detergent purposes. (For Modes of Application, see Index in *The Natural Method of Healing*. In case of obstinate constipation we refer also to Enemata "Constipation" further, "Convalescence," and "Medicine, Opinions of Medical Men on Taking.")*

If, therefore, a member of your family falls ill, apply with confidence the universal remedy, the steam bath in bed, and with the aid of the other healing agents mentioned here (fresh air, etc.), you will be successful in most cases.

But to give the reader a better idea of the subject, and a more general survey of the comprehensive heading "Bad Health," I will give some special instructions on this subject.

FEVER

Treatment of the acute, i.e., inflammatory diseases, attended by fever. The first thing to do is to examine the patient, whether his temperature is higher than usual (normal is 98.6° F/37° C). With the hand, feel his head, chest, stomach, feet; where the heat is greatest, there is the seat of the disease and the inflammation.

Either sponge bath of the whole body with tepid water (73° to 81° F / 23° to 27° C,) is applied in the first place, or a lukewarm bath (88°

---

*Bilz refers throughout this article to methods found in his book, *The Natural Method of Healing* (1898). —Ed.

F / 31° C) and the patient then put to bed; or steam bath applied in bed, or some fever treatment* a cool enema is likewise administered at once. For it is an inviolable principle, when combating disease, not to apply treatment to a single part of the body only, but at the same time to the whole of it.

If, during the examination of the body, as directed above, the greatest amount of heat and pain should be found to exist in the throat, pointing to croup or diphtheria; or in the chest, indicating inflammation of the lungs; or in the sides, suggesting pleuritic; or in the abdomen, indicating intestinal inflammation of some kind—then a soothing compress or pad should be put on the affected part. If the head should be hot, combined with violent headache—symptoms which may point to inflammation of the brain or its membranes—cool compresses are placed round the head. Together with these cool compresses or pad around or on the throat, chest, stomach, head, etc., which should be changed when warm, a derivative treatment must, particularly if the pain does not diminish, be applied at the same time. It consists in stimulating packs for foot and leg and calf, also partial packs, etc.; for cold feet a hot water bottle, wrapped in a wet cloth, may also be applied to them, or a foot steam bath given previously. Or instead of the derivative treatment, a steam bath in bed may be given, with a thick extra compress round the affected part. Duration half an hour to an hour, as it agrees with the patient. This application is continued (or if agreeable, it may be altered with some other fever treatment), and repeated as long as the heat (the fever and pain) greatly increase. The greater the heat, the thicker and wetter the cooling or soothing compresses or pads, and the more frequently they must be changed.

VIOLENT ABDOMINAL PAINS

If there is costiveness, apply treatment given under "Enemata" and "Constipation." If there are violent pains in the intestines, etc., warm or hot compresses should be applied frequently, especially if the pain in the stomach does not diminish. In all diseases with attendant fever, keep the window always open, and sometimes the door, too; the couch [bed] should be cool, and feather duvets avoided as much as possible; the diet must be cool and non-stimulating. If the patient shivers, vigorous dry or wet rubbing must be applied; and afterwards a dry pack, or a steam bath in bed instead. If he perspires in this, it should be succeeded by a bath (86° to 88° F /30° to 31° C). If after this treatment a rash appears (the purples, smallpox, or pustules, denoting scarlatina, measles, etc.), it may be considered a very favorable sign, because with them the morbid matter in the body is generally thrown off, and the illness assumes a mild character.

In order to entirely remove all foreign substances from the system, it is advisable to give the patient affected with the purples or the smallpox a few more steam baths in bed, or stimulating three-quarter or full packs, in which he will perspire gently; and to follow up with a bath.

In smallpox, constantly apply compresses to the face to prevent the troublesome itching which causes the patient to scratch his face, resulting in its being pitted. For further information we refer to an article on smallpox.

MOUTH INFLAMMATION

Inflammation of the cavities of the mouth and gullet, and exudation of morbid matters from them, i.e. croup, etc. are treated with cooling compresses round the throat, to be changed every fifteen minutes; or according to necessity, coupled with a detergent or derivative treatment and gargling with tepid water (68° to 77° F / 20° to 25° C) every hour.

As already mentioned, steam baths in bed, duration from one hour to an hour and a half, together with thick throat compresses (73° F / 23° C) are most efficacious. In this complaint it is also essential to give cooling, non-stimulating diet, frequent gargling or drinking of moderately cold water, nose baths, mild pure air for breathing, detergent enemas, massage of the neck and back (slapping the back). Care should be taken to keep the feet invariably warm.

CHRONIC, PROTRACTED DISEASES

For the cure of chronic diseases, of whatever kind, a strengthening or, according to the case, a regenerative treatment, is of primary importance, in addition to the often mentioned steam baths applied in bed. A perfectly equal distribution of the first things to be aimed at should the patient's feet be constantly cold, rubbing of the feet with a wet towel must be resorted to as a remedy; in addition to foot steam baths, foot baths, followed by walking exercise, walking barefoot, etc.

CHRONIC CONSTIPATION

Chronic constipation must be removed by fruit diet and whole-meal bread, as well as by the frequent and regular enemas and massage of the stomach, and hip baths combined with massage of the stomach.

SKIN

Further, in chronic complaints great attention should be paid to the skin. Wet rubbing of the whole body with cool water (73° to 77° F / 23° to 25° C) or a lukewarm bath (86° to 90° F / 30° to 32° C) must be applied daily. For weakly people or persons not used to water, the water may be taken from two to four degrees warmer. Always begin with water that is not too cold and lower the temperature very gradually.

The system of a chronically affected patient having been approved by the above means, a more regulated treatment may be entered upon for the purpose of strengthening the affected organs and removing from the system the morbid matter and all impure substances existing in the blood. This is only accomplished by sweating cures, such as steam baths in bed, stimulating packs, etc. The patient must perspire gently and often very gently indeed. Excess must always be avoided. Do not try to force perspiration; it will come of its own accord at the proper time.

The stimulating abdominal compress, if continually used at night for a length of time, will of itself eliminate a great quantity of morbid matter from the body. Many a chronic sufferer has been restored to health by it alone. Indeed, most astonishing results are obtained by it. This compress, i.e. the sheet, must be washed thoroughly in warm water and rinsed in cold every day; and every week it should be washed with soap and boiled and dried in the open air, in order that every atom of discharged matter may be removed. Breathing exercises, curative gymnastics, and massage must also be employed. Many chronic complaints may be treated with the regenerative, sometimes with the preliminary treatment. Enemas, besides being applied in constipation, should also be given for derivative purposes.

If, after a lengthening application of steam or sweating packs or compresses, etc., eruptions such as abscesses, herpes, etc., should appear, they may be looked upon as favorable symptoms.

CHRONIC HEAD AND BRAIN DISORDERS

For chronic affections of the head or brain, which may perhaps be of a gouty or rheumatic nature, compresses round the head (more or less wet, as the patient's feelings prompts), to be changed more or less frequently, together with head douches may be combined with derivative treatment. In the same way, head baths, steam baths for the head, nose, forehead, and mouth baths; as well as gargling (77° to 90° F / 25° to 32° C); dry, and wet full packs; followed by bath are all highly beneficial.

CHRONIC EYE DISEASES

In chronic affections of the eyes, the following applications are advised: eyebaths (73° to 89° F / 23° to 32° C) opening and shutting the eyes in the water, gentle massage in water, massage of the eyes and throat, throat compresses, washing the eyes, bathing the head or back of head, and derivative treatment, as well as abdominal compresses at night. Nonstimulating diet. The patient would also do well to have a sweat pack occasionally; see "Sweating Cure". For chronic congestion of blood in the head, apply now and then cool rubbing of the feet, and stimulating packs of the legs and feet at night; as well as derivative hip baths.

Chronic Ear Diseases

In chronic diseases of the ear use frequent gentle injections with tepid water; head baths and head steam baths; ear baths and ear steam baths; neck compresses, massage of the throat; masticate vigorously (hard crusts of bread); and, after the injections, put at night wet cotton-wool into the ear.

Eruptions, Abscesses Of The Head

In abscesses or eruptions on the head, or in the face, apply stimulating, dissolving, local compresses; stimulating or dry full or three-quarter packs; or steam baths for the purpose of perspiring. A bath or wet rubbing of the whole body daily; detergent or derivative treatments as well.

Chronic Throat Diseases

In chronic diseases of the throat (internal or external), wash the throat frequently with cool water and expose it to the air. Further, apply local stimulating compresses, tepid gargling, bathing the mouth, and detergent treatment. Also a steam bath in bed now and then is beneficial, besides other sweating cures. Massage of the throat for internal affections.

Chronic Chest And Lung Diseases

In chronic affections of the chest or lungs, e.g. chronic catarrh of the lungs, etc., with viscid expectoration, apply daily one or two gentle wet rubbings of the whole body; or bath, stimulating trunk and leg packs at night (the latter only if the other should not suit the patient), trunk and shoulder pack in bed during the day. Repeated gargling, drawing water up the nose, breathing exercise; and a sip of water taken after every fit of coughing. Derivative treatment; bathe the mouth, and apply wet or dry full or three-quarter packs for the purpose of perspiring, or give steam bath in bed. Fresh air, and sleep with the window open.

Breast Tumors

Induration of the breast, use stimulating, dissolving compresses on the place, made of linen folded many times. When the tumor opens, put wet lint on it and wash it, and wash it with tepid water frequently. Above all, we recommend either a three-quarter steam bath, or a steam bath for the breast.

CONSUMPTION

Chronic pulmonary diseases (consumption) are treated with soothing compresses on the chest, occasionally also with gently stimulating packs, or bed steam baths, if they agree with the patient; bathing the whole body with lukewarm water (86° to 90° F / 30° to 32° C). However, if the latter prove too exciting for patients who are very ill, they should not be persisted in.

Stimulating packs for the feet, calves, thighs or legs. Plenty of mild, pure air, particularly forest air. Breathe through the nose, sleep with the window open, practice breathing exercises, and adopt a strictly non-stimulating diet (drink the juice of stewed fruit).

STOMACH, LIVER, INTESTINES, KIDNEY, GALL BLADDER CHRONIC DISORDERS

Stimulating trunk packs or stomach compresses at night, with stimulating leg packs, cool lavations of the regions of the stomach, liver, intestines, etc. Douche for the stomach, hip baths with the massage of the abdomen, steam baths in bed, or else stimulating full or three-quarters packs with extra compresses on the affected part; massage either of the affected part or of the whole body.

CHRONIC AFFECTION OF THE SEXUAL ORGANS

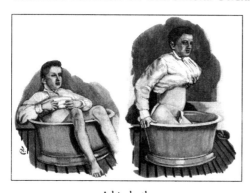

A hip bath

Tepid hip baths (66° to 80° F/19° to 27° C), stimulating stomach compresses at night, and stimulating or soothing T pack; now and then stimulating full packs, or steam baths in bed, with extra compresses on the genitals. Besides these, local treatment is advised for females in the form of injections [vaginal douches] (77° to 81° F / 25° to 27° C), partial baths (77° to 90° F / 25° to 32° C) from two to four daily, and also stimulating compresses on sore places, e.g., for men under the prepuce, etc. For this purpose prepared wet cotton wool or linen is employed, to be changed or removed as soon as it gets dry or the patient's feeling prompts its renewal or removal. This, however, has to be done very cautiously, so as not to injure the freshly formed skin under it; the compress is either softened by wetting it, or the under layer is left on and wetted by putting a fresh layer of lint on it.

The main requirement in these cases is a strict, non-stimulating diet, and abstention from sexual excitement.

Leucorrhea And Hemorrhage

In "the whites" (*fluor albus*), cleanliness must be established by injections, rinsing or washing out, and several hip baths daily (81° F / 27° C). To allow the water to enter readily, the vagina should be distended. Stimulating stomach compress at night, and a wet cloth passed between the legs.

In protracted hemorrhage of the womb, hip baths are always the best remedy. They should be of a temperature of 73° F / 23° C, and last from ten to fifteen minutes; by the gradual addition of cold water, they are reduced to the temperature of spring water, about 46° to 54° F / 8° to 12° C.

Legs

In paralysis and swelling of the knee, lengthy cool or cold knee affusions are applied, or cooling compresses round it, as well as stimulating packs of the thighs or leg, with the same kind of compresses on the knee. Also steam baths with cool lavations to follow are of great effect. Further, occasional stimulating full packs with extra compresses round the knee, or local stimulating packs and massage are recommended.

In chronic ulcers on the legs and feet, etc., keeping the wounds clean is of great importance. Next bathe them a long time in water of 77° to 81° F / 25° to 27° C, continually pouring water on the wounds and ulcers, either with a vessel or with the hands. In doing so, the limb has to be held up outside the water; stimulating packs of the affected parts. Sun baths to the affected parts and a tepid bath or affusion afterwards. When walking out or taking indoor exercise in cold weather a rag with Vaseline on it should be applied. For the pack (lukewarm water, 77° to 86° F / 25° to 29° C is used) the sheet should not be wrung too dry and extra damped lint is put on the ulcer. It should be changed according to the patient's feeling, i.e., as soon as he feels the pack to be inconvenient.

Further, a stimulating full or three-quarters pack applied now and then, or a steam bath in bed, with extra compress on the ulcer, are of benefit. Strictly non-stimulating diet and fresh air. In severe cases, a regenerative, or a preliminary treatment.

Paralysis Of The Limbs

Repeat cold frictions of the limb with bare hands dipped in cold water, then stimulating local packs, succeeded by cold wet rubbing, partial steam baths, full steam baths, full packs, etc., both dry and wet sweating packs, to be changed as the patient's feeling suggests. Kneipp douches after getting thoroughly warm. The treatment most agreeable to the patient should always be chosen. Wet rubbing of the whole body, sun baths with lukewarm or cooler douche baths, affusions, friction baths, massage, and curative gymnastics, also applications of the Faradic interrupted current are all of great benefit.

SPRAINS, STRAINS, AND DISLOCATIONS

Rest for the injured limb, cooling or soothing compresses; or cold water dropping on the sprained part, or holding it in cold water for some time. In dislocations, the limb must first be set. Stimulating compresses to be applied afterwards, but only if agreeable to the patient. Massage is especially effective here. It consists in gentle, concentrated rubbing, but at first not near the inflamed part, beginning by rubbing gently and then gradually more firmly. When tendons are torn, rub in every direction.

ABSCESSES

For abscesses of every kind, it is best to apply stimulating compresses.* The harder the abscesses and the tighter the skin, the thicker the wet linen cloth must be laid on. Most beneficial also is an occasional stimulating three-quarter or full pack, or a steam bath in bed with extra compress on the abscess. Strictly non-stimulating diet. It is only under the hard skin, e.g., of the hand or the soles of the feet, that an incision may be made to relieve the abscess. In all other places, they open of their own accord when they have matured, in consequence of these stimulating compresses. Exceptions are, however, made occasionally with very young children, or when the pains are excessive; a light prick with a needle, or a slight cut in the abscess is sufficient to help the matter to discharge and thus give relief. After it is opened, gentle pressure of the abscess will aid the discharge, and tepid water may then be dropped on it, and the pus washed off. Wet lint is again put on it before another stimulating compress is applied.

It should be mentioned that sun baths, massage, curative gymnastics, and dietetic, regenerative, or preliminary treatment are of great value in many chronic diseases. No less important also is attention to a gentle action of the skin, according to the patient's condition, good air in and out of doors, sleeping with the windows open, daily opening of the bowels (enemas for constipation and cleansing). Mixed, plain, or invalid diet, suitable to the patient's strength, and breathing exercises in the pulmonary diseases, etc.

---

*Stimulating compresses implies a cold compress. —*Ed.*

Lastly, do not forget that every compress, pack bath, etc., has to be changed or removed at once, if it becomes inconvenient to the patient. If the application is on that account discontinued, a cool, tepid or lukewarm sponge both of the parts before treated should follow.

The following plaster can also be recommended for ordinary boils and ulcers to which a wet compress cannot always be applied during the daytime. Dissolve equal quantities of pitch, turpentine, and oxicrocius over a very moderate fire, and spread it thinly on a piece of linen—this is the ordinary red pitch plaster.

We have now mentioned the diseases human flesh is heir to, and given practical hints for their cure, so that everybody, though he may not know the disease, nor its name, can help to avert or to soothe it in case of need. At the same time, we must point out that all the different applications, which we have enumerated above, must never be continued one after the other too frequently, so as to cause weakness and prostration instead of giving strength and recovery of health, but moderation must be observed with regard to them. It has always to be born in mind that it is Nature only (the vital, preserving, healing force, residing within us) that cures the disease, and that we can only assist Nature by these applications.

Pauses also have to be made sometimes in wearisome, chronic diseases that can only be healed slowly, in order that the patient may recoup a little. For the all-important point in the cure of diseases is to give tone to the system, and keep it strengthened, so that the innate vital force may the better be able to eject all morbid matter from the body, and thus conquer the disease. The patient must therefore study himself in this respect.

If the reader acts conscientiously according to the manner indicated, and gradually makes himself more conversant with the character of the Natural Method of Healing, he will soon experience the beneficial results of it and acknowledge what a blessing that system really is, and he will gradually rid himself of the monstrous error that healing is only possible from medical science, and exclaim with me, "Thank God, I have at length vanquished this error, this fatal prejudice, which has sacrificed health and life and caused endless expense."

—Bilz, *The Natural Method of Healing*

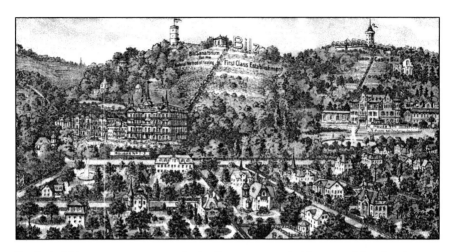

Friedrich Bilz' success using water for healing was rewarded by an indebted and grateful patient with the gifting of four immense palatial buildings that would become the Bilz Sanitorium in Dresden-Radebeul, Germany.

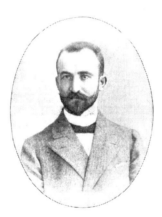

Otto Wagner,
Director of the Bilz Sanitorium

In acute attacks of illness, attended with fever, the patient is kept in the steam bath for from half an hour to one hour, but above all, only as long as he feels comfortable, and until the fever has again obtained the upper hand. It should be followed either by a lukewarm bath (88° F/31° C), or by wet rubbing of the whole body in tepid water (73° F/23° C).

In acute cases (when there is a fever), the linen sheet should not be wrung so dry as in chronic cases.

If, therefore, a member of your family falls ill, apply with confidence the universal remedy, the steam bath in bed, and with the aid of the other healing agents mentioned here (fresh air, etc.), you will be successful in most cases.

For it is an inviolable principle, when combating disease, not to apply treatment to a single part of the body only, but at the same time to the whole of it.

If the patient shivers, vigorous dry or wet rubbing must be applied; and afterwards a dry pack, or a steam bath in bed instead.

A perfectly equal distribution of the first things to be aimed at should the patient's feet be constantly cold, rubbing of the feet with a wet towel must be resorted to as a remedy; in addition to foot steam baths, foot baths, followed by walking exercise, walking barefoot, etc.

Always begin with water that is not too cold and lower the temperature very gradually.

Do not try to force perspiration; it will come of its own accord at the proper time.

The stimulating abdominal compress, if continually used at night for a length of time, will of itself eliminate a great quantity of morbid matter from the body; and many a chronic sufferer has been restored to health by it alone.

At the same time we must point out that all the different applications, which we have enumerated above, must never be continued one after the other too frequently, so as to cause weakness and prostration instead of giving strength and recovery of health, but moderation must be observed with regard to them.

The Natural Bath*

by Adolf Just, Jungborn, Stapelburg, Harz, Germany.
Translated from the German by Benedict Lust
The Kneipp Water Cure Monthly, II (11), 315-317. (1901)

Since I look only to Nature when I want to know the right thing to do for my health and my well-being, I always find that everything that I have recognized as strictly natural, that is, as thoroughly in the spirit of Nature, has on trial always proved itself to be the right thing entirely. Where Nature is accurately observed, experiments to prove the correctness of a procedure are superfluous. When Nature's intentions are perfectly understood we can at once confidently rely upon them as correct, just as primitive man and the animals in the free state have always eaten and bathed without first convincing themselves of the right way by experiment. This has likewise been shown by the natural bath.

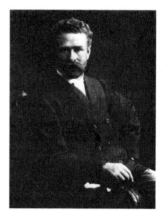

Adolf Just (1859-1936)

After the first bath of this kind, I at once felt benefited and refreshed in a way that I had never experienced from any other water application. Almost all who besides myself have tried this new bath have been surprised by its agreeable and positively good effects.** All experienced a very strong but pleasant sensation of coolness, and after the bath a much better and more agreeable bodily warmth. The points that were especially commented on were the exceedingly stimulated digestion, warm feet for the entire day, increased action of the skin as shown by a slight perspiration, unusual vivacity and cheerfulness, remarkable vigor, and other favorable manifestations.

---

*The original title of this article was "Return to Nature". Benedict Lust had used material from Adolf Just's book, *Return to Nature* which he had translated into English with the help of his brother-in-law, Reverend Albert Stroebele. —Ed.

**Only a few were frightened by the healing crises brought on by the baths. In one person, for instance, who suffered from chronic lung trouble, a lung trouble put in its appearance after a few days: the chronic ailment had become acute, a most favorable sign. The same person also declared that sun baths did not agree with him, that they gave him pains in the body, while these pains only showed that the foreign matter (disease germs) in his body were being loosened by the sun, preliminary to being thrown off. Patients who show such little appreciation of Nature and her healing forces, will probably never regain their health. —Adolf Just.

I could here mention innumerable reports that I have received concerning the efficacy of the bath, both by letter and by word of mouth, the latter always with a happy, beaming face. But I send it into the world simply on its own merits and without flourish of trumpets.

Whoever understands Nature and knows that everything which is in the spirit of Nature and according to her dictates must result in the greatest blessing for mankind, will welcome this bath, and to him it will bring blessing and happiness in abundance. Let those who care nothing for all-wise Nature and everything for the "science" of men, of sick men, and who flounder from one error to another, scorn and deride it!

In sending my bath into the world, I wish to give it only a few directions on the way. I disapprove, on the whole, of the warming of the water: it is against Nature.* It is not so difficult to sit with only the posterior and the feet in entirely cold water, once the abdomen and sexual organs have been washed and rubbed, the interior especially of the abdomen has been cooled off, and the blood is once more driven towards the extremities. But for those who cannot stand it very long in winter, which does not easily happen, one can take a very short bath, or even dispense with it altogether. In this case we have still another resource, namely, going naked, or the earth compress on the abdomen, of which I shall speak more in detail later.

The water ought not to be too deep, about as deep as the width of the bather's hand; for adults at most three inches. The rubbing and the exercise after the bath must not be executed according to any definite rules, or any system of massage, or gymnastics, but entirely according to one's own feeling and inclination.

Whoever has the opportunity (and the opportunity can always be found if it is only sought) can take his bath in the open. Man originally had to take his bath in the open, and in the open he must again take it regularly, if he is to derive the full benefits of it, just as food partaken in fresh air always tastes better, and does more good than when it is eaten in the room and in impure air.

Women can discontinue their bath during their monthly periods. The other remedies of Nature, however—walking barefooted, the air and light baths, earth compress, etc.; women need not avoid during this period. They are especially benefited at that time.

The bath can always be taken in rivers (near the shore when they are deep), in brooks and small ponds.

In the room, if it is heated, the windows can always remain open to some extent. The early morning, or at least the forenoon, when one has

---

*In order not to discourage beginners, they may be allowed to warm the water a little or to take the bath in a warm room. —Adolf Just.

not yet broken one's fast, or has eaten very little, is the best time for the bath.

All fishes (water animals) try to avoid the air, while all air creatures take great pains not to get their bodies into the water, and while taking their bath, as little as their bodily structures will allow. Man is the highest light and air creature. If the air should suddenly be entirely withheld, he could live for only a very short time. Even if only a small part of the air is withheld, he at once loses vitality and is weakened, just as the fish begins to die when he is taken out of his element, the water. But now the body is almost entirely immersed in water during a full bath, and the skin, through which the body ordinarily absorbs quite a considerable quantity of air, can neither absorb nor throw off the bad, used-up air. The body is, therefore, weakened and injured by a full bath. If the full bath lasts only a very short time, perhaps only several seconds, the benefit which the body derives from the cooling, for which a few seconds suffice, may be somewhat greater than the harm done by depriving it of air. If the full bath lasts five, ten, fifteen minutes and longer, as is customary in our bathing institutions, it is always very injurious. If we deprive a part of the body or separate organs of air, for instance, the hands by means of leather gloves, these are always injured and lamed. In our sitz baths, hitherto, the abdominal organs were always surrounded by water from all sides. These were therefore shut off from the air and rendered more or less inactive, so that they could not work in the right way during the bath. Thus, the effect of these baths was essentially weakened. Neither was the water thrown over the entire abdominal surface in the sitz bath, and there was no rubbing.* In the natural bath everything that interferes with the full effect of former water applications is done away with, and this is the explanation of the great results that are only now being achieved by water.

It is to be hoped that the natural bath will now be welcomed by the public at large, by rich and poor, by high and low, and carry to old and young the blessing and well-being which the kind mother, Nature, has always intended to shed upon mankind with lavish hands. Let no one say that he does not need the natural bath because he is well. For it is plainly not the first intention of Nature to cure diseases by the bath, but rather to keep her creatures well, bright and happy.

As winter succeeds autumn and night the day, according to stern natural law, so man, leading an unnatural mode of life, breathing impure air, using tobacco, alcohol, coffee, etc., must fall a victim to disease. This does not always manifest itself in the form of what is called disease nowadays, but disease is nevertheless present and will make itself felt plainly enough.

---

*Adolf Just's natural bath involves a lot of rubbing and movement while in the bath, in order to warm the body and improve circulation. —Ed.

The child in school is inattentive and indolent and learns his lessons with difficulty. Often he is ill-bred and becomes a prey to sin and vice. He is punished, often severely enough. But the poor fellow is in fact only ill and suffers his punishment innocently. The husband and father is unkind, harsh, and often even brutal toward his wife and children, toward those whom he loves. Later he is filled with remorse, not knowing that only his nerves have been overheated by the use of alcohol, tobacco, and other modern poisons, and that he too is ill.

Others are directly driven on to the path of vice and crime. They are put into houses of correction and penitentiaries, instead of being cured and made whole.

The young wife becomes whimsical, irritable, and hysterical.

> With the cestus loosed—away
> Flies illusion from the heart.

Conjugal happiness is not realized, as had been expected, and the heaven dreamed of in reality turns into hell. The young girl who entered wedlock with the fairest qualities and sacred heart, an angel, becomes a vixen. But do not reproach her, poor thing, for the unnatural life which married people almost always lead bears fruit and demands as its first victim the wife.

The plants and animals of the forest, in the state of Nature (not the plants of the fields), retain their health, beauty, youthfulness and goodness up to a certain period, fixed for the individuals of the same species, when they die suddenly, with only a few exceptions which here again have been caused by man's interference with Nature.

Among men in modern times, one becomes shortsighted in childhood, another hard of hearing, one loses his teeth, another his hair, many suffer from nervous troubles, and even are enveloped by mental darkness. The young girl who is a celebrated beauty today, suddenly falls away, grows thin and pale, or becomes bloated and ruddy soon after her marriage, and appears offensively homely to the man whom she had so recently charmed.

Many people are favorably situated, but nevertheless give themselves no end of care and trouble. Even millionaires are sometimes troubled by the care for food.

> Care at the bottom of the heart is lurking:
> Her secret pangs in silence working,
> She, restless, rocks herself, disturbing joy and rest.
> We dread the blows we never feel,
> And what we never lose is yet by us lamented!

> —Goethe, Faust

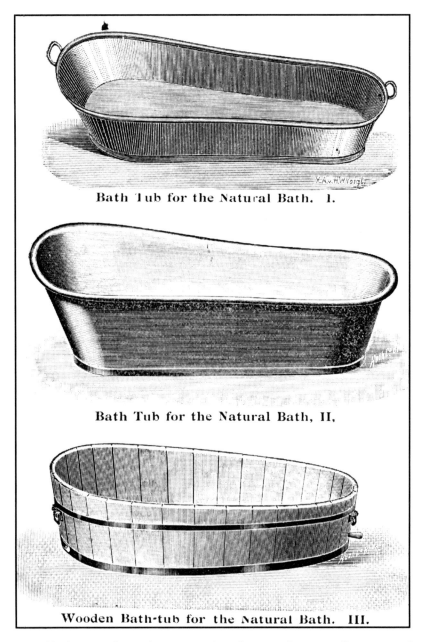

Bath Tub for the Natural Bath. I.

Bath Tub for the Natural Bath, II,

Wooden Bath-tub for the Natural Bath. III.

Natural baths were taken in three to six inches of water in these specially constructed shallow bath tubs.

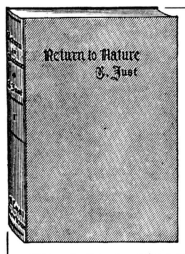
Cherished as one of the seminal books for the early Naturopaths, Adolf Just's book *Return to Nature* (1901) was tranlated into English by Benedict Lust with the aid of his brother-in-law, Reverend Albert Stroebele.

When Nature's intentions are perfectly understood, we can at once confidently rely upon them as correct, just as primitive man and the animals in the free state have always eaten and bathed without first convincing themselves of the right way by experiment. This has likewise been shown by the natural bath.

Almost all who besides myself have tried this new bath have been surprised by its agreeable and positively good effects. All experienced a very strong but pleasant sensation of coolness, and after the bath a much better and more agreeable bodily warmth.

The water ought not to be too deep, about as deep as the width of the bather's hand; for adults at most three inches.

Man originally had to take his bath in the open, and in the open he must again take it regularly, if he is to derive the full benefits of it, just as food partaken in fresh air always tastes better, and does more good than when it is eaten in the room and in impure air.

Women can discontinue their bath during their monthly periods. The other remedies of Nature, however—walking barefooted, the air and light baths, earth compress, etc.; women need not avoid during this period.

Let no one say that he does not need the natural bath, because he is well. For it is plainly not the first intention of Nature to cure diseases by the bath, but rather to keep her creatures well, bright and happy.

1902

In Memoriam Elise Amend

The Neck Bandage
Benedict Lust

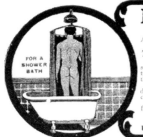

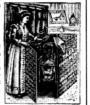
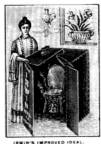

These ads illustrate the enthusiasm for Water Cure

In Memoriam Elise Amend

by Benedict Lust

The Naturopath and Herald of Health, III (7), 294.

On June 25th, 1902, a staunch adherent to the Kneipp cure movement passed away in the person of Miss Elise Amend, who owned the New York Kneippianum at 1931 Madison Ave., New York City, and also a summer branch at Poughkeepsie, New York.

Elise Amend was a graduate of Wörishofen and has personally successfully treated and cured many hundreds of sufferers. She was well liked by her patients and highly esteemed by her colleagues. Her work will be carried on, as heretofore by Miss Dina Amend, who will continue the good work begun by Elise Amend, whose memory will long be cherished by everybody who had the good fortune to know her personally.

THE NECK BANDAGE

by Benedict Lust

The Naturopath and Herald of Health, III (12), 493-494. (1902)

This bandage, as its name implies, is applied only to the neck. Take a wet thick soft towel or bandage of from four to six folds and with it encircle the throat closely, beginning below the ear and under the chin; and over this is a dry cloth evenly wound.

The effect of this bandage is to extract foul matter from the throat and to draw the superfluous heat from it. It must not be kept on too long without removing it because it develops heat so rapidly and when this becomes too intense more harm than good is done.

It affects not only the head but also the body, guiding the blood downwards and cutting off the excess flow. What would otherwise go into the head will be repressed by this bandage; but if it be too hot, the blood and secretions are drawn from both the body and the head into the throat.

For example, a person having a swollen throat wished to reduce it by means of the neck bandage. He felt so great relief from it that he kept it on a long time believing that the longer he did so, the greater good. However, his throat daily grew worse and he could not effect a cure. At length when it became as bad as possible, he came to me and poured out his complaints.

I answered him shortly: "If you attract matter from your body and head into your throat, of course it will be swollen. If you wish to reduce this, lay a very cold cloth round the throat which will contract, but as soon as warmth is generated, expansion takes place and cancels the good already done. If you want cold to diminish heat, then you must renew your bandage every quarter of an hour and continue it for an hour or an hour and a half. In this way only will your throat be cured.

In case of a rush of blood to the head the neck bandage will be of no avail. I should employ rather a foot or thigh bandage or a wet cloth on the stomach—in fact, one must work from below to draw the blood from above.

The neck bandage can and does draw the blood from the head to the throat, but it must not stay there and the only way of getting rid of what has been drawn into it is by constantly renewing the bandage. In inflammation of the throat, the neck bandage may be employed with great advantage. If, however, it be applied ignorantly or carelessly, the mischief will be increased. The neck bandage gets hot quickly and draws the blood rapidly towards the throat thereby increasing the inflammation.

Should it so happen that the heat or the inflammation is increased by employing the neck bandage, then on no account must it be kept on longer than ten minutes without renewal, and the water should be as cold

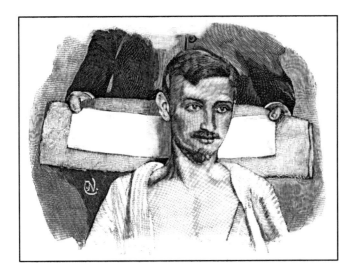

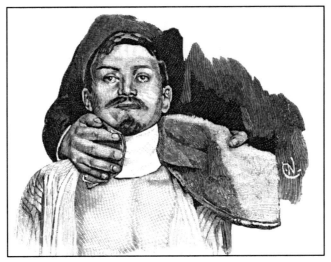

The neck bandage or compress

as possible into which the cloth is dipped. It would be still better to lay a six-fold cloth on the stomach which would rapidly develop an increased warmth and so relieve the inflammation in the throat. It would be of benefit also to have a bandage from the foot to the knee which would draw the blood from the head to the feet. There are cases in which the neck bandage must be warm and not cold. For example, in quinsy [peritonsillar abscess] one applies the bandage as hot as the patient can bear it, in order to work upon the coagulated blood to separate and disperse it and by a rapid interchange of matter to ward off the danger.

The principle is the same as in blood poisoning—the hot bandage prevents the spread of inflammation and eliminates the foul matter.

In diphtheria where a rapid accumulation of matter forms, the flow of blood to the throat is prevented by a frequent change of the cold bandage. For this reason, the warm bandage must be renewed every ten or twenty minutes, with cold applications.

The neck bandage is especially used in obstructions and swellings of throat or head.

One might suppose that goiters would be very easily removed by the application of the neck bandage. This is not my opinion, which is that this result can be obtained only by making the bandage of short duration and soaking them three or four times, one after the other, after they have been wound round the neck for ten minutes. If the bandage becomes warm, the goiter increases rather than diminishes because the blood flows to it still more and produces swelling in the throat.

A freshly caught cold in the throat or chest may, by means of the neck bandage, be cured within an hour if the neck bandage be changed every eight or ten minutes. It is very important that the patient making use of the neck bandage should be in bed and remain there quietly, because with every movement comes air and this must be strictly kept from the throat.

The full benefit of this bandage can only be secured if it is laid on the neck properly and with knowledge.

The effect of this bandage is to extract foul matter from the throat and to draw the superfluous heat from it.

If you want cold to diminish heat, then you must renew your bandage every quarter of an hour and continue it for an hour or an hour and a half.

The neck bandage can and does draw the blood from the head to the throat, but it must not stay there and the only way of getting rid of what has been drawn into it is by constantly renewing the bandage.

It would be still better to lay a six-fold cloth on the stomach which would rapidly develop an increased warmth and so relieve the inflammation in the throat.

A freshly caught cold in the throat or chest may, by means of the neck bandage, be cured within an hour if the neck bandage be changed every eight or ten minutes

1903

DRINKING COLD WATER

WATER APPLICATIONS

ON THE DIFFERENT EFFECTS OF COLD WATER
DR. ALFRED BAUMGARTEN

HYDROPATHY, HYDROTHERAPY AND WATER CURE

MEANS OF HARDENING FOR CHILDREN AND ADULTS
BENEDICT LUST

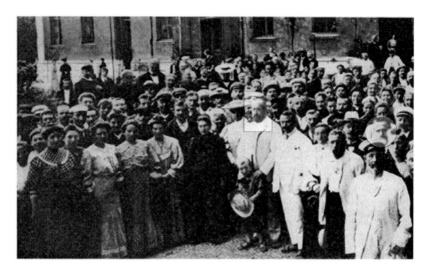

Dr. Baumgarten was one of the doctors who studied at Wörishofen with Kneipp. After Kneipp's death in 1897, Baumgarten helped oversee patients at Wörishofen. He lectured and wrote on Hydrotherapy. Dr. Baumgarten (highlighted) is in the front row behind the young boy. Benedict Lust (highlighted in circle) is seen standing to the immediate right of the man in the white hat in the second row on the bottom right.

DRINKING COLD WATER

by Dr. Alfred Baumgarten

The Naturopath and Herald of Health, IV (3), 48-51. (1903)

W hat is the definition of a douche? We define a douche as an application in which large quantities of cold (flowing) water at a low
temperature are permitted to come in contact with certain portions of
the body, and this quantity of water having no pressure, exercises only
a thermal influence. The ordinary douche is void of mechanism, unlike
that employed in the needle douche, but the same effect is brought about
by the flow of cold water applied so as to form a sheet over the portion
of the body treated. What conclusions are we to draw from the above?
As a result of the cold water applied in the above manner, humors or
impurities of the body are congested as long as the flow of water continues. Respiration ceases for the moment, the blood rebounds, its circulation is accelerated and finally the whole nervous system is influenced.
This nervous influence varies with each individual. Take, for instance, the
knee douche; some people are not affected at all by this. Others again are
affected to such a degree that it takes moral and physical persuasion to
keep them at it.

I had occasion this noon to apply the knee douche to a man who
had tried it some ten or fifteen times on himself. "Every time," he said,
"that I applied the douche, the blood would course to my head with
such rapidity that I often thought some blood vessel would burst." Is
this the possible or probable result of the knee douche? Certainly.
If you will but remember what I have said in my preceding treatise, you
will easily comprehend this. If cold water will act on the skin and capillarize* in such a manner that the blood in place of going to the interior
organs will suddenly rebound and rush to the head, it is evident that a
feeling of congestion at that particular portion is experienced. This holds
true with those of a nervous disposition. From this we must conclude that
the effect of the douches is entirely too severe for the nervous.

That flowing water will consume a greater quantity of heat from the
body than standing water is not open to dispute, for I have demonstrated
and proved this fact repeatedly. If, for instance, you will immerse your
arm into a basin filled with cold water, keeping it there for two minutes,
then take the same quantity of water and let it flow down over the arm,
you will find the temperature of the standing water lower than that of the
flowing. These observations are important in so far as they go to prove
that which we wish to prove, i.e., that cold douches are more efficacious
than all other cold water applications.

---

*We can only speculate on Dr. Baumgarten's use of the word, "capillarize" to mean vaso-
constriction and vasodilation of the capillaries that occur during the primary and secondary reactions of cold water applications. —*Ed.*

The system of treating by douches dates back to 300 B.C. A certain passage found in the works of Hippocrates reads thus: "So any portion of your body pain you, be influenced or swollen, take your cold water, pour it over the sick part and the pain will cease." Such are the directions of Hippocrates for the cure of gout and rheumatism. Others have attempted the same in later years. So the Englishman Floyer, Schwertner (1730), Dr. Johann S. Hahn (1738), Professor Oertel (1830). Also, Priessnitz occasionally employed douches. But the present combination of douches put into a system by Kneipp has not been attempted before. Every douche has a particular office or function to perform, which, as need and circumstances warrant, we call to our assistance. All this sounds very feasible indeed, but often matters are difficult and the process for a thorough cure is long and tedious.

I will now endeavor to prove that the cold Water Cure is not a matter of fiction or fantastic, and that it is entirely free from so-called suggestion. Many have said that certain cures wrought in Wörishofen had little to do with cold water, but must be attributed solely to the imposing personality of Father Kneipp.

Another class of people is prone to think that religion plays an important part in our cures or that the dignity of Father Kneipp as priest and God's representative influenced many cases. I can assert that these are two entirely different things. The priest Kneipp and the water doctor Kneipp were two separate functionaries embodied in the one man, but who were entirely independent of each other. Anyone who asserts that laying on of hands, curing by prayers, etc., are used here is falsifying the truth knowingly or unknowingly. If done knowingly, we are compelled to call this vile calumny and the person should be made to retract.

I therefore wish to draw attention to the fact that all means used here are strictly natural means and not as some newspapers put it at all, weird and supernatural.

Sometimes, if in the course of conversation in a European report, you declare your intention of going to Wörishofen, a sad pitying glance would meet you and accompanied, perhaps, by the ejaculation "All a humbug!" "The Rev. Father Kneipp will come, spread his hands over you, and murmur a few words; then you are douched with cold water, and that's the whole process."

I most sincerely pity all those having such or similar ideas at Kneipp's treatment. No man has ever been more systematic in his cold water application than Father Kneipp.

Taking up the thread of our subject again, we have seen how the cold douches improve our circulation, stimulate the nervous system, increase the appetite, and lend vigor and energy to all functions of the body. It is the general claim that under certain conditions the douches are sometimes injurious. One patient, for instance, will, during the course of treatment, lose his sleep, another his appetite, and another will grow nervous. Some go into hysterics, while still others complain of stomach disorders, etc. Now, one should be prepared to experience the one or the other of all these symptoms and many others while under treatment. All these symptoms are but the indication of a crisis.

The general condition of patients during treatment seems to be this: for the first few days they feel invigorated, delighted, rejuvenated and they solemnly denounce all drugs and patent medicines. After five or six days of treatment have elapsed the symptoms mentioned above make their appearance. "That tired feeling," "awful headache," "loss of appetite," are coming on, and then comes the cry, "We have been deceived, the cure is not what we thought it to be". In short, courage fails them entirely. This is what we call the crisis, which, according to the will power and the disease of the individual, will be more or less severe. Even the healthy are not exempt from this. Let me quote an example. Some three years ago, a French gentleman came to me with the request for a few douches just to satisfy his curiosity and to entertain his friends on arriving at home. I kindly requested him to come during office hours, and I would then give the necessary directions. At the appointed hour he came. I examined him, but on the whole found little out of order. Directions were accordingly given and he went his way. After the lapse of eight or ten days he returned. Dropping himself in a chair he murmured: "This cure is a humbug. What are your directions to effect? I came here to learn all about your cure, but your directions are simply nonsensical." "That's immaterial," I replied, "you go and do as directed." Sullenly he went his way. After the eighth day he again returned. Dropping himself into a rocker, he exclaimed.

> This is a d--- cure. Why every bone and muscle in my body seems
> to be strained. The worst trouncing would have no other effect.
> I am under the impression that with your wise directions I have
> contracted muscular rheumatism or something similar.

Now what should have caused this? It was simply the stimulating influence of cold water on his system. All the dormant impurities lodged here and there had been shaken up thoroughly. I explained matters to him and he left with renewed courage. After four weeks, he returned to say "Good-bye." He was in the best of humor, his cheeks were flushed and he declared he never felt better or stronger in all his life.

I relate this because many sick persons are under the impression that the Water Cure is too harsh for them, that it would weaken them too much, if it already affects the healthy to such a degree. They need have no fear, for not everyone is affected in this way; neither are severe applications applied to those who are already weak from disease and exhaustion.

What constitutes the dreaded crisis? In the first place, severe colds and then diarrhea which appears suddenly after going over to symptoms of cholera. Also, muscular pains often thought to be rheumatism, general stiffness and entire depression. The symptom most in evidence, however, is insomnia. Nearly every nervous person undergoing treatment will experience this. Many, on retiring, sleep at once. But after a few hours' rest, they suddenly start up, continuing awake for the remainder of the night. With certain individuals this excitement causes absolute insomnia. With others, especially those belonging to the stout class, somnolence will set in. They will constantly complain of a tired, drowsy feeling, a desire for sleep, etc. These, in short, are a few of the symptoms appearing during the crisis. They vary with each individual and each disease. Courage and resolution, therefore, are necessary when these things come upon us.

The crisis is a natural result and an absolute necessity! Why? When the body for a long time continues to go through the regular routine of everyday life and is then suddenly side-tracked, cleansed, washed, invigorated and strengthened, it is evident that a reaction must set in. The vitality still left will unite with the cold water in expelling the impurities from the system. The crisis is not at all injurious; on the contrary it is an indication that Nature is reviving and that she is asserting her rights. I know of parties who have had a crisis three or four times during one cure.

Another addition and partner to the crisis are cutaneous eruptions. In regard to these, I wish to state that the more numerous these eruptions are the more certain are we of a thorough cure. If these eruptions are numerous, then the excretion of waste matter is also great and the system can brace up and regain strength. To exemplify this, we will assume a case of poisoning by mercury. There are numerous diseases treated with this poison, some with good results, others with utter failure; we will, however, not discuss this question here. What we do know and can assert is this: mercury applied and rubbed into the skin has permeated the entire body being afterward found in metal form in the bones. No poisoning could be more thorough than this. Now it is evident that the system must make the greatest effort to eliminate a poison so deeply rooted. If, then, cutaneous humors, boils, etc., appear, it should be a cause of satisfaction to us, for then we are certain that the poisons can be eliminated.

In ordinary, everyday life we meet with persons thus afflicted, and friends will say their road to health is a severe illness during which this poisonous matter will be brought out. And the fact is that if such persons are stricken with typhoid and similar diseases, they are, for the most part, healthier and more robust after than before the disease. The same process also takes place during the late cure and these symptoms should, as said before, be a cause of satisfaction to us. It would be of little value, however, if these eruptions and boils were brought to the surface by artificial means. Let Nature have her course and let her assert her rights. It is not necessary that they appear in every case; that is entirely dependent on the individual and the disease in question.

I now wish to say a few words on drinking cold water.

The whole human race has come to the conclusion that a beverage of some kind is necessary.

The Bavarian minus his beer is a vacuum, the Englishman wanting ale or porter will fade away; thus every country or sections thereof have their own peculiar beverage. I am of the opinion that a certain quantity of liquid is absolutely necessary for the body. On the other hand, we should choose that liquid which is purest and which will be of greatest value to the body. The best liquid is, without doubt, God's purest beverage "Water." Good spring or well water takes the first place on the list. In order to have constant supply of spring or well water, we should not hesitate to devise means and ways of getting and keeping it. Water, in order to retain the oxygen, must be kept in wooden or stone vessels well covered. Dr. Hufeland, 1820 to 1830, in speaking of cold water, says: "With every draught of the pure element we take a stimulus, a renewed vigor is imported to our whole being." I endorse this fully and wish to add that the more we accustom ourselves to use water exclusively, the more will we learn to appreciate it as our best friend.

Drinking of water has also another advantage. It insures a full purse, for water is not only cheaper than any other beverage, but by drinking it we also gain for our future both in capital and in health.

I do not condemn beer and wine, for in my opinion an occasional glass of beer is not only useful, but in some diseases even necessary. Those, however, who, in their younger days have accustomed their stomach, their heart and their palate to the stimulating influence of alcohol, so that in their opinion they now cannot exist for half a day without indulging, will in sickness and disease find the beat of their heart to be but faint, and if the excess is continued, the heart will refuse to perform its functions at last. These are only a few advantages of drinking cold water. It is not necessary that large quantities be consumed. I know of places where forty to sixty glasses are consumed in one day. This is nonsense, pure and simple. Bread and water, the well-known meal of the prisoner, is not so poor as many fancy; it contains sufficient nourishment for any person. Take those who have created sensations all over the country by their protracted fasts. They subsisted on water and water only. We see from this that water is also nutritive, for it contains many extracts taken in its course through the earth. Those under constant mental strain will know the value of cold water. Water drinkers reach a high age, retain clear, bright, and unclouded brain.

A man accustomed to long hours at his desk will take tea or coffee to stimulate him, but suddenly he finds himself wrecked—he has overestimated his strength. Those, however, who partake only of water will work better, longer, more successfully.

Do not permit yourself to be led by others to believe that assertion that alcohol is nourishing or strengthening. No, it is simply oil in a flame which for the moment will burn furiously but in a short time leave only the ashes as a remnant of all it had been. When drinking cold water, we know exactly how far our physical powers can go, for water will not deceive us.

What is the definition of a douche? We define a douche as an application in which large quantities of cold (flowing) water at a low temperature, are permitted to come in contact with certain portions of the body, and this quantity of water having no pressure, exercises only a thermal influence.

These observations are important in so far as they go to prove that which we wish to prove, i.e., that cold douches are more efficacious than all other cold water applications.

What constitutes the dreaded crisis? In the first place severe colds, then diarrhea which appears suddenly after going over to symptoms of cholera. Also muscular pains often thought to be rheumatism, general stiffness and entire depression. The symptom most in evidence, however, is insomnia.

The crisis is not at all injurious, on the contrary it is an indication that Nature is reviving and that she is asserting her rights.

Another addition and partner to the crisis are cutaneous eruptions. In regard to these, I wish to state that the more numerous these eruptions are the more certain are we of a thorough cure.

On the other hand, we should choose that liquid which is purest and which will be of greatest value to the body. The best liquid is, without doubt, God's purest beverage "Water."

Drinking of water has also another advantage. It insures a full purse, for water is not only cheaper than any other beverage, but by drinking it we also gain for our future both in capital and in health.

When drinking cold water, we know exactly how far our physical powers can go, for water will not deceive us.

WATER APPLICATIONS

by Dr. Alfred Baumgarten, Wörishofen

The Naturopath and Herald of Health, IV (5), 124-126. (1903)

Applications of cold water as directed by Reverend Sebastian Kneipp consist in douches, baths, entire and partial ablutions, entire and partial packs. It is, therefore, all important to know just how each separate application will act on the skin and the entire system. We must, so to say, see the process going on in the interior man.

Doubtless there are many thousands who through ignorance, neglect, prejudice etc., will not admit that simple cold water applied to the skin can affect such wondrous cures. Many ask themselves, how can it be possible that water only touching the skin, can affect the interior and can bring about such changes in the system?

We will now consider what effect the exterior application has on the interior organs. First and foremost, we will recall the well-known physical law: "Heat expands, cold contracts." Starting from this principle then, it necessarily follows that the pores and cells of the skin contracts when cold water is applied, and what are the results?

Every man of brain will ask at once, why? And the science which answers this "why" is called physiology. It is one of the exact sciences; and just this science proves and upholds every principle of the Kneipp cure.

The cold water acting on the skin will influence the little blood cells which by their contraction force the blood to the interior and main arteries.

What will now happen to the skin? When the blood flows to the interior, you will notice that the skin turns a deathly pale, but if the flow of water continues, the skin will soon turn red again, for the one who applies the water knows that he must let water flow until the skin has regained this tint.

What further process takes place? By the cold a spasm of the capillary ducts takes place, forcing the blood to the interior. This spasm generally lasts but a short time, some 70 to 80 seconds according to the state and condition of the individual. Now then, after these 70 to 80 seconds have passed, these small capillary blood vessels which before had contracted, again expand and the blood rushes to the surface. This in short is the whole process on the skin of the body. Three things can be observed in the above process. First, the opening of the pores permitting the skin to take in oxygen; secondly, the loss of heat through the skin; thirdly, a refreshing sensation permeating the whole body.

How can and does the skin inhale, as it were, the oxygen in the air?

When breathing, a person inflates the lungs with the air of the surrounding atmosphere, and by this process oxygen combines with the blood. Oxygen, as we know, is a certain gas and is the most potent factor in all functions of the human body and its organs. The larger the quantity of oxygen in the blood, the better its quality. If, then, the blood comes to the surface and the skin takes in oxygen through its pores, what is the result of this process? The results remain identically the same as those brought about by breathing through the lungs. The capillaries being enlarged, the blood comes into contact with the air and this process is of the utmost importance for regaining health.

If the physician will tell you that your blood is poor, that you have bad blood, scrofulous blood, in short that you are predisposed to all the diseases of the blood that are known, what is to be done? A campaign against the accumulation of foreign matter in the system must be instituted at once. The impurities must be driven out of the system, and a new and healthy blood must be created.

Oxygen as you are aware is the nourishment of the blood. The larger the quantity of oxygen in the body, the healthier the person. The respiration of the skin is therefore all important when cold water applications are made. The douches afford the best means of instituting, aiding and increasing this respiration of the skin.

The reaction so much spoken of in the Water Cure is nothing more than a rush of blood to and from the inner organs which in coming to the skin gives it the peculiar red coloration. The impression that with the first reddening of the skin all is well, is erroneous. While dressing immediately after the water application, an agreeable comfortable heat develops; this however, is soon succeeded by a chill which at times is pretty severe. Anyone having taken water applications will have experienced the truth of my assertion. This feeling of warmth succeeded by chills is the consecutive ebullition of the blood from the exterior to the interior and vice versa. During these ebullitions opportunity is afforded to the blood to take in a supply of oxygen.

It is for this reason that the douches and cold baths are of such value to the blood. Oxygen destroys the morbid matter in the system. This in a few words explains the whole process.

The art, however, is to find out the proper application for each individual case.*

Another feature of all cold water applications is the loss of heat of the body. When taking a body with the temperature about 98° to 100° F/37° to 38° C, for such is the normal warmth of the body, and pouring over this body water at 45° to 59° F/7° to 15° C, it is evident that some heat from the body will be absorbed by the water.

---

*Dr. Baumgarten's book, *Die Kneipp'sche Hydrotherapie* (1909), provided guidance in the application of Kneipp's therapies. See page 209. —*Ed.*

It is this question which has commanded my attention in the last few months. I have taken a tub covered by a grading of wood. Having placed a patient on this graded tub, I applied the cold water for a douche. I also measured the quantity and temperature of the water both before and after the application, and I was able to compute what percentage of heat had been withdrawn from the body. This is what one would call practical physiology for the purpose of supporting a system.

I have continued these experiments with several colleagues and we are now able to say just how each douche acts on the body and the heart, and how much warmth is taken from the body.

We have found that after a hip douche, the temperature of the water had been raised by one degree. Putting this into formula, I am able to compute just how much heat is thus taken out of the body and what amount of vitality is lost by this heat. It is now evident that this is not so simple as might appear but that close and accurate study is essential. Since I have found that simplicity and observance of natural laws are the main spring in Father Kneipp's system, I am prepared to say that this form of treatment with cold water has come to remain with present and future generations. No system is so accurate and so certain of success as this one.

I have just said that a certain percentage of warmth is withdrawn from the body. Is this withdrawn to remain? No! The Creator in His providence and wisdom has ordained that no power or vitality in the motion of the universe shall be lost but only converted into another.

If, therefore, we lose a percentage of warmth by the cold water, the activity of the heart and the cold feeling stimulate the system to produce new warmth and that is the point we desire to arrive at. Our object is to increase natural warmth, for the better the oven is heated the better is the diffusion of heat. Thirdly, cold water applications are advantageous because they leave behind that light, invigorated, rejuvenated feeling. Now, what causes this? Our skin is interwoven with many little nerves, the presence of which is brought home to us when we cut, pierce or otherwise injure the skin. In the same manner in which these nerves can be afflicted by cutting, piercing etc., so are they also affected by cold water and after the irrigation is over, there remains this invigorated feeling which is known to everyone who has taken cold baths.

If the whole process is viewed in this light, it must certainly be evident to us that cold water can and will achieve great results.

Finally, I wish to draw attention to the marvelous effect which is produced by the cold water on the circulation of the blood. The mass of blood rushing and flowing to and from the organs displaces and mingles with greater masses of blood. The larger the displacement and the oftener it occurs, the more improved will the circulation in general be. When the heart has attained that condition in which it is able to supply with blood every part of the body from extremity to extremity, then we can say that the circulation is perfect. Before concluding, I wish to touch upon one very important point. Before any application, make it your business to be thoroughly warm, and after the application also do not stand idle but exercise, or walk until normal warmth has again set in. The purpose of this is evidently clear to you.

The cold cannot influence a cold body in any other way but to increase the cold. It is therefore necessary that contraries be present, otherwise the desired effect is not obtained. The skin of the patient must be warm for then when the cold water touches it, the sudden change of temperature brings about the physiological process of which we have been speaking.

We now hope that all possible doubt as to the efficacy of cold water has been removed. Let everyone, whatever his ailment be, draw his own conclusion as to what benefits may be derived from above.

No matter what the disease is, whether it be the stomach, nerves, kidneys, lungs, or liver, all must agree that an increase of good healthy blood is a most potent factor in uprooting disease. Doubtless, no one will assert that harm has come to any person whose skin has been hardened and stimulated to action and secretion by the various water applications.

Finally, cold water applications stimulate the appetite in a marvelous manner. Many have found that their pocket books were entirely too small for the demands of their stomachs.

Taking all in all, we must say that cold water will in every case improve and stimulate the whole constitution and that we are able to cure most diseases and relieve others which are incurable by the simple applications of cold water.

Often we have been confronted with questions such as: "Why do you followers of Kneipp's theories in Wörishofen claim absolute and certain cure for all diseases?" If we present the facts to ourselves in proper light, we must say that with the few healing factors at our disposal we can and have achieved more than those who have 500 and more different healing factors (i. e. drugs) of which barely 300 have been thoroughly studied and tested. Aside of this, there are many little things in the Water Cure which are of considerable momentum, such as simple mode of living, exercise in the open air, proper clothing, diet, etc.

My duty, therefore, is to show you how cold water acts in general and what results may be obtained thereby. To this end, I have taken the experience of all of us and principally that of the Rev. Father Kneipp, and to the above I add my own experiments in behalf of the Rev. Father Kneipp's system.

DIE KNEIPP'SCHE
HYDROTHERAPIE

::   VON   ::
ALFRED BAUMGARTEN
:: DR. MED. UND PRAKT. ARZT ::

MIT 109 HOLZSCHNITTEN 13 ZINKÄTZUNGEN
78 TABELLEN UND 567 SPHYGMOGRAMMEN

WÖRISHOFEN
BUCHDRUCKEREI UND VERLAGS-ANSTALT WÖRISHOFEN
1909

Dr. Albert Baumgarten, devoted to Kneipp's work wrote a German book, *Die Kneipp'sche Hydrotherapie* (1909), which substantiated the validity and mechanisms of Hydrotherapy with scientific experiments and research.

When the blood flows to the interior you will notice that the skin turns a deathly pale, but if the flow of water continues, the skin will soon turn red again, for the one who applies the water knows that he must let water flow until the skin has regained this tint.

This spasm generally lasts but a short time, some 70 to 80 seconds according to the state and condition of the individual. Now then, after these 70 to 80 seconds have passed, these small capillary blood vessels which before had contracted, again expand and the blood rushes to the surface.

If the physician will tell you that your blood is poor, that you have bad blood, scrofulous blood, in short that you are predisposed to all the diseases of the blood that are known, what is to be done? A campaign against the accumulation of foreign matter in the system must be instituted at once.

The reaction so much spoken of in the Water Cure is nothing more than a rush of blood to and from the inner organs which in coming to the skin gives it the peculiar red coloration.

Since I have found that simplicity and observance of natural laws are the main spring in Father Kneipp's system, I am prepared to say that this form of treatment with cold water has come to remain with present and future generations. No system is so accurate and so certain of success as this one.

If, therefore, we lose a percentage of warmth by the cold water, the activity of the heart and the cold feeling stimulate the system to produce new warmth and that is the point we desire to arrive at.

Thirdly, cold water applications are advantageous because they leave behind that light, invigorated, rejuvenated feeling.

Finally, I wish to draw attention to the marvelous effect which is produced by the cold water on the circulation of the blood. The mass of blood rushing and flowing to and from the organs displaces and mingles with greater masses of blood.

Before any application, make it your business to be thoroughly warm, and after the application also do not stand idle but exercise, or walk until normal warmth has again set in.

The skin of the patient must be warm for then, when the cold water touches it the sudden change of temperature brings about the physiological process of which we have been speaking.

On The Different Effects Of Cold Water

by Dr. Alfred Baumgarten

The Naturopath and Herald of Health, IV (7), 184-185. (1903)

Our next consideration will be what we are to do in order to have fresh water for our applications.

Many are in the habit of preparing water in the evening for use the following morning. Now that it is a mistake. During the night, the gases escape and the water loses a great percentage of its freshness and efficacy. If water must be prepared the evening before, it is best to do this in wooden tubs with proper lids for them; then the water should also be kept in a cool place. Water will keep best in vessels or tubs prepared of clay.

I know of persons who had some made for this special purpose and who found that the water will keep its temperature for a longer period than it would in any other vessel.

Water in its effects upon the skin and the body is one of the best but in the hands of the inexperienced, one of the worst healing factors. On first glance, Water Cure seems very simple and many are tempted to boast that they can apply the water treatment as well and efficiently as the next man. This is a mistake. The order of the various applications is a potent factor and requires a close study and years of experience to be able to adopt them to individual cases.

How does the cold water act on the human skin and body during a Kneipp cure? In the first place, it acts by its coldness. When giving an upper douche to a person, you cover the surface of the back for one or two minutes with a sheet of water thus preventing transpiration; the blood is forced into the interior, the skin is cooled to about 46° F/8° C, stimulating its activity thereby. Following this up more closely we must note at first the temperature of the water at various seasons.

On pouring a sheet of water of 80° F/27° C, over the body we notice an immediate change in the color of the skin, a deep pale pink. The blood now courses to the interior. The cells of the skin are taken by spasm which subsides in a short time. Soon again we notice the skin turning red, the blood has returned.

The effect of a Kneipp douche is, therefore, a spasmodic opening and closing of the pores of the skin, thus restoring perfect circulation.

You will now ask what purpose or effect will be experienced from these phenomena? The blood when coming to the surface of the skin will take up a new supply of oxygen which means nourishment to the blood. This coursing in and out of the blood opens all the little outlets of the skin permitting its taking up of oxygen, this is the respiration of the skin. When passing through a pine forest you will notice that the air permeated by the peculiar odor will act very soothing on the respiratory organs. The same process takes place on the skin when giving a douche according to Kneipp's theories.

Kneipp's greatest merit consists therein that he has arranged his douches in such a manner that even the weakest and most delicate can undergo treatment, and that we no longer need to call the Water Cure a "horse-cure" when we can achieve such great results with the most simple means.

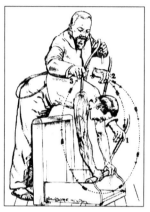

The arm douche, using a hose

Take, for example, the arm douche. Under personal observation study and experiments, I have found the arm douche to be very efficacious for heart failure. But how can the simple arm douche be of avail in heart failure you will ask? The effect is thus: by douching the arm, the blood is drawn from the weakened heart to the extremities, thereby easing that vital organ and affording ease also to the respiratory organs. The same process takes place in other organs of the body according to the part douched. It is, therefore, not an easy matter to direct the various applications without some knowledge of the various diseases, also of anatomy.

It was often said the Kneipp's applications and his whole mode of treatment were too short to be beneficial. This at first seems true. Kneipp had 30 to 40 years experience—with eyes fabulously trained to read the diseases at sight, thus doing away with all examination. A man, thus, trained will see at once what others cannot detect after hours of physical examination. This was one of the remarkable traits of Kneipp: that his quick and searching eye could detect at once. Of course, he was not infallible. *Errare humanum est* was as well applied to him as to others, but in the majority of cases, his diagnosis was correct.

For the benefit of those inclined to be a little doubtful in regard to what I have written above, I will now relate an occurrence which will strengthen my assertions. While I was staying at Wörishofen helping Kneipp during consultation hours, a family from Paris, with several grown up children at home, came with the request that I present their case to the Reverend Prelate, he being too busy for a chat with them. They gave me photos and diagnosis of those at home, and these I presented to the prelate after consultation hours. The diagnosis I kept, giving only the photos, four in number. To my utter surprise every symptom contained in the diagnosis I held was recognized and called out by Kneipp on looking at the photos. I have never told this in public, because it was always said that Kneipp was too rash and never thorough enough. But with all his rashness, he succeeded in astounding the medical profession. This much about the efficacy of the cold water.

There still remain a few words which I would like to say, and that is in regard to the herb called yarrow. This herb taken in tea or extract form cannot be surpassed as a food for impoverished blood. Especially our growing up female generation ought to take note of this and use it constantly for nothing will build up the system quicker than good blood.

The order of the various applications is a potent factor and requires a close study and years of experience to be able to adopt them to individual cases.

When giving an upper douche to a person, you cover the surface of the back for one or two minutes with a sheet of water thus preventing transpiration; the blood is forced into the interior, the skin is cooled to about 46° F/8° C, stimulating its activity thereby.

On pouring a sheet of water of 80° F/27° C, over the body we notice an immediate change in the color of the skin, a deep pale pink. The blood now courses to the interior.

The blood when coming to the surface of the skin will take up a new supply of oxygen which means nourishment to the blood. This coursing in and out of the blood opens all the little outlets of the skin permitting its taking up of oxygen, this is the respiration of the skin.

Kneipp's greatest merit consists therein that he has arranged his douches in such a manner that even the weakest and most delicate can undergo treatment, and that we no longer need to call the Water Cure a "horse-cure" when we can achieve such great results with the most simple means.

Under personal observation study and experiments, I have found the arm douche to be very efficacious for heart failure. But how can the simple arm douche be of avail in heart failure you will ask?

A man thus trained will see at once what others cannot detect after hours of physical examination. This was one of the remarkable traits of Kneipp: that his quick and searching eye could detect at once.

HYDROPATHY, HYDROTHERAPY AND WATER CURE*

by Benedict Lust

The Naturopath and Herald of Health, IV (10), 286-287. (1903)

Hydropathy, Hydrotherapy and Water Cure have a cold and forbidding sound. It usually has also a chilling and depressing effect. For example, a certain establishment in New York City is wont to prescribe cold sitz baths of forty-five minutes to the most bloodless, anemic, shivering, and neurotic. And through the perversions of Water Cure, not through its principles, the tender shrinking invalid revolts from it as harsh, disagreeable and harmful.

Now Naturopathy believes in cold water, and Naturopathy's apostles take a cold douche or plunge or an Adolf Just [natural] bath, at least once daily. Nature was, is, and always will be before Hydropathy. Any regime, whatsoever, that outrages your natural instinct is both unnatural and undesirable. Unmitigated Water Cure demands a robust constitution and a fairly vital condition. Modified Water Cure appeals with infinite gentleness to the delicate child and the sensitive woman.

Moreover, there are attendant advantages in Hydropathy that its materialistic prescriber fails to consider. Chronic invalids are essentially limp and lifeless. Their credulity in outside medicaments and machinations has made them repeated prey to pseudo-healers, only to leave them in disappointment, doubt, and discouragement. They are much in the condition of the heathen who has outgrown fetish-worship and has not yet developed spirit sufficiently to grasp God worship.

Now to such cerebrate invertebrates, Physical Culture decrees "Exercise, or die." And Dietetics announces, "You must study proteins and hydrocarbons and carbohydrates, in their relation to gastric, hepatic, and intestinal derangements." And Mental Science proclaims, "All is good, all is Wisdom, all is Power; be perfect forthwith."

Hydrotherapy whispers "Be still, and let me heal you." And the contrast is most soothing and satisfying. It has a sort of cure-you-while-you-wait idea that is peculiarly pleasing to the American mentality. Understand, we posit Water Cure as initial, not final. It must be supplemented by Physical Culture, Mental Culture, and a host of higher agencies. As a purely physical and preparatory measure, it is unsurpassed.

Then, too, water is the symbol of purity. A man may have brain and be a brute, intellect and be a roué, civilized and be a degenerate. But foul food, foul drink, foul habits, and foul thoughts cannot long resist the wooing of the purest power in Nature.

---

*This article was the fifth in a series entitled "Health Incarnate; A Naturopathic Silhouette". —Ed.

In deference to the many ardent disciples of Father Kneipp, and inconsideration of its inherent worth, the following extract from *Practical Guide for Father Sebastian Kneipp's Method of Cure* is presented without alteration. The complete works of Father Kneipp are essential to adequate conception and practical application of his principles. And the study of his life and system will be a revelation to those who imagine the Kneipp Cure is "walking barefoot in the morning dew."

EFFECTS OF THE WATER CURE

A pure and unremitted Water Cure is disadvantageous or even dangerous in cases of:

1. organic heart complaints;
2. organic or chronic, severe and far-advanced stages of lung complaints;
3. nervous sufferers who have brain trouble;
4. complaints that result from injury to the spine;
5. recurring epileptic fits in persons who are already imbecile;
6. general and advanced stages of dropsy;
7. great degeneration in the cells and tissues;
8. patients whose physical condition is too much enfeebled by age or disease, hence no longer capable of reaction.

Only the expert naturopathic physician can be trusted to prescribe mild water applications in above cases.

Let this be carefully noted, and let it not be believed that every disease can be cured by water, or only by water. There are many maladies in which a cure can be effected only if all factors of Naturopathy are applied intelligently to suit the case, and especially certain dietary rules; or indeed, not at all.

Promise of the best results, however, is held out by the Water Cure, in cases of:

1. all acute (violent) inflammations, like croup, erysipelas, diphtheria, pneumonia, acute inflammatory rheumatism, scarlet fever, measles, smallpox, typhus, etc.;
2. injuries;
3. gout and rheumatism;
4. chronic stomach troubles;
5. liver, spleen and kidney inflammations;
6. diseases of the skin, gland troubles and syphilis;
7. nervous diseases that proceed from an over-excited brain;
8. all diseases in which interruptions and disturbances of the circulation are distinctive symptoms and;

9. excessive use of certain medications such as morphine, hydrate of chloral, mercury, etc.

AIDS IN THE WATER CURE

Aids in Water Cure include: Kneipp's herbs and food remedies prepared from them, correct diet, air and exercise.

The best medicines are certainly those that are not poisons, and hence do not harm, as fortunately is the case with so many medicinal plants. (See list of Kneipp remedies.)

*Correct diet consists in the right choice of articles of food. A mixed diet is certainly the best: vegetable or plant foods, and animal or meat foods. Among the former we class farinaceous cereal (bread), leguminous plants (peas, beans, lentils); and among the latter are meat, fish, fat, butter, cheese, eggs, and milk. Fruit, beer, wine, coffee and spices are luxuries, which partaken of moderately, are not very harmful, and even useful in certain diseases and for old people.

Pure air, and a rational use of the lungs, coupled with sufficient exercise out of doors, and in the house, are fundamental rules for good health.

Now Naturopathy believes in cold water, and Naturopathy's apostles take a cold douche or plunge or Adolf Just [natural] bath, at least once daily.

Understand, we posit Water Cure as initial, not final. It must be supplemented by Physical Culture, Mental Culture, and a host of higher agencies. As a purely physical and preparatory measure, it is unsurpassed.

Let this be carefully noted, and let it not be believed that every disease can be cured by water, or only by water.

---

*Naturopathy does not concur wholly with this classification. —*Benedict Lust.*

Means Of Hardening For Children And Adults*

by Benedict Lust

The Naturopath and Herald of Health, IV (11), 313-322. (1903)

Healthy persons can strengthen their bodies, that is to say, harden them, render them better able to resist attacks of disease, and less sensitive to draught and changes of temperature by a correct care of the skin and body. Accordingly, children ought to be quickly washed every day all over the body (in a room whose temperature is about 60° to 66° F/16° to 19° C with water of about 71° to 80° F/22° to 27° C), not dried off, and then put into bed for about ten minutes, or immediately dressed so that they may run about and take some exercise. Also, children may daily be dipped up to under their arms in cold water for two seconds.

Adults, before going to bed (even in the bed) or after rising, should wash the upper half of the body, front and back, and arms and legs with a coarse linen towel dipped into cold water and then wrung, which process is to last no longer than a minute. If warm tub baths are taken, which should not last longer than five minutes, they must always be followed by a rapid, cold ablution, after which, if the body is not dried off, exercise must be taken, as after all cold showers, until the skin is quite warm again. River baths ought not to last longer than six minutes, in order that the body may not be deprived of too much warmth. Cold sitting baths ought not to last longer than two or three minutes, and cold whole baths in tubs not longer than several seconds (often just in and out). Walking barefoot in wet grass, on wet stones, in newly fallen snow, in cold water, are all good means of hardening.

The weaker or more debilitated the organism of a person is, the milder and fewer in number must the water applications at first be. With individuals of this kind, only such degree of cold ablutions should be resorted to as anyone can bear, they must not last too long and no cold showers or baths be taken, as long as there is any feeling of chilliness or deficient warmth. An organism that is unable readily to replace the warmth of which the cold water has deprived it, must become gradually inured to it and strengthened by ablutions of tepid and cooler water. Many of the bandages are equally efficacious whether made with warm or cold water.

Shower baths must be given so long till the skin reddens, hence reacts, and a feeling of warmth ensues, which is effected more quickly by cold water than that of higher temperature. Just as ablutions, shower baths and bandages should be applied only when the body is warm, so after

---

*Health Incarnate; Naturopathic Silhouette, VI was the original title for this article. —Ed.

these ablutions etc., exercise must always be taken in order to quickly regain an even bodily temperature.

Our great master says, "A moderate application of water is the best" which means that all water applications should not be made too frequently and too vigorously.

During menstruation, only whole ablutions and upper shower baths are allowed.

According to Kneipp, all diseases are due to bad formation of the blood for blood is the sap of life.

Water has the power:
1. to dissolve the morbid matters in the blood,
2. to evacuate what is dissolved,
3. to strengthen anew the enfeebled organism,
4. to restore a regular circulation.

The cold Water Cure and KNEIPP REMEDIES have the following effects:
1. They increase the activity of the entire organism, thereby increase the consumption of combustible matter, promote the circulation of the blood, distribute an even bodily warmth, heighten the activity of the nervous system, and therefore all of them results of a more rapid interchange of matter.
2. They promote the excretions of and evaporations of the skin.
3. Make one less sensitive to draughts and changes of temperature.

APPLICATIONS THAT DISSOLVE MORBID MATTERS

HEAD VAPORS

The head vapor is applied for catarrh, head troubles, ringing in the ears, oppression to the chest, inflammations of the eye that are due to colds, rheumatism, of the neck, etc. It is generally applied twice, for a period of twenty minutes each. A vessel, provided with a cover, is filled ¾ with boiling water, placed on a low chair in a warm room, and the patient sits down before it, with upper half of his body uncovered. The head

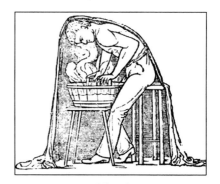

Kneipp's head vapor

and neck are now held over the vessel, which together with the upper half of the body is closely but loosely enveloped in a large woolen blanket. The cover of the vessel is raised and the vapors are allowed to take effect for 20 minutes. The blanket is then removed and the whole upper body washed off with fresh water and dried. Then exercise is taken in the warm room until the skin regains the normal temperature.

Foot Vapors

The foot vapor is made in like manner, and after a lapse of ten minutes, a hot brick may be put into the water to heighten the effect; the vessel or tub is placed on the floor, and a piece of board laid across the top; on this the patient, seated on a chair before it, with lower half of body uncovered, places his feet, and wraps all in a woolen blanket. Finally the feet are quickly washed off with cold water.

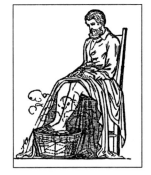

Kneipp's foot vapor: the feet and legs are covered snuggly with a woolen blanket to hold in the heat and vapor.

Herbal Vapor Baths

The close-stool vapor bath is prepared by putting oat straw, shavegrass or hay flower extract into boiling water, and sitting with uncovered lower half of trunk over the vapors for 20 minutes. Afterwards, a whole ablution is taken and the patient exercises in the room, or goes to bed until the normal warmth of the body is restored.

In this same manner vapors are applied to other parts of the body, for instance, to the arms in case of rheumatism, etc.

Warm Herbal Baths

Warm baths are made with an addition of salt and charcoal, hay flowers, oat straw, pine sprigs, malt husks, etc. (The Extracts may be used instead.)

The warm foot bath must not have a higher temperature than 77° to 79° F/25° to 26° C and is to last from 15 to 30 minutes. The feet are immersed as far as the calves. The herbs are covered with the boiling water, which is then allowed to cool to the required temperature.

The warm sitting bath is made by pouring boiling water over the herbs, letting them boil five minutes, and pouring all into a sitting bath tub that contains warm water; then when this cools to a temperature of 77° to 82° F/25°to 28° C, [the patient] sits in it (without the feet, and the water level reaching to the navel) for 10 to 15 minutes.

The warm whole bath has the purpose to increase the body temperature and to dissolve and evacuate morbid matter. It is taken like the cold water bath, but with warm water.

Warm part baths for other parts of the body include hand or arm bath taken like the foot bath.

The head bath is taken by first holding the upper part of the head in cold water for ½ minute, then from five to seven minutes in warm water of 77° F / 25° C, supplying water with the hand all the time, then drying well and remaining in the room till the hair is perfectly dry.

The eye bath is taken by dipping forehead and eyes for ½ minutes into warm water (77° F / 25° C) to which some of Kneipp's eye water has been added, repeating this five times. Finally, the eyes are washed with fresh water.

APPLICATIONS TO EVACUATE THE DISSOLVED MORBID MATTER

HEAD AND NECK BANDAGE

The head bandage is excellent in cases of rheumatic headache, tetters [itchy skin, such as eczema], and diseases of the scalp. Face and head are first washed in cold water without drying. The head is then carefully wrapped in a linen cloth that has been dipped into water and wrung, and over this a woolen cloth is closely folded. After 20 minutes, the linen cloth is dipped again and this kept up for an hour, after which head and face are quickly washed in cold water and carefully dried.

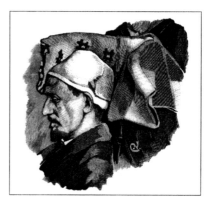

Head and Neck Bandage

The neck bandage is applied in a similar manner, the wet cloth being wound several times around the neck and a flannel band put over it. The wet bandage should be changed every 20 to 40 minutes for the length of time prescribed. Never allow the bandage to remain without changing more than 40 minutes or even overnight.

FOOT BANDAGE

Cotton socks or stockings are dipped into cold water to which one-third its quantity in vinegar has been added. Drawn over the feet a woolen cloth wrapped around them, after which to bed for one to two hours. This foot bandage takes fatigue out of the feet and induces sleep.

LOWER BANDAGE

A sheet folded twice is dipped into a cooled down decoction of hay flowers, oat straw, or pine sprigs, well wrung, and then wrapped round the body from under the arms to the tips of the feet. A woolen cloth or blanket is wound around this, after which the patient is put to bed for one to one and half hours. This is an excellent remedy in cases of gout, rheumatism, kidney troubles and cramps.

SHAWL BANDAGE

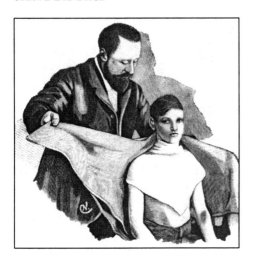

A napkin (linen cloth about 40 inches square) folded over into triangular shape is dipped into cold water, well wrung, put on over the back and crossed on the breast, and covered by a woolen cloth. The patient then goes to bed for one to one and half hours. Greatly to be recommended in cases of throat or chest catarrh and diphtheria.

The Shawl

WET SHIRT

The patient stands in a tub, clad only in his shirt, cold water is poured quickly over him; he is then wrapped in a blanket and goes to bed for one to one and half hours. When salt is put into the water, this is called the salt shirt. Very good for obstructions of the blood, cramps, nervous disorders, St. Vitus dance.

SPANISH MANTLE

The Spanish mantle or largest bandage is a long gown of coarse linen with wide sleeves, reaching to the feet. The patient puts on the wet mantle, and enveloped in a large woolen blanket, goes to bed, where he rests, well covered from one to two hours. It is an excellent remedy for gout, mucous and typhus fever. Younger persons dip the Spanish mantle into a cold decoction of hay flowers, and older people into one that is warm.

SHORT BANDAGE*

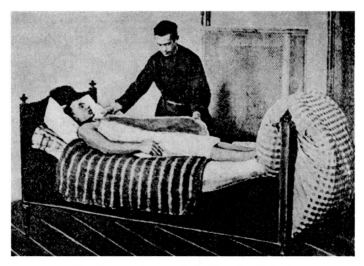

The short bandage applied with patient in bed.

The short or smaller bandage is a coarse sheet folded over four to six times so that its breadth is from the arms to the thighs. It is the most frequently used, and can be applied either cold or warm, by dipping the sheet into a cold or warm decoction of hay flowers, or in a mixture of water and vinegar. Of course, the blanket is wrapped over it and then to bed for one to one and half hours, well covered. As a final measure, women may rub the abdomen with some camphor oil. This bandage proves efficacious in most disorders, notably such which still remain a mystery, where it often serves as a sort of revelation.

COMPRESSES

While bandages are swathed around the whole body, compresses are merely poultices of coarse linen folded to several thicknesses, dipped into

---

*Benedict Lust wrote on the Short Pack in February issue, 1900 in *The Kneipp Water Cure Monthly:* "Healthy people should apply a short package [bandage] once every week or at least every fortnight to prevent sickness. The short package is a means to cleanse liver and kidneys, to free the bowels of winds, gases and superfluous water. Dropsy, heart and stomach complains are unknown to the friends of the short package. Many sleep many a night enveloped in the short package and enjoy thereby and excellent rest until morning. Against phlegm of the stomach, diseases of the heart and lungs, against various complaints of the head and throat, the short package [bandage] finds its manifold applications. "Whenever I am in doubt about a complaint," Father Kneipp wrote, "or if I want to ascertain the exact of the disease, the short package [bandage] is always my true friend and best advisor." (Lust, 1900, 20) —*Ed.*

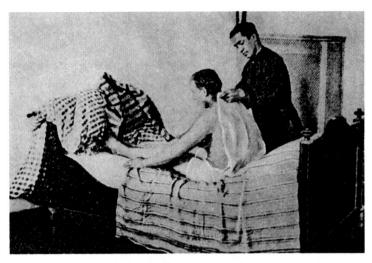

Back compress

warm or cold water, well wrung and laid directly over the suffering parts, being covered with a woolen cloth. These compresses are renewed every half hour and continued from one to two hours, the patient meanwhile lying well-covered in bed. According to their varying purpose, we distinguish:

Upper Compress

The upper compress, which extends from the neck over the chest and entire abdomen.

Under Compress

The under compress, which extends from the cervical vertebra down the entire back, to which end a blanket is first placed in the bed, and upon this the wet linen cloth. The patient lies on this, draws the blanket around him, then covers himself well with extra bed covers. N.B. For these upper and under compresses a coarse linen sheet folded at least 10 times is used, and this, as a rule, remains lying for an hour and need not be renewed.

Upper and under compresses may be taken simultaneously or in succession.

Abdomen Compress

The compress on the abdomen is applied from the stomach down over the entire abdomen, and taken either in cold water and vinegar, or warm in a decoction of hay flowers, shave grass or oat straw, renewing every half hour.

HARDENING APPLICATIONS FOR BLOOD CIRCULATION

SHOWER BATHS (GUSHES)

There must be no drying after any shower baths. The water at first should have a temperature of 60° to 65° F / 16° to 18° C, and the shower baths be taken in a warm (that is, not cold) room.

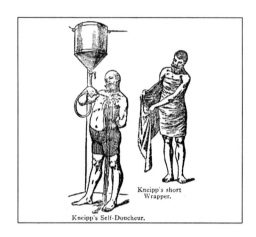

KNEE SHOWER OR GUSH

The knee shower, which is always given in connection with an upper shower bath, is taken with the legs being uncovered to the knees, the patient seated in a chair, and the feet placed in a tub. The shower is given by means of a watering can from the toes to the knees. The first can is applied to both feet simultaneously, the second can specially to the calves and knee [and delivered] in such a way that the water runs evenly down over the feet. The third or last can is to be poured two or three times directly over the feet. At first, three cans are taken; later from four to six.

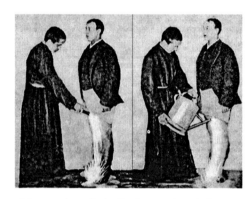

A knee gush applied with a hose and a watering can

UPPER SHOWER OR GUSH

First, the upper body is quickly uncovered and warmth is sought in exercise, then both arms are supported on a tub in such a way that the upper body is almost horizontal. Someone else must now pour a can of cold water from the right shoulder down that side of the back and back again, on the other side up the left shoulder, carefully avoiding wetting the spine. At first, one can, then from two to three cans may be given, while healthy persons can stand as many as five cans, that is to say, till reaction sets in, indicated by the reddening of the skin and increased warmth of the parts wetted. Finally, the chest is quickly washed, the clothes put on without drying of the body and exercise taken until the body is evenly warm again.

BACK SHOWER OR GUSH

The patient fully uncovered sits in the bath tub on a board laid crosswise over it, and has the water poured over him as in the upper shower bath, the whole lasting only from 15 to 30 seconds at first, never more than one to two minutes at most. The chest during this time is washed with the water running from the shoulders.

THIGH OR LOWER SHOWER

The shower for the thighs or lower shower is applied like the knee shower, with this difference that here the region of the kidneys, and the abdomen are included.

WHOLE SHOWER BATH

The bather stands in the tub fully undressed and the water is poured over him, beginning at the feet, then down both sides of the back avoiding the spine and likewise down the chest. Two to six cans of water are used, according to the susceptibility of the bather or the temperature of the cold water.

N.B. Besides these shower baths, there is the head gush, which is taken by evenly pouring the contents of a half of one can over the entire head, then thoroughly drying it. The face and eye gush are also frequently applied as substitutes for the face and eye bath. The eye gush must be applied very mildly, the spray of water on each eye lasting only a second.

COLD BATHS

Duration one to three to six seconds, later on 30 to 60 seconds at most.

COLD HALF BATH

The bather sits down, feet and all, in a bath tub filled with cold water reaching up to the navel.

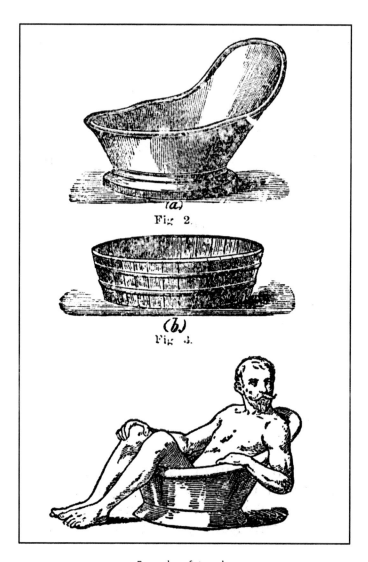

Examples of sitz tubs

COLD SITTING BATH

The bather sits down in a sitting bath or small tub, the feet remaining outside, the water reaching the navel.

COLD WHOLE BATH

The bather sits down in a bathtub, the water reaching to the armpits, and after the bath does not dry himself. As for all cold ablutions, baths and showers, the body must be comfortably warm before and after taking the bath. The normal warmth is regained by exercise in a room whose temperature is not too low.

COLD ABLUTIONS

These are often effectually employed in such cases where the patient cannot stand the cold baths and showers, or very poorly at best. They must not last longer than one to two minutes. The best time for taking them is in the morning directly on rising, and the patient may then retire back to bed for a few moments or take exercise until the normal bodily warmth is regained. The ablutions may also be taken before going to bed, or even in a bed in a room that is not too cold.

Vinegar diluted by three times its quantity of water can be employed for these ablutions. Take a coarse rough towel, dip it in cold water, wring, and quickly wash chest, abdomen and legs, then dip again, wash the back and finally the arms. There must be no chill present before the ablution.

Ablutions of certain parts of the body are called part ablutions, of the entire body, whole ablutions.

WALKING BAREFOOTED

Walking barefooted is as excellent a means for hardening as for diverting heat from the upper body and head. Persons who suffer from excessive sweating of the feet ought not to walk barefooted too long. After walking barefooted, dry stockings and shoes must always be put on, and exercise taken. There should be no pauses of standing still during the walk.

1. Walking in wet grass should be done on soft, good turf, wet by dew, rain or sprinkling, and last 15 to 45 minutes.
2. Walking on wet stones should last from three to five minutes; with healthy persons of 15 minutes.
3. Walking in newly fallen snow should last three to four minutes, and not be done in a cutting wind; best of all in the spring.
4. Walking in autumn hoar-frost should not last longer than three to four minutes.
5. Walking in water is done by walking up to the calves in water for one to three to five minutes, either in running water or in the bathtub.
6. Walking in sandals is a pleasant and excellent means of hardening.

Accordingly, children ought to be quickly washed every day all over the body, (in a room whose temperature is about 60° to 66° F / 16° to 19° C with water of about 71° to 80° F / 22° to 27° C, not dried off, and then put into bed for about ten minutes, or immediately dressed that they may run about and take some exercise.

Cold sitting baths ought not to last longer than two or three minutes, and cold whole baths in tubs not longer than several seconds (often just in and out).

Shower baths must be given so long till the skin reddens, hence reacts, and a feeling of warmth ensues, which is effected more quickly by cold water than that of higher temperature.

During menstruation only whole ablutions and upper shower baths are allowed.

While bandages are swathed around the whole body, compresses are merely poultices of coarse linen folded to several thicknesses, dipped into warm or cold water, well wrung and laid directly over the suffering parts, being covered with a woolen cloth.

There must be no drying after any shower baths.

At first, one can, then from two to three cans may be given, while healthy persons can stand as many as five cans, that is to say, till reaction sets in, indicated by the reddening of the skin and increased warmth of the parts wetted.

Walking barefooted is as excellent a means for hardening as for diverting heat from the upper body and head.

1904

HEALTH INCARNATE
BENEDICT LUST

THE KNEE DOUCHE
DR. ALFRED BAUMGARTEN

FATHER KNIEPP AND HIS METHODS
BENEDICT LUST

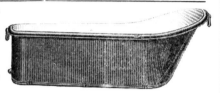
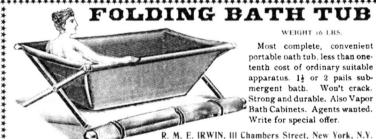
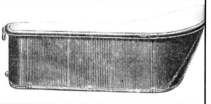
These ads of various bath tubs were found in the Lust's magazines from 1899 to 1902. If available today, the sitz bath tub or any of the bath tubs would would be an amazing purchase.

Health Incarnate

by Benedict Lust

The Naturopath and Herald of Health, V (1), 4-7. (1904)

A Naturopathic Silhouette, VII

The chapter on Hydrotherapy cannot find more fitting conclusion and consummation than tribute to Louis Kuhne, pioneer hydropathist and serotherapist.* His works, *Facial Diagnosis* and *New Science of Healing*, have revealed virgin realms prognostic, etiologic and prophylactic. The causes, conditions and treatment of disease hitherto unexplained, he has beautifully and conclusively disclosed, and his life study has been a basal factor to Naturopathy.

Posthumous honor, after a martyr's death,** is beginning to bear faint recognition of the incomparable service rendered mankind, and when you read and digest his books you will join the vast army of New Therapeutists [therapists], whose tremendous advance is but the prolongation of the ideas of Kuhne.

Hydropathy ill-applied is not simply disagreeable, it is decidedly dangerous. And it is essential to note the following suggestions:

1. *Cold water should never touch cold flesh.*

    Exercise, massage, warm applications or other circulation quickeners must precede. Profuse perspiration is the best preparation for a quick cold bath.

2. *Reaction must always follow.*

    If it does not, shorten or modify application, or omit altogether. Flesh brushes and friction towels*** are a valuable adjunct in arousing circulation before the bath.

3. *Every warm ablution necessitates succeeding cold.*

    Just a dash—a few seconds plunge or spray or douche. Melcher's shower yoke is perhaps the best apparatus for the purpose, though, a bowl or bucket is quite sufficient.

---

*Benedict Lust referred to Louis Kuhne as a Serotherapist which we would think of as someone who administers serum from an infected animal prepared for vaccine production. I have not found any evidence that Kuhne was using serums in his Water Cure practice. —Ed.

**Alluding to Louis Kuhne (1835-1901) as a martyr, Benedict Lust suggested that Kuhne did not receive fitting recognition for his achievements during his lifetime.

***Massage Rollers, Massage Vibrators, Muscle Beaters, Flesh Brushes and the like are indispensable in digestive and circulatory disorders. Naturopathy commends especially the Massage Rollers of Dr. Forest and others. —*Benedict Lust.*

4. *Artificial drying after a bath is not advisable.*

   The best plan is to cover up tight between blankets for a few minutes, the next best to don underclothing and exercise vigorously,
   the next to dry by hand-rub and evaporation, the least salutary
   is wiping dry and rubbing until red. This is directly opposed to
   the common belief; the philosophy of it is explained by Father
   Kneipp and other Hydropathists.

5. *All apertures, doors, windows, etc., should be closed during
   bath.*

   About the only time for a closed window.

6. *Bathing should precede eating by not less than an hour, and follow it by not less than three.*

   This suggests the early morning and the late evening—the former
   for the daily cold plunge, the latter for the weekly or semi-weekly
   hot lather. Cold water tonifies for the day's work, hot soothes for
   the night's slumber.

7. *A cabinet bath should be taken by sedentary persons at least once
   a month.*

   For this purpose Robinson's Cabinet is admirable, as also Irwin's
   and the Betz. Naturopathy never advises and seldom counte-
   nances the Turkish bath.

8. *Imported castile soap is the best for general purposes.*

   Ivory is a close second; tar, oatmeal, gluten and like special soaps
   are excellent if pure.* Kneipp's tormentil and herbal soaps are
   the only medicated preparations Naturopathy commends; these
   do not claim cosmetic effects on the skin.

9. *Vinegar, oil, milk, mud and many special baths akin to Hydropathy are often temporarily superior to water.*

   This applies especially to invalids not yet able for the unadulterated water cure.

10. *The Internal Bath is always preferable to cathartics, pills and
    purgatives.*

    The J. B. L. Cascade and the Forest New Method Syringe are
    probably the best flushing instruments. A rectal tube and foun-
    tain syringe are often adequate. Colon lavage should never be

---

*Ivory soap has as its branding, 97% pure which means that it is 97% pure white.
In order to obtain this level of whiteness, mercury has been implicated in the making of
Ivory soap. —Ed.

taken save under experienced direction and it should not become habitual.

11. *Menstruation, rheumatism, heart affection, neurasthenia, dropsy and other special conditions forbid the indiscriminate use of water.*

In general, an effective course of treatment necessitates sanatorium supervision at the naturopathic institute or some similar establishment. We shall be glad to recommend to you naturopathic sanitaria in various countries and cities of the world.

12. *Hydropathy means perseverance.*

If you expect complete renovation in a day or a week or a month, the Water Cure is not for you. It never heals save from the source, and that means following the back-track of long repeated errors. The rationale of the whole treatment is fully explained in the works of Kneipp, Just, Kuhne and others.

13. *Hydropathy is not alone for the ailing.*

If you want nerve force, digestive vigor, sex power and the typical tokens of superb manhood and womanhood, water rightly used will do locally what no other single agency can.

Take an occasional morning walk barefoot in the dew, or a splash in a rain storm, or a cold sitz, or a Kneipp application. And above all, a cool dash every morning.

Kinesitherapy [sic] is a less attractive name than Physical Culture, but more expressive. Bodily beauty does not require sinews of steel, muscles of whipcord, endurance of the adamant, much less does health exact them. While the pretty biceps of a professional athlete is a happy contrast to the muscular atrophy of the average American, Naturopathy does not deify the physical. The therapeutic function of exercise preceded and underlies the aesthetics, and is essentially different in motive and movement.

It is impracticable to present here the naturopathic view of all the diverse systems of exercise, from the dainty grace of Del Sarte and Emerson to the strenuous force of Swoboda and Macfadden.* But the Naturopathic criterion may be indicated very briefly. We reject all movements having any other object in view than the vivifying of the vital processes. These include muscle stretching and tensing for the circulation and assimi-

---

*François Delsarte's work focused on the intricate relationship between movement and emotion inspiring modern dancers such as Isadora Duncan. Dr. Emerson, a teacher and philosopher, pioneered the art of self expression. Alois Swoboda and Bernarr Macfadden were key figures in the Physical Culture movement championing physical exercise for everyone. —Ed.

lation, nerve relaxation for poise and repose, skin friction and stimulation for elimination and alimentation, organ movement and manipulation for digestion, secretion, excretion, palpitation and lung exercises for life-power. The latter will be considered under Pneumatotherapy.

The matter of exercisers is the first to claim attention. Their choice and use depend upon the stage of mental development of the user. Such a distinction is not commonly made outside of Naturopathy, but a little thought will prove its claim.

Externals of any kind are the measure of a man's limitations. In therapeutics, faith in a patent medicine characterizes a mental weakling. In thought, dependence on environment and circumstance is indicative of shriveled will. In religion, the worship of a fetish or a charm or a form proclaims intellectual bondage. In fact, the physical and psychic are always complementary, preponderance of the one involving deficiency of the other.

Now there are just two ways to tense a muscle—by outer resistance and by inner concentration. The man whose brain is rudimentary and his body uncontrolled requires apparatus-work in large and frequent allotments. He is usually of vital temperament, with anabolic powers far in excess of catabolic. Prone to corpulency and averse to mentality he delights in an exerciser as a child shakes a rattle. For him the wall-exerciser is undoubtable beneficial. The beginner also in body building need's something to play with.

The great majority of American invalids are nervously dyspeptic, emaciated, anemic and excessively motive-mental in temperament. For them the ordinary exercises are positively harmful. They are self-reliant and inherently kinetic; the very thought of depending on a machine of wood and rubber is distasteful in the extreme. Moreover, the spasmodic jerk of the concern wears away the little flesh remaining; its movements seldom reach the vital organs most needing attention, and it is altogether unsuited for such cases. Movements demanding *correlation of mind with muscle* are the only satisfactory ones, and such need no apparatus but a brain and a body.

Certain appliances for the body, however, are decided vitalizers, and not to be confused with mere muscle-makers, and or flesh reducers. Massage rollers, massage vibrators, muscle beaters, flesh brushes and the like are indispensable in digestive and circulatory disorders. Naturopathy commends especially the massage rollers of Dr. Forest and others.

Exercise of any sort to be re-creative must be recreational. And it is a physiological and psychic fact that baseball on a blistering August day may be highly beneficial, whereas digging potatoes might produce a raging headache. If you regard exercise as an unavoidable bugbear, if you perform it perfunctorily with no motive but the fear of disease, if you cannot take pride in the growing beauty and symmetry and suppleness of your body, in short, if you deem activity a duty, not a delight, no amount of calisthenics or gymnastics or exercisers can make you what you can and ought to be. But if you keep one ideal of physical strength and beauty indelibly graven on your mental vision, if you put every particle of your energy and concentration and determination into the realizing of that ideal, if you feel health radiating a tiny bit more each day, and if you see the greatest desire of your life approaching attainment because of a better and purer and stronger body, then you are beginning to know and value the electric thrills of right activity.

Weary tomes have been spun out on the necessity of exercise, and we do not propose a repetition here. It is sufficient that Naturopathy makes Kinesitherapy the third factor in Natural Healing.

Suggestions:

1. *Never take vigorous exercise less than a half-hour before or three hours after eating.*

   Gentle walking, with deep breathing, in the open air is the only movement allowed immediately following meals. Perfect quiet is usually better.

2. *Never exercise to the point of exhaustion.*

   A wholesome weariness is often the best daily means of correcting nervous and dietetic errors. Fatigue is never beneficial.

3. *Always begin with extremities.*

   Congestion at the centers is the rule in chronic ailments, frigid hands and feet invariably accompanying digestive and circulatory derangement. In massage, friction bath, etc., the same rule applies; begin with the feet and work toward the center.

4. *Wear absolutely no clothing, or at most a single thickness.*

   The one exception is that of corpulency, which may don heavy sweaters to induce perspiration.

5. *See to it that the outside air is freely circulating, or has just been so.*

   Oxidation is the chief purpose of exercise; fetid air poisons rather than purifies, and does it in direct proportion to depth of breathing and vigor of moving.

6. *Follow every exercise period with a touch of cold water.*

   Extremities need not be wet—just a pint or two dashed on chest, back and sex organs is amply sufficient.

7. *For vitalizing specialize in body-work.*

   Exercise without apparatus is best, with the exception of massage rollers, vibrators and muscle beaters.

8. *Make the morning movements chiefly stretching, bending, twisting, massaging; let the heavy work just precede retiring.*

The objects of exercise are assimilation and circulation. Most nervous dyspeptics forget this fact and make the period of chief activity devolve on an empty stomach. As a result, they dissipate nerve-force instead of food-force, and wrongly attribute the consequent depression to the act of activity.

9. *Take your own exercise alone.*

The misunderstanding and diverting and ridiculing of others is distinctly subversive. And if you are the right kind of man, perfect body-building will become to you a part of the day's sacred silence.

10. *If possible join a gymnasium.*

Once a week or so forget your dignity, your cares, and your ultra-refinement and be simply an animal ready for a frolic with the youngest boy. In lieu of a gymnasium, a punching bag and boxing glove are quite satisfactory.

11. *Keep before you in every movement the ideal image of perfect form.*

Imagine to yourself how you will look and feel and be with that chest broadened, those muscles hardened, those arms filled out, that face rounded; and don't be satisfied till each day proves, before the mirror, a tiny bit more of symmetry and beauty.

12. *Form the habit of flexing and tensing the muscles several times during the day.*

You can do it walking or sitting or lying, when you know how, and learn to delight in the resulting thrill of power.

13. *Make the greatest longing of your life the basis of body-building.*

If you have no ambition, get one. A beautiful body as an only and ultimate aim will never come. But if the glorifying germs of dissatisfaction have taken possession of you, increasing strength will not let you lapse back into the inert state of contented animalism that characterizes the professional athlete. It will rather be an incentive for mental and moral achievement—the sure sequence of the psycho-physical.

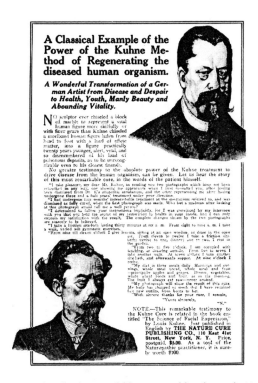

Louis Kuhne wrote two books that would be revered by the early Naturopaths: *The New Science of Healing* (1891) and *The Science of Facial Expression* (1897).

His [Louis Kuhne's] works, Facial Diagnosis and New Science of Healing, *have revealed virgin realms prognostic, etiologic and prophylactic. The causes, conditions and treatment of disease hitherto unexplained, he has beautifully and conclusively disclosed, and his life study has been a basal factor to Naturopathy.*

Hydropathy ill-applied is not simply disagreeable, it is decidedly dangerous.

Follow every exercise period with a touch of cold water.

The great majority of American invalids are nervously dyspeptic, emaciated, anemic and excessively motive-mental in temperament.

THE KNEE DOUCHE

by Dr. Alfred Baumgarten, Wörishofen

The Naturopath and Herald of Health, V (1), 7-10. (1904)

I n two preceding lectures we have spoken on the various effects and
results of the Water Cure. We are now prepared to take up each single
douche, consider its effects and the various modes of applying the douche.
We will first consider the simple, comparatively insignificant knee douche.
Many will ask, only a knee douche? What effect can a knee douche have?
I want to say right here that the knee douche is as good in its place as any
of the larger applications, and to despise it evidences a lack of insight and
appreciation for what it has done to others.

A knee douche is defined as follows: an application of cold flowing
water from the kneecap to the feet, applied in such a manner as to form
a flowing sheet of water over the whole lower leg. There are two points
especially emphasized here, viz., flowing water and evenness of application. In the beginning, the douches were all administered by Kneipp himself with a watering can. All know what a watering can is. We also know
that a small spout is generally attached to the can. It is evident then that
the whole stream issuing from the spout to the can was used by Kneipp in
applying his douches, and furthermore that no pressure was used. These
are two important factors.

In a controversy with Dr. Clement Nieman, this gentleman claims

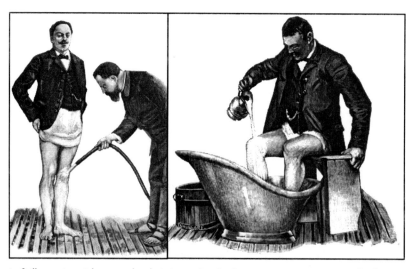

Left illustration: A knee gush administered with a hose or a watering can. Right illustration: a knee gush applied by the patient.

that Kneipp's douches existed long before Kneipp was born, and therefore are nothing new to the world, Priessnitz having applied them already. I want to say this: I have been to the [Priessnitz] springs and have personally investigated the matter. The water for the douches at the springs is led through the spouts having a fall of ten to twelve feet. The Kneipp douches, however, are given without pressure. After some time when success crowned the efforts of Reverend Kneipp, the can was no longer used, and the hose was adopted. The hose in general use is the size used for garden purposes. The knee douche can be applied in two different postures. The patient may be seated or he may stand. If the patient stands, we begin at the heel, slowly rising up the calf of the leg, returning to the heel; then the other leg is treated similarly. It is perfectly immaterial whether the right or left leg is to be treated first; it is simply done to give a start. Why begin at the heel? The reason is this one: the calf of the leg being composed of various muscles and flesh is less sensitive than the shin. Every bone is enclosed by a very sensitive skin. It is for this reason that we begin operations at the heel. It would be equally as well for one to begin at the front if the patient is not too sensitive. The water must then be applied evenly until, after sixty to one hundred seconds, then the reaction will set in.

I presume that all know what is meant by reaction. The blood returning to the exterior vessels, filling them while expanded colors the skin a deep red. Evidently, this coloration varies with the individual, according to his or her physical condition. If the patient is to be seated during the treatment, as often is the case with such who are very weak, he will be seated on a chair with a large basin in front of him to place his feet in and also to receive the water used. When giving the knee douche to weak patients sitting on chairs or on the edge of the bed, it is well to raise the column of water at the side of the shin, that portion of the leg being not so sensitive. If the column of water is rightly applied you will note that it encircles the whole of the leg like a stocking, and especially if the person be seated and the water applied above the kneecap. Those desiring to learn the art of applying the douche must have exceptional flexibility of arm and wrist, and a quick eye to perceive the greatest coloration of the skin. This is essential.

The duration of the knee douche in both forms should be from sixty to one hundred seconds, and if necessary even longer, according to the condition of the individual.

What effect does the knee douche produce? The effect of the douche is two-fold. Firstly, its influence on the blood; secondly, its influence on the nervous system. How does it affect the blood? The blood in the legs will rise to the upper portion of the body. After a short time the contracted vessels will again expand, permitting the flow of blood to the extremities and reaction takes place. This reaction continues for some time if not interrupted by drying off with a towel. The most important feature in the whole treatment is to let Nature work of her own accord, only assisting and stimulating her for action by the influence of cold water. This being done, Nature will then work of her own accord. Her work, if not influenced and interrupted by us, will be sure, reliable and beyond criticism. This, then, in short, is the effect of the blood circulation coursing to and from the extremities douched. Another effect is the absorption of heat, cooling the blood and lowering the general temperature of the body. This absorption of heat is not without good results. I have instituted repeated experiments, endeavoring to find just how much heat is absorbed by the knee douche. I will not go into details here; suffice it to say that the knee douche is the best remedy for increase of natural warmth. Therefore, cold water properly applied generated warmth. At first a severe chill is experienced, but increased circulation and reaction produce a comfortable warmth. The best underwear, therefore, is cold water. Away with your woolens and your flannels.

The knee douche also influences the whole nervous system. You will find in the words of Kneipp that he repeatedly refers to the knee douche and states how men, strong, robust, have crouched like children and have yelled when it was applied. This is correct! Applying the flow of cold water above the kneecap, you will often experience a sensation as though rheumatic pains were passing through the legs and joints. Whence and why is this? The cause for this is found in the fact that at the knee joint a large number of very sensitive nerve fibres are concentrated, this being the largest joint of the human body.

The knee douche acts as a tonic on the whole system. It revives, invigorates, and gives new life and energy. The laborer returning from his day's toil will place his sore and tired feet in cold water; immediate relief comes, that tired feeling is gone, he feels himself refreshed and strengthened. So it is with the knee douche. This douche is the best remedy for that tired, worn-out feeling. There is one thing often occurring with the knee douche which must not be overlooked here. [Nervous or hypersensitive] persons will experience a rush of blood to the head. Many are compelled to abandon the douche entirely on this account.

Why is this? The action of the skin and of the fibres under it will be as entirely nervous one, and the blood vessels contracting and expanding are all nervous actions originating and influenced by the nerve center. If, then, a person is inclined to be very sensitive and nervous it is evident that the rush of blood to the head will be greater than with the average normal person. A person otherwise normal will feel the soothing effect on his entire system. With a nervous person, however, the reaction will set in more rapidly and more vigorously and thus, the blood driven up from the extremity, will rebound and fill the brain as with a congestion. These are the causes why some nervous, blood-impoverished persons cannot take these douches or even go barefooted into cold water without violent shock to their nervous system. The knee douche is a great healing factor in diseases such as podagra [gout of the feet], rheumatism, gout, etc. Podogra generally appears in the toes of the left or right foot, which becomes swollen and highly inflamed. In such cases, the afflicted suffers intense pain and has a high temperature. Whatever he may take, it will not alleviate his suffering. In such cases, the knee douche is a Godsend means of relief. I have repeatedly observed that nothing will cure, or even relieve podogra as quickly as the knee douche. Only this noon, I met a gentleman who informed me that he was a sufferer from podogra for years. Often he would remain in bed for two or three months until he employed the knee douche, finding not only relief but absolute cure.

Also with muscular rheumatism the douche is of great help. Muscular rheumatism is a dangerous and painful disease. It mostly begins at the right knee, accompanied by high fever, absolutely inability to move, and severe pain. The suffering is often so great that every breath will be painful.

To such sufferers the knee douche should be applied regardless of protests, for only then will the pains disappear. But often the sufferer is unable to move or bend the knee. What is to be done then? You will take a napkin or small towel; tie this around the ankle of the sick limb, also one above the kneecap, then place a flat dish under the limb, and in this matter you can apply the water evenly over the limb. This is the method used in severe cases. If the patient is able to move the knee but a little, it is always better to apply on the person in a sitting posture. There is no known remedy which will relieve the pain quicker than the knee douche on the inflamed limb. It is important to draw attention to this since a great number see certain death in such a treatment. I can assure them, however, that there is absolutely no danger. In more than a hundred different cases I have had success, and even in such where heart trouble was dominant.

But how often may the knee douche be applied? It is not to be used too often. Cold water applied to one particular portion of the body too frequently causes an unusual flow of blood in that direction; a number of chyliferous vessels* form so that the whole contains more blood than normal circulation could put there. This may do more harm than good. For this reason you will find the great variety in all of Father Kneipp's directions.

How can we apply the knee douche at home? Anyone having a gar-

---

*This reference to chyliferous vessels refers to lymph vessels. —Ed.

den hose, bathtub and running water can apply the douche. Those who are not in possession of a hose can use a can or some other vessel in applying the douche. We can, therefore, under the ordinary circumstances apply the douche at all times and places.

In conclusion, I wish to draw your attention to the fact that the knee douche should not be applied too long, and always ends when the skin reddens.

What effect can a knee douche have? I want to say right here that the knee douche is as good in its place as any of the larger applications, and to despise it evidences a lack of insight and appreciation for what it has done to others.

A knee douche is defined as follows: An application of cold flowing water from the kneecap to the feet, applied in such a manner as to form a flowing sheet of water over the whole lower leg.

If the patient stand we begin at the heel, slowly rising up the calf of the leg, returning to the heel; then the other leg is treated similarly.

Why begin at the heel? The reason is this one: the calf of the leg being composed of various muscles and flesh, it is less sensitive than the shin.

The water must then be applied evenly until, after sixty to one hundred seconds, then the reaction will set in.

I presume that all know what is meant by reaction. The blood returning to the exterior vessels, filling them while expanded, colors the skin a deep red. Evidently, this col-oration varies with the individual, according to his or her physical condition.

If the column of water is rightly applied you will note that it encircles the whole of the leg like a stocking, and especially if the person be seated and the water applied above the knee-cap.

This reaction continues for some time if not interrupted by drying off with a towel. The most important feature in the whole treatment is to let Nature work of her own accord, only assisting and stimulating her for action by the influence of cold water.

I will not go into details here; suffice it to say that the knee douche is the best remedy for increase of natural warmth.

You will find in the words of Kneipp that he repeatedly refers to the knee douche and states how men, strong, robust, have crouched like children, and have yelled when it was applied. This is correct!

The knee douche acts as a tonic on the whole system. It revives, invigorates, and gives new life and energy.

These are the causes why some nervous, blood-impoverished persons cannot take these douches or even go bare feet into cold water without violent shock to their nervous system.

In conclusion I wish to draw your attention to the fact that the knee douche should not be applied too long, and always ends when the skin reddens.

FATHER KNEIPP AND HIS METHODS

by Benedict Lust

The Naturopath and Herald of Health, V (7), 145-149. (1904)

Being the substance of an address delivered on April 14th, 1904, at the Cosmological Center, 36 W. 27th St., New York City.

A number of years ago, a young man then twenty-two years of age went back to Germany to die of consumption—*given up* by all the medical men who had had anything to do with him.* He had tried Homeopathy and Allopathy, and other methods, but without result.

The young man went to Wörishofen in Bavaria and saw Father Kneipp. The good Father looked him over, heard all he had to say, and at the conclusion of the interview said, "I don't know whether I can put you together again or not, but I will see what we can do." The young man started to take the cure, and his health began to improve from the very start. In eight months he was in the enjoyment of perfect health.

When he proved in his own experience the value of Father Kneipp's treatment for himself, he determined to devote his life to transmitting to others the benefits of the system of healing that had done so much for him. He set to work to study that system, and told Father Kneipp that he should go back to America and teach the people there how to cure disease by means of it. The Father slapped him on the back heartily and said, "Follow the system in America!"

That young man was myself. I can truly say that I have faithfully fulfilled my promise to the very utmost of my ability. (Incidentally, it may be said that Mr. Lust is a tall, well-built, vigorous man, with bright eyes, clear complexion and every outward evidence of superabundant good health, high animal spirits, and physical vigor. Nobody, to look at him, would have the least idea that he had ever had a day's sickness in his life—much less that he had ever been as sick as he described in his address. As a living advertisement of the virtues of the Kneipp system of healing, it would be very hard to improve upon Mr. Lust himself.—Reporter.)

Father Kneipp was a man of very simple life, but he possessed a large share of personal magnetism that created confidence and love and made people willing to obey him promptly and unquestioningly. As can be seen

---

*Benedict Lust, 20 years old, arrived in New York City in 1892. The culmination of long hours of work as a first class waiter at the Savoy Hotel and a trolley car accident during his visit to the Chicago World Fair in the following year in 1893 were some of the factors that precipitated the need for medical care. Lust sought the help of Father Kneipp in 1894 and after his return to New York City began his publications dedicated to Kneipp's Water Cure in 1896. He was 24 years old when he embarked on his new career as publisher. —Ed.

by his portraits, his face was full of character. It was distinguished by the size of his nose, and the distance between the nose and the lips. He was a tall man with a sturdy, robust figure and his manner of speaking sounded rather rough to the ears of city people.

He was born and brought up in the country, and had but few educational advantages. He desired to be a priest very early in his life, but he only realized that wish by hard work and by enlisting the sympathy of a priest, who gave him valuable aid. He worked so hard at his studies that his health gave way after three years at high school and he was sent home to die, the doctors telling him they had no hope of his recovery.

At this time a book fell into his hands that had been written on the Priessnitz Water Cure—the father of hydrotherapy—or healing by means of water.*

Father Kneipp did not originate water curing, but he modernized and improved the practice found already in existence. Fifteen years ago people were much stronger than they are now, and could withstand much more vigorous treatment. Kneipp, in those days, practiced what was called the "horse cure", so called because of the strength of constitution needed to stand the applications. He himself broke the ice in the Danube for four weeks to give himself the treatment prescribed by [Hahn], and feeling none the worse at the end of that time—though no marked improvement was manifest—he returned to college to resume his studies. There, he earned the title of the "water doctor", and practiced his methods on the other students, mostly at the fountain in the courtyard late at night after the professors had gone to bed. There, he effected two cures that were so successful that he made lifelong friends of his grateful patients, who helped him a great deal after he became a priest.

At first when he became a priest, he devoted himself to the duties of his parish but he could not help trying to cure people whom he found to be sick. Several times these efforts conflicted with his official duties as a priest, and once even he found himself under arrest.

In Munich a judge said to him, "You are trying to make criminals: nobody needs the Water Cure." Father Kneipp replied, "You need it yourself; for I can see that you will be a dead man in six months." And the event proved that Father Kneipp's words were true.

In another court, the judge asked him: "Can you cure rheumatism?" "Yes, I can!" The next day he came to the establishment to take the cure.

―――

*The book, *The Effect of Water Unto and Into the Human Body"* (1738), written by Johann Siegmund Hahn, M.D., influenced Sebastian Kneipp in pursuit of his own health. Although Benedict Lust cited Priessnitz as the author of the book, Priessnitz (1799–1851) and Hahn (1696 –1773) did not live at the same time. Priessnitz was illiterate and did not leave behind any written documents. —*Ed.*

The success of the treatment soon made it popular and such heavy demands were made upon him that the Bishop forbade his doing any more of this work. He did his best to obey for a time, until an incident happened that decided all his future life.

One night, he was sent for to treat a woman said to be dying. He sent back word that he could not come. Again the summons came, and again he refused. About eleven o'clock he went to bed, but found himself unable to sleep for thinking of the woman, and of the possibility of her dying because he had refused to go to her assistance. At last he got up, saying, "I'm going to see the woman, and stick to the work of curing the sick from this time on."

That night settled the question of his practicing, and his success soon proved that God had called him to heal the sick by his methods. In 1886 he published the German edition of his book, *My Water Cure*, so that readers could cure themselves at home without coming to him. But instead of lessening the number of people visiting him for advice, it greatly increased them. Wörishofen was filled with strangers from all parts of Europe. Hotels were built, and the out-of-the-way village became a town of 24,000 inhabitants.

The agents used in Kneipp's healing methods are air, light, sunshine, and diet, as well as water. Primarily, the Kneipp methods are intended to prevent sickness by keeping well people in good health, to cause robust persons to live plain, simple lives, and to harden the constitution by means of the natural agents just named—not by means of drugs and medicines. Father Kneipp's book gives full directions for both, the preservation of health and the cure of sickness. The book has been translated into fifty-two languages, and in the German language alone, 136 editions have been issued.

ABLUTIONS

To an average normally healthy man Kneipp would say: "Keep your constitution hardened and robust, and protected against the weather, so that you do not become sensitive to cold." He prescribed washings and ablutions, and not sponge baths as people usually take them.

A beginner should just take cold water out of a basin and apply it quickly to the arms, chest and upper part of the body, and then put on the clothing at once—without drying the skin with a towel. Next day, the other parts of the body should be treated in the same way, but no towel must be used before putting on the clothes again. The body must always be kept warm and exercise must be taken at once so as to promote and sustain quick reaction of the skin.

BATHS

After a while a half bath may be taken. Get into a bath tub half full of cold water, sit in it while you count to "4", get out quickly, and dress immediately, without using a towel. The use of a towel causes the body to lose warmth. Water left on the skin retains warmth as it is evaporated by the heat of the body. Coarse underwear should be worn, as fine garments stick to the body and prevent the air from having free access to the skin; therefore, the material should be of coarse linen or cotton. This half bath may be taken about three times a week.

No item of treatment should be continued long enough for the system to *get used* to it because then it will fail to produce good effects. Therefore, it is wise to change the order of different details of treatment taken, or omitting some for a while and then resuming. This principle holds good in all applications of the Water Cure.

A full bath is like the half bath, except that all the body is submerged.

DOUCHES

Among other applications that can be used at home are douches. These are not shower baths (in which water comes down from above or around the patient), but can be given by a watering can or a hose with one and a half inch opening. The water just runs over the skin, but is not directed against the body with any force.

The first of these is the knee douche. This is very useful for drawing the blood from the head and strengthening nervous patients; also to induce sleep in cases of insomnia.

The application begins at the heel, and goes upward at the back of the leg to the knee. The water is applied until the skin gets red; it is stopped then, in order to avoid the loss of heat and vitality.

Then there are hip douches; back douches (very useful for strengthening the back and the spinal cord), chest douches, and douches for various other parts of the body, the mode being the same in all cases, and no towel being used before clothing is resumed.

The lightning gush is like the douche, except that force is applied to the water, the attendant holding the hose about six feet from the patient.

Cold water applications always produce heat and increase vitality, and the different douches cause better metabolism, or assimilation of food. Therefore, patients need more food, more rest and more exercise while taking them. People who are working every day should not take more than two or three a week.

Kneipp did not oppose all steam baths. Properly applied they will relieve cold in the head and the chest or the limbs, but he put herbs in the water of the vapor baths and thereby made them more effective. Every warm application should, however, be followed by a cold douche or other method of treatment.

PACKS

The principal is a wet sheet wound round the body from the arms to the knees, the water used being cold for a strong patient, but warm for a weak one. It should be kept on for half or three-quarter's of an hour. It is very useful for dissolving impurities of the system, and causing it to excrete morbid matter. It should always be applied with care.

The Spanish mantle covers the body, the patient being wrapped in a sheet and put to bed. It produces a good sweat, and the patient should be washed down with cold water afterwards.

For sore throat, neck bandages wet with cold water, may be used; they must be renewed every ten minutes. The bandages must never be allowed to remain on after they get warm, and no air must be permitted to get between the skin and the bandage.

A good way to cure a cold is by a half bath, taken three or four times a day, with cold water alone. The trouble is not really with the nose or the throat in itself, but exists all over the body, although it may be more manifest in these special organs. The impurities in the system are unable to escape by the pores of the skin, and therefore try to get out in that form of phlegm, etc., through the membranes. Vapor baths are good, and so are packs, but the half bath, previously described, is the simplest method.

DIET

Kneipp was not a vegetarian or a fruitarian, but his system is a kind of bridge from the old system of diet to these new ones. He never told anyone to give up anything all at once. If a man were in the habit of drinking fifteen glasses of beer a day, he would reduce the number to seven; if ten cigars were smoked a day, he would make it five; three meat meals a day would be cut down to one. To people used to taking much medicine, he would give herb teas of various kinds.

One of his principles was to get city people out of the city into the country. He had a marvelous capacity for handling people, and managing them so as to make them do what he wanted.

He was one of the busiest men in the whole German Empire, and often had 4,000 people to hear him when he lectured. I had four interviews with him altogether; one of them at five o'clock in the morning.

He stood up for a mixed diet of meat and vegetables; he ate meat himself but recognized that vegetarianism was good, if the dietary were properly arranged. Father Kneipp drank two or three glasses of beer in a year, but he was not a crank on the subject of intoxicants.

He was against the use of white flour declaring that the best part of the wheat was removed in the milling. He believed in soups made of cereals with vegetable or milk stock, but not in soups made from meat; also in plenty of sauerkraut.

Father Kneipp died at the age of 76 from overwork. He usually worked from 4 a.m. till 11 p.m. every day in the week. For the last few years of his life, he certainly did not take proper care of himself. Still it must be borne in mind that he had been "given up by the doctors" at the age of 28.

As a priest, he possessed private means, so that he was not obliged to treat people for money, and he did not care for money at all, in itself. One of the Rothschild's offered him 50,000 florins if he would go to Vienna to treat him, and he refused to go, not even answering the letter. He traveled in Germany and Italy and went to Paris once, where he effected some marvelous cures. In one year he cured the Archduke Joseph of Austria of a kidney disease of thirty-six years' standing. As a token of his gratitude the Archduke gave 150,000 florins for a public park in Wörishofen.

Father Kneipp established six institutions of healing and philanthropy. He built a children's asylum in 1892, where 3,000 "incurable" cases have been treated by nature methods, and a building for old men and old women, to which only the poor were admitted. There are institutions at a distance from the city for certain diseases such as cancer.

The Father was very democratic in all his ways. Each person who visited him received a number as they entered the waiting room, and no rank or social position would procure any advancement over the poorest person who had previously arrived.

A certain princess staying at a hotel sent four or five messages by servants for him to visit her, but without result. She then sent a lady-in-waiting, who told the Father that she held this position in the princess's household. Instead of being impressed with the dignity of the messenger, however, he said: "Oh, I call that a servant girl; when I am through with all these other people, I will come, and not before!"

An Austrian prince, on leaving Wörishofen after a successful course of treatment, called on the Father as he left the town and handed him a purse of gold for a present. He took it and put it into his deep pocket. A little while after a poor Romanian woman came to ask him to give her the money to get home again to Bucharest. He dived down into his pocket and handed her the purse that he had just received from the Archduke, which contained 800 Marks.

Since Father Kneipp took up the Nature Cure, about 250 health movements along similar lines have been started, some of which have done much good. None, however, was as good as his, which has been taken up by even the medical world in Europe. And in all parts of America are to be found institutions in which Kneipp's system of healing is worked out in greater or less detail.

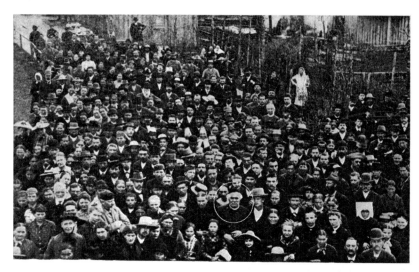

Photo of a large group of patients returning from a lecture given by Father Kneipp (in circle).

A number of years ago, a young man then twenty-two years of age, went back to Germany to die of consumption—given up by all the medical men who had had anything to do with him.

Father Kneipp was a man of very simple life, but he possessed a large share of personal magnetism that created confidence and love and made people willing to obey him promptly and unquestioningly.

About eleven o'clock he went to bed, but found himself unable to sleep for thinking of the woman, and of the possibility of her dying because he had refused to go to her assistance. At last he got up, saying, "I'm going to see the woman, and stick to the work of curing the sick from this time on."

Father Kneipp's book gives full directions for both, the preservation of health and the cure of sickness. The book has been translated into fifty-two languages, and in the German language alone, 136 editions have been issued.

A beginner should just take cold water out of a basin and apply it quickly to the arms, chest and upper part of the body, and then put on the clothing at once—without drying the skin with a towel.

No item of treatment should be continued long enough for the system to get used to it because then it will fail to produce good effects. Therefore it is wise to change the order of different details of treatment taken, or omitting some for a while and then taking again.

The first of these is the knee douche. This is very useful for drawing the blood from the head and strengthening nervous patients; also to induce sleep in cases of insomnia.

The water is applied until the skin gets red; it is stopped then, in order to avoid the loss of heat and vitality.

Every warm application should, however, be followed by a cold douche or other method of treatment.

The bandages must never be allowed to remain on after they get warm, and no air must be permitted to get between the skin and the bandage.

One of his principles was to get city people out of the city into the country. He had a marvelous capacity for handling people, and managing them so as to make them do what he wanted.

Father Kneipp died at the age of 76 from overwork. He usually worked from 4 a.m. till 11 p.m. every day in the week.

In one year he cured the Archduke Joseph of Austria of a kidney disease of thirty-six years' standing. As a token of his gratitude the Archduke gave 150,000 florins for a public park in Wörishofen.

Father Kneipp established six institutions of healing and philanthropy. He built a children's asylum in 1892, where 3,000 "incurable" cases have been treated by nature methods, and another building for old men and old women, to which only the poor were admitted.

Each person who visited him [Father Kneipp] received a number as he entered the waiting apartment, and no rank or social position would procure any advancement over the poorest person who had previously arrived.

1905

DOES HYDROTHERAPY REQUIRE REFORM?
BENEDICT LUST

THE COMPRESSES
T. HARTMANN

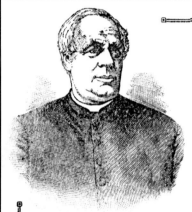
Benedict Lust published ads for the sale of Kneipp books throughout his years as publisher of *The Naturopath*.

Does Hydrotherapy Require Reform?

by Benedict Lust

The Naturopath and Herald of Health, VI (3), 70-71. (1905)

There appeared an article under this title in the *German Medical Paper* written by Dr. A. Schleicher of Bozen Gries, which may also interest our readers. Dr. A. Schleicher, who has been practicing the Water Cure for twenty years, in this article starts from the biological principle formulated by Professors Schulz and Arndt of Greifswald, according to which slight stimulants incite vitality, medium strong ones increase it, strong ones check it, and very strong ones suppress it. The said professors at first applied this idea to the use of medicines and had arrived at the remarkable conclusion that, according to this law, there is much truth in the opinion of the Homeopaths who, with their small and insignificant stimulating medicines, declared to be able to obtain the opposite of what the Allopaths obtain with the same means in large and baneful quantities. Thus, for instance, the Allopath with their large doses of rhubarb, bring on diarrhea, while the Homeopaths, with apparently small doses of the same rhubarb, cure certain forms of diarrhea.

Now, Dr. Schleicher declares, that this Schultz-Arndt law also holds good for Hydrotherapy, although so far it has not received due attention in this respect.* In Water Cure, also, it is better to remain at slight and medium strong stimulants, in preference to more strong ones. The representatives of the old Priessnitz method have often violated this important biological law and therefore, met with frequent failures. The Kneipp method, however, pays due consideration to this law in every respect.** The water curist should only bear in mind the stimulation of the heat of the body; stimulation caused by hard rubbing and pressing (as this is the case with the cold rubbings of the Priessnitz school) should be eliminated in the water treatment and replaced by massage. The most important principle of a reformed Hydrotherapy should be: to take the temperature neither too warm nor too cold, but in accordance with the reaction of the individual. The application should always be a short one:

---

*The Schultz-Arndt law has been recently revived with the Hormesis theory, prevalent in Natural Medicine. —*Ed.*

**As a devoted follower of Kneipp, Benedict Lust sometimes comes across as a blind follower. Although, Priessnitz' methods can be construed as intense and the duration of treatments long in comparison to Kneipp's, I cannot fault Priessnitz in his methodologies. Priessnitz' patients were often labelled as incurables, and having this prognosis delivered by medical doctors invariably meant that the patient's medical treatment employed grossly toxic doses of mercury in the form of calomel. Priessnitz saved the lives of many of these poisoned patients that would otherwise face horrific deaths. —*Ed.*.

the form of application is never to be hurtful, rough and unpleasant. The slight stimulants consist of washing and not rubbing the body. The latter is to be discarded, as the stimulation by rubbing is too strong and not uniform. While only one part of the body is rubbed warm thereby, the other part remains cold. There is frequently no reaction after the rubbing, consequently, it often causes colds. It is different with mild washings which always result in a healthy reaction.

As medium-strong stimulants, the half baths and gushes on the knee, thigh, chest and back increase vitality and are pleasantly accepted by patients. They offer the advantage that quite cold water can be used in their application and the reaction takes place in a uniform way. "The reform Hydrotherapy has nothing to fear." Dr. Schleicher writes literally in his paper, "to accept the cold water gushes, used by the natural physician Father Kneipp as remedies. Why not take the good things where they are to be found?" Dr. Schleicher recommends, just as useful and effective, barefoot walking, in wet grass and in the bath tub, the value of which is still not sufficiently recognized by many water sanitaria.

Anyhow, in using water applications, the following points should not be neglected. First, the exposing of the warm body to the cold application should be of short duration (which Priessnitz and his followers still do not sufficiently consider)* and in the second place that neither the cold water application nor an exposing of the body to such should be made when the patient is shivering. If necessary, the cold water application is to be proceeded by a warming of the body. For the latter, Dr. Schleicher particularly recommends the sun baths made so popular by Rikli of Veldes. It seems to me also of great importance what Dr. Schleicher mentions about the number and repetition of such applications, as much is to be desired in this respect.

I know, for instance, a Kneipp physician whose patients, without exception had to subject themselves four times a day to gush applications. It must be made a principle that a thorough reaction must take place before a new application is given; but this reaction does not come as soon as we are often apt to think it does. Sometimes an entire stopping of the cure is necessary. In any case, the organism must be given time to relax. As to the packings and wrappings, Dr. Schleicher expresses himself that the entire packing of the body (full pack) is no longer used, although, in my opinion the Spanish mantle sometimes gives great benefit. The part packings for throat, chest, trunk, feet, etc., will always remain good; but their duration should be limited to such an extent as not to be

---

*Priessnitz' treatments were long in comparison to Kneipp's, however both men always followed the rule that the body needed to be warm before cold water applications were applied. This inference that Lust states to the contrary is a misunderstanding by Lust. It seemed that Priessnitz and Kneipp achieved similar success using quite different methods. —Ed.

made unpleasant to the patient. The so-called Priessnitz wrapping has proven to be a very stimulating one, but it also should never be applied for more than three hours. The time has passed where Neptune's girdle is worn day and night.

We are very glad to see in Dr. Schleicher a protector of our good cause, and we are especially pleased that he has succeeded in finding sympathizers at a place where there is little understanding and still less interest for the new system and its followers.

"An eye to see Nature, a heart to feel Nature,
and the courage to follow Nature."

—*Benedict Lust, 1905, 71*

Dr. A. Schleicher, who has been practicing the Water Cure for twenty years, in this article starts from the biological principle, formulated by Professors Schulz and Arndt of Greifswald, according to which slight stimulants incite vitality, medium strong ones increase it, strong ones check it and very strong ones suppress it.

Now, Dr. Schleicher declares, this Schultz-Arndt law also holds good for Hydrotherapy, although so far it has not received due attention in this respect.

It must be made a principle that a thorough reaction must take place before a new application is given; but this reaction does not come as soon as we are often apt to think it does.

The Compresses

by T. Hartmann

The Naturopath and Herald of Health, VI (12), 372-378. (1905)

The compresses open the pores; and by this process all morbid matter will be expelled from the system. Whatever comes out is absorbed by the damp cloth; of this fact everybody may convince himself, if he washes the linen cloth used as compress. It is necessary to wash every compress after it has been used. Besides, each patient ought to have his own.

The large packs are applied in the following way: a woolen blanket is spread on the bed, and on this a cold wet sheet is laid. The patient lies down on it. He is first thoroughly wrapped up in the wet sheet so that no air may enter; then he is wrapped in a woolen blanket in the same way and then he is covered with a comforter.

The linen used for the pack should be very coarse. The coarser it is, the more porous it will be, and the better can steam permeate it. If the linen is wet, the pores close. This is the reason why linen, especially, has come into bad reputation among the better class. (A linen highly recommended by Father Kneipp, the Prior of the Convent in Wörishofen, and by many physicians who have studied this treatment, is a kind of tricot linen, known as Kneipp linen-mesh.) Fine linen is of no use at all here; the very coarsest should be taken. The coarser the thread the better; the linen must neither be new nor stiff; if it is, it will not attach itself to the body.

Packs should always be cold. Warm ones produce scarcely any effect at all; they may only be used for babies.

In the case of hay flower packs,* I make an exception because these are dissolving. I apply them for swollen hands and feet, or I make these packs of oat straw which always dissolve the most obdurate gouty swelling. Tea of oat straw or fir branches is excellent for gout. In order to make these packs, hay flowers or oat straw are steeped in boiling water, wherein they remain for some time, and then the linen cloth is wetted in this decoction. The more the fir twigs are permeated with resin, the quicker the gout will be cured. Patients troubled with this disease ought to take this treatment in spring. The fir twigs have to be gathered, skinned and boiled in water and the decoction is ready. Packs in which salt water or vinegar is used also produce good effect; they open the pores and produce warmth very quickly. There is scarcely any difference at all between vinegar or salt water. Of course the packs must not drip when they are put on any painful part.

It is also necessary that the body be thoroughly warm before any pack is applied. If, for instance, the feet are cold, the blood will not circulate.

―――●

*Hay flowers refers to the dried plant material found at the bottom of a hay stack. —Ed.

Therefore, it is necessary that the patient first makes himself warm by exercise! If he is to be too weak to do so, he must first warm himself in bed, then take the packs and rest again.

While wrapped up, one must remain quiet in bed without changing his position. Besides, one must neither eat, nor drink, nor talk because the entrance of the least air from outside would impair the effect of the method. If the patient falls asleep, which usually happens after the first or the second pack, he may be assured of good results and must not be disturbed. When awake the pack must be removed. The first reaction is the best. If the patient cannot fall asleep, he ought to remain one or two hours in the packing.

Sweating is not at all necessary; indeed, if it occurs, the pack has not been well arranged. Nor is it necessary to remain for hours in the wet sheets. The less time the application takes, the better the effect.

If the pack has been removed, the patient should remain in bed for fifteen or thirty minutes or take a walk. Should the patient perspire—which is not to be expected—he ought to take a wash or a bath.

As a rule, the patient remains from one-half to two hours in the pack; this depends, however, entirely on the constitution of the individual. For delicate people, one-half hour is sufficient; strong persons must have one and a half to two hours. This process, repeated from time to time, opens the pores and cleanses the skin.

Packs for the largest part of the body should be taken twice a week, and only for a few weeks. Anemic people cannot take this cure, but old people and children are benefited by it. I know people who take a pack regularly every two or three weeks, and they feel well.

There are different kinds of packs:

1) the Spanish mantle which covers the whole body;
2) the short pack, or wet shirt;
3) the head, throat, arm, hand and foot pack, and the shawl.

SPANISH MANTLE

The Spanish mantle has its name from a Spanish priest who applied it very often. It is a long shirt with sleeves reaching to the feet. In front the mantle is open, it is closed by a tight fitting collar. The material is of coarse linen. The patient puts on the mantle, then lies down on the bed on which a woolen blanket has been spread. In this he is wrapped up tightly. He is then

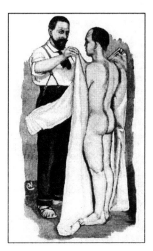

A robe used in the Spanish mantle.

covered with a down quilt or another warm cover. In these wraps he remains from one to two or three hours. The Spanish mantle may be used longer than other packs because the whole body lies in a pleasant vapor. The covering must not be too hot, lest too much heat be produced. After each application the mantle must be washed thoroughly. Everyone who uses these applications would do well to have his own mantle; one is sufficient for a life time. If only the pores have to be opened, the mantle may be dipped in cold water; but if a greater irritation of the skin be desired, it should be wetted in salt water. If hay flowers, oat straw or fir branches are used, the last named are most effective against gout; the pack must be thoroughly hot. If the patient falls asleep, he should not be disturbed, but as soon as he wakes he must be taken out of these wraps.

The Spanish mantle will especially be appreciated by stout people, by those who take little exercise and those who are inclined to gout, fever and pulmonary inflammation. It will be found excellent in the early stages of typhoid fever.

LOWER PACK

The lower pack begins under the armpits and reaches to the toes. A flannel blanket is spread over the bed, and over this the wet sheet. The patient lies down; his legs are first wrapped up separately in the wet sheet, and then in the woolen blanket; not both together, or the wet sheet would not attach itself to the body. The feet, too, must be wrapped up carefully, or they will not become warm.

Those who have nobody to wait upon them, may put on wet drawers which reach to the feet, and then wrap themselves up in the woolen blanket.

SHORT PACK

The short pack begins also under the arm, and reaches to the knees. Over the wet sheet a dry one is put and then the woolen blanket. The night gown is not taken off, or the arms and the upper part of the body would feel cold. The dampness of the wet sheet passes over to the dry one; the morbid matter of the body is absorbed by the wet cloth, which has then the same effect as a compound lead plaster.* The dry cloth becomes wetter than the wet one; if the dry sheet remains dry, this method produces no effect at all.

Blood poisoning is frequently caused by the running of a nail or a splinter into the flesh. Put a pitch-plaster on it, draw out the morbid matter and—blood poisoning will not happen. But in these days pitch

---

*Compound lead plasters were made of lead carbonate mixed with either ammoniac, galbanum, or turpentine to soothe burns and dermatitis. —*Ed.*

has gone out of style. The other day a woman ran a needle into her finger. She called on me— "the tinker," as some people call me. I applied a pitch-plaster, and within a few days the needle came out. It is a great pity that people no longer believe in pitch.

Weak people should have the short pack from an hour to an hour and a half; strong people may go on for two hours. Weak people may take it once a week; strong ones twice or even three times a week, but they should never take them for more than two weeks running.

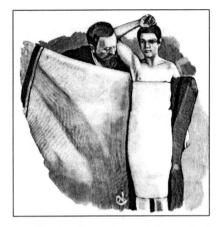

The short pack can also easily be applied without assistance from a bath attendant.

The short pack begins at the upper part of the body. It is excellent for erysipelas. It is also to be recommended for children; wrap them up in this way and they will sleep all night.

THE SHIRT

A coarse shirt is dipped into cold water and then applied in the same way as described before. An excellent effect will be attained by taking a full gush or douche over the wet shirt, then wrap up and go to bed. For children the shirt is to be preferred to the Spanish mantle.

THE HEAD PACK

First the head is wetted by washing or by pouring water over it. Then it is wrapped up in a wet cloth so that only the face remains free; if not made airtight, rheumatism may follow. Nor must the application be too long, or congestion may be caused.

THE SHAWL

The shawl is also a kind of throat pack. The damp cloth hangs in three points over the back; in front the points are brought together, and then covered with a woolen shawl. This must not become hot, or blood would rush to that place.

ARM AND HAND PACK

A person's arm is often bitten by an insect, or hurt in some way and— blood poisoning is produced. In such cases, packs of hay flowers will be the best. In cases of bruises, the pack is put into cold water and vinegar.

Hay flowers cannot be too highly recommended; many an operation has been prevented by their application.

Foot packs are excellent for those people who suffer from insomnia, especially when caused by blood going to the head.

SAUERKRAUT AS A MEDICINE

Sauerkraut is so well known as an article of food that we need hardly waste any words about it. It is, however, less known as a medicine.

By means of quite simple, so-called "home" remedies, if we take them in time, we can frequently prevent dangerous diseases, or at least greatly modify them. Among such home remedies, sauerkraut takes the first place, as it is not only a healing remedy, but also a preventive of sickness.

Sauerkraut is applied internally and externally. In the first place, it strengthens and settles the stomach if too much is not eaten. It is best to take small quantities, but eat it frequently. Used in that way it is a nourishing article of diet. Sauerkraut water also settles the stomach when out of order. In the East, particularly in Serbia, if one has "indulged" too much, he can find sauerkraut water as well as wine, in every saloon. The price for both beverages is the same. People, who have been in the unfortunate position of experiencing unpleasant effects from drinking too much, assure us most positively that a glass of sauerkraut water thoroughly settles the stomach in a short time. Among the followers of Naturopathy, of course, nobody will ever have occasion to use sauerkraut water for such "pains", but it is certainly well to be acquainted with the fact. Two tablespoons, taken in the morning half an hour before breakfast, will strengthen the stomach considerably.

Externally, sauerkraut can be usefully applied as a poultice, particularly for fresh wounds, old ulcerating cancers, inflammation, injuries, headaches and lumbago, as also for contusions and certain ear troubles. Applied in this way it hastens the bringing of an ulcer to a head, reducing the pain during this time.

SO SOLST DU KNEIPPEN!

About two years ago I became acquainted with the Kneipp cure, and as I found out that its originator frequently hits the nail on the head, says and proves so many things about which nobody had thought before, I became a real "Kneipp follower" in every respect. For example, I not only resorted to water applications, but dressed myself according to Kneipp, and abstained from alcohol (I had also read Forel, Bunge, and others on this subject), etc. I had always been a friend of water because it had done me much good. Since my birth, I have suffered from constipation (which was inherited), and during my school days I had an evacuation only every three to eight days (very seldom more frequently than once in two or three days) without, however, suffering any pain. Later on, my bowels moved more frequently (once in every two or three days, or four, at the most), but I had hemorrhoids. I have tried everything possible. I took exercises to stimulate the bowels, according to Schreber's lessons for indoor exercises. I kneaded, beat and rubbed the abdomen every day for six months, and increased this treatment gradually, but without success. Sometimes during or after the treatment, I felt some action but it produced no effect. The only thing that gave me relief was a simple enema with water (which I, however, seldom used).

By chance a small booklet came to my hand, in which a patient mentioned how he had been relieved from such trouble by drinking fresh spring water. This induced me to try it to see whether this would not help me too. In any case, it could do me no harm, unless it might increase the temperature in the abdomen and dam up the bowels. I continued my water drinking cure for some time, and since have had regular evacuations. Otherwise, I did not change my living in any way and besides other indulgences ate twice a day quite a good deal of meat (a quantity which would be poison for many young men!) with wine, as is customary with the well-to-do classes. The cure consisted of daily drinking water, regularly two hours after dinner, beginning with one or two wine glasses taken in swallows and increasing this to one quart in from twenty to thirty minutes. After that, I took outdoor exercise for half or three-quarters of an hour. While the much recommended gymnastics and all other remedies, including bodily exercise, had no effect, water did all that I needed without any other help.

Frequently, when I recommended for constipation drinking water by the spoonful every hour, many laugh at it disbelievingly, while others have not the perseverance to continue long enough to effect a cure.

In Schreber's lessons for indoor gymnastics, I also read that one can prolong life from ten to twenty years by daily washing of the body with cold water. I followed this advice, but had to give it up. I did not do it the right way, and rubbed myself too much. But now I am glad to have come across the benefactor, Father Kneipp, who teaches the right method. I only was somewhat disappointed not to find in the book, *So Shalt Thou Live* (*So solt ihr leben*), a proper statement on the value of eggs. I had known people who were indebted to eggs for their health and strength and even my own mother had, after great loss of blood in an operation, recovered with unusual rapidity by an almost exclusive diet of raw beaten eggs. But I asked myself, have not similar results been obtained by a Kneipp milk cure, by taking milk by the spoonful and adopting other suitable Kneipp diet? And I was not disappointed. Because the principle thing with sick people is to give proper nourishment to the sick or weakened stomach;

to give less at a time but more frequently. Years ago, I suffered from stomach and bowel catarrh due to much sitting, mental overwork and lack of exercise. But in from one to two weeks I was all right again by eating oatmeal every one or two hours. Sometimes, I ate too much of it at the persuasion of my parents, who thought I would thus gain strength more quickly; but Nature rebelled every time, and I always feel angry when sick people are forced to eat.

I was much interested in the article on "Salt," in the book *The Way to Live*. Salt is doubly harmful; firstly, by its stimulation, and secondly, because the thirst it causes is so often quenched by harmful things (wine, beer, coffee, tea or liquors with water), instead of using pure innocent water, which many people nowadays think is "flat".

Superficial critics sometimes admit the effectiveness of Kneipp's gushes, but usually do not refer to his medicines at all. Most of the herbs recommended by Kneipp are known to the older people of the country, though they are seldom if ever, used; folk would rather take more "up-to-date", medical prescriptions. But Kneipp has also made good discoveries in regard to his medicines. Besides the excretive oil, which I still remember, I want only to mention, fenugreek. If we ask a druggist what *Foenum graecum* is used for, he will say for cattle. A pharmacist even told me that this product was used for cattle vermin. Kneipp has, by discovering this remedy, deserved greater fame than a dozen medical professors by their apparently epoch-making inventions. How much study is wasted on disinfectants and, finally, how little use they are, particularly in treating wounds! A short time ago, I heard several country women talking to each other, and one said: "How terrible the place smells of carbolic acid in the hospital," to which another one replied in her wisdom: "Well, but that not only cleanses the wounds, but the air too." Most physicians think carbolic acid an indispensable article—and in this respect they all agree. Its only virtue is that it has a terrific odor, but when applied to wounds or ulcerations its benefit is doubtful, and its use may, indeed, be harmful. About the effect of *Foenum graecum*, Kneipp's books and a trial will give the best information.

As to hardening the constitution of children, rich people are now paying more attention to it. In most cases they do not start right and with regard to strengthening them they only go as far as limiting or prohibiting the use of liquors. In respect to clothing, they naturally go with the fashion. Many people cannot overcome their prejudice against linen underwear, and cold water, particularly during the cool and cold seasons, etc. A short time ago, on a hot day, I met a boy with naked legs, woolen socks, and warm felt shoes and with the upper part of the body heavily clad and wearing a thick cap. I naturally asked myself whether his parents were of sound mind; and yet he was the child of rich people! In the country, however, one will find here and there a country woman living successfully after Kneipp's theories with her big and little children.

Bathing in ice cold streams was formerly considered conducive to health and some old people assert that is has cured them of many diseases. When I, as a child, went bathing they kept me and others often back, fearing we might hurt ourselves. It was said that many diseases had been washed off in the stream. Now, this cold stream is too cold for both and young, and they tremble if only mention is made of it, and they stared at me when I assured them that I had bathed in it up to November and started again in March.

If I mention the following incident, it is only to draw the attention of sufferers to the fact that if they want to take a Kneipp treatment they should go to a real Kneipp adherent; i.e., to one who not only uses Kneipp's applications and Kneipp's prescriptions, but who makes them follow religiously all his other rules as to applications, diet, etc.

In visiting my native village, I suggested to an old factory workman who could not do work on account of his swollen left leg, that he should try the Kneipp cure which would surely help him. I did this because the physician by whom he had been treated for some time, and who had experimented with all the medicines he knew, could not do him any good. About three months later, I was told that the man was almost at death's door. I enquired of the physician who had treated him and tried everything, even bleeding, leeches, etc., and he described the man's condition as very serious, although he was not dead.

I then went to the man himself. He was exceedingly weak and thin, had no appetite, complained of pressure on the chest, which increased by midnight and then decreased. The urine came out in drops or partly remained in the bladder; the stool was rather irregular; sometimes the patient had passed blood for days; but his pulse was satisfactory. I had not really any hope of being able to cure him, but I was satisfied if I could lessen his suffering, and besides, I was very curious to see what a strictly carried out Kneipp cure would do for him. I started with a washing (water and vinegar) of the entire body, very weak knee gushes, and hay flower wrappings. Besides daily washings of the entire body, I applied alternately very weak limb, back and upper body gushes, half baths, short wrappings and wrappings of the lower part of the body. I gave him every day spoonfuls of rosemary wine; I forbade him to take the excellent claret and other things which the physician had recommended. I only permitted a certain tea which the physician had praised for weeks for its merit, and which was the last remedy that had done any good, and this because I found that it was Wühlhuber 2.* I was surprised at this, because the

---

*Wühlhuber 1 and 2 are herbal formulas created by Father Kneipp. —*Ed.*

physician had never wanted to know anything about Kneipp, and had said before me that it were better for Kneipp to keep quiet and not spoil the business of other people; also that a priest had tried to induce him to go to Kneipp and to see a tea, invented and prepared by Kneipp, highly praised, that had had a wonderful effect on a dropsical child. The smell of *Foenum graecum*, which came from the tea bag, startled me (it looked too much like Kneipp) and induced me to examine this tea more closely and then I discovered that it was pure unadulterated Wühlhuber 2.

The physician thought that the sick leg should be cured first. He had maltreated it badly by frequent injections of little tubes, with the result that it gave the patient a great deal of pain. He knew that the leg, besides water, also contained clogged blood. Lymph and lymphatic mucus could be readily felt by pressing with the hand. But I wanted, first of all, to strengthen the patient generally, and stimulate a greater activity of his system; then the leg would get well. So I ordered a strict and strengthening diet: milk by the spoonful, broth, etc. With drinking water by the spoonful, a regular movement of the bowels was obtained. If necessary, I also ordered small quantities of shavegrass (Zinnkrautthee) with juniper berries, and later wormwood with sage. On the seventh day of the cure they wrote me that the bad leg, in which every action of the skin and partly also circulation of the blood had ceased for more than four months, had come to life again and perspired considerably and further, that violent burning had been felt at the heel. I recommended washing the heel and the perspiring leg with vinegar and water at certain times. Then I consulted an energetic and enthusiastic follower of Kneipp whom I knew well, and the treatment was continued according to his directions.

The condition of the patient improved, the ailing leg returned to its normal condition, so that after two or three weeks the swelling had entirely disappeared and the leg was the same as the other one, although before there was a difference of ten to twelve centimeters in the size of the calf of the leg. Later on, the patient would leave the bed for a few hours, and even go down stairs in order to sun himself outside. The patient felt quite well, although he was weak. As my suggestions particularly with regard to diet were never entirely followed, and gradually less and less attention was paid to them, I finally withdrew altogether. Nine months later the invalid passed away.

Although the patient had a very unhealthy occupation and was rather fond of spirits (in which, however, he did not overindulge), I was fully convinced that he could have prolonged his life by several years if he had conscientiously and carefully carried out the directions given him.

The linen used for the pack should be very coarse. The coarser it is, the more porous it will be, and the better can steam permeate it.

In the case of hay flower packs, I make an exception because these are dissolving. I apply them for swollen hands and feet, or I make these packs of oat straw which always dissolve the most obdurate gouty swelling.

Packs in which salt water or vinegar is used also produce good effect; they open the pores and produce warmth very quickly. . . . Of course the packs must not drip when they are put on any painful part.

If the patient falls asleep which, usually, happens after the first or the second pack, he may be assured of good results and must not be disturbed.

Sweating is not at all necessary; indeed, if it occurs, the pack has not been well arranged. Nor is it necessary to remain for hours in the wet sheets.

The Spanish mantle may be used longer than other packs because the whole body lies in a pleasant vapor.

If hay flowers, oat straw or fir branches are used, the last named are most effective against gout; the pack must be thoroughly hot.

Among such home remedies, sauerkraut takes the first place, as it is not only a healing remedy, but also a preventive of sickness.

People who have been in the unfortunate position of experiencing unpleasant effects from drinking too much, assure us most positively that a glass of sauerkraut water thoroughly settles the stomach in a short time.

Externally, sauerkraut can be usefully applied as a poultice, particularly for fresh wounds, old ulcerating cancers, inflammation, injuries, headaches and lumbago, as also for contusions and certain ear troubles.

Frequently, when I recommended for constipation drinking water by the spoonful every hour, many laugh at it disbelievingly, while others have not the perseverance to continue long enough to effect a cure.

Superficial critics sometimes admit the effectiveness of Kneipp's gushes, but usually do not refer to his medicines at all. Most of the herbs recommended by Kneipp are known to the older people of the country, though they are seldom if ever, used; folk would rather take more "up-to-date," medical prescriptions.

1906

THE EFFECT OF KNEIPP'S TREATMENT ON DISEASES
BENEDICT LUST

Kneipp's linen mesh established a new standard for underwear; a huge improvement from the woolen undergarments that were used.

THE EFFECT OF KNEIPP'S TREATMENT ON DISEASES

by Benedict Lust

The Naturopath and Herald of Health, VII (2), 74-75. (1906)

How does Kneipp's treatment affect patients? By the applications of water, which have to be made twice a day, the quality of the blood will be improved.

If, as Dr. Virchow says, blood is not a liquid but a living organ—a statement we all endorse—this organ must be nourished well and in the right way. The blood is nourished, that is, made sound and healthy by keeping all the functions of the body in working order; and this is done by the inhaling of oxygen. The more oxygen the blood contains, the more vital it is, and the healthier and stronger is the individual.

How is oxygen imparted to the blood? By breathing. The more good air is inhaled by the individual, the better and stronger will be his blood. We do not consider here the breathing through the lungs, the mechanism of which is well known to everybody, but Kneipp's treatment which, by its water applications affects the inhaling of the skin which is almost entirely neglected by the medical sciences. During the reaction of Kneipp's water applications, blood-waves are continually driven out of the body to the surface of the skin, and by this process the capillaries are enlarged and prepared to absorb the oxygen in the air. The more blood-waves appear on the surface of the skin, the more oxygen is imparted to the blood which, then, will be better fitted to resist morbid or contagious matter: be these acria [sic] of the humoral pathology, or the bacilli of the modern medical conception.

The next essential feature is the nourishment of the body. The lymph or chyle passing into the blood, consists of the assimilated substances, formed by the chyme. The lymphatic ducts enter the blood, keep it at the normal temperature and influence its quality.

It stands to reason that we must be careful in taking in oxygen. At the same time we must also be mindful to take only such substances which will keep the blood in a pure and healthy condition.

Here the water applications will be of good service in producing the right distribution of blood. A cold hip bath will drive the blood into the lower limbs. By the steady application of water on one and the same place, the blood will remain in that part. If I have, for instance, congestion of blood to the head, the blood should be drawn to the lower part of the body. This is not so easy as it may appear. In taking knee, hip, or half baths, one has also to reckon with the reaction, that is, a blood wave which moves from the skin to the interior. This blood wave will be the stronger, the larger the part of the body is which is covered with water, and consequently, the greater the force by which the blood wave is driven back into the body. If only hip or half baths were applied, the reaction would aggravate the condition of the patient instead of ameliorating it. In this case the chest and the back have to be treated to cold ablutions; then the reaction will appear in the lungs and the abdomen which is especially affected by chest ablutions. As soon as the body has become used to these ablutions, the circulation of the blood will be equalized. Then the full bath may be used and by cold compresses on the abdomen much blood will be drawn to the middle of the body. This is another important factor in the regulation of the blood.

As an illustration, I may mention an abscess on the leg. Father Kneipp considers an abscess as a ventilator or provision for the secretion of the bad humors and impurities of the blood which must be dissolved and thrown off. This accomplished, the abscess is likewise cured.

This treatment begins with mild ablutions which are intensified every day and applied to the upper as well as the lower parts. Light compresses are added to draw out all the sick matter from the abdomen which, according to Father Kneipp, is the chief seat of the evil. The abscess itself is not treated except by bandaging to protect it against impurities. If the excretion from the abscess is not sufficiently profuse, it may be increased by compresses made of hay flowers.

The cure will be effected slowly; the abscess has disappeared without having caused any internal suffering. By the water application, the blood has become richer in oxygen and, consequently, the sore has been healed.

In any fever the effect will be the same; only the applications are used in a lesser degree. Baths and ablutions will drive out the fever and strengthen the patient. Although a reaction may take place, it will never be of any serious consequences.

A patient suffering from influenza, treated every hour according to Kneipp's method to a very cold ablution, the skin not being dried but covered quickly, will be cured within a short time. If I only recall to mind the tortures to which not only I but also other influenza patients have submitted, as antipyrin, antifebrin, and calomel teas, nothing to say of wine and alcohols, I am happy now I know how to treat myself next time I get influenza.

Kneipp's ablutions always produce soothing effects. The best illustration of this statement is that of acute articular rheumatism. When symptoms of typical swelling, and flush of the right knee joint, accompanied with a great deal of pain and high fever became apparent, I at once take the watering pot and pour ice-cold water over the knee of the patient. Unrelentingly I pour it over the painful swollen joint and soon make the amazing observation that the pain abates, and even to such a degree, that the patient, who at first yelled when the knee was only slightly touched, is now able to bend the knee without the least sensation of pain. He believes himself to be cured. But this is a mistake. In about two hours, when the soothing effect of the water has passed, the pain will return and even in the left knee. I then repeat the same process; this time on both knees. This cure should be repeated every two hours. Even when all joints were affected by rheumatism, I have cured the patient with cold ablutions within four weeks. The patient, an anemic young girl of sixteen years, was able after four weeks of treatment to run barefooted with the other children of the Orphans' Asylum of which she was an inmate.

Such results cannot be contradicted by a pitiful shrug of the shoulders of an M.D., but he must admit that Kneipp's method has been of good effect in such acute diseases as those just cited. Whoever will try it may easily convince himself of the truth of this statement. Father Kneipp's method heals thoroughly, without leaving any traces of sickness or resulting in blindness or deafness, as often happens when treated by means of drugs.

As soon as the body has become used to these ablutions, the circulation of the blood will be equalized. Then the full bath may be used and by cold compresses on the abdomen much blood will be drawn to the middle of the body. This is another important factor in the regulation of the blood.

This treatment begins with mild ablutions which are intensified every day and applied to the upper as well as the lower parts; light compresses are added to draw out all the sick matter from the abdomen which, according to Father Kneipp, is the chief seat of the evil.

A patient suffering from influenza, treated every hour according to Kneipp's method to a very cold ablution, the skin not being dried but covered quickly will be cured within a short time.

Kneipp's ablutions always produce soothing effects. The best illustration of this statement is that of acute articular rheumatism.

Unrelentingly I pour it over the painful swollen joint and soon make the amazing observation that the pain abates, and even to such a degree, that the patient, who at first yelled, when the knee was only slightly touched, is now able to bend the knee without the least sensation of pain.

1907

The Importance Of Ablutions In Natural Healing
Benedict Lust

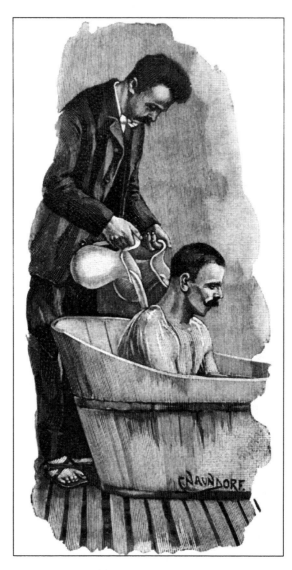

An ablution using jugs of water

THE IMPORTANCE OF ABLUTIONS IN NATURAL HEALING

by Benedict Lust

The Naturopath and Herald of Health, VIII (9), 261-262. (1907)

Nobody has yet realized the full value of a correct ablution. Much washing is done with and without soap, with warm water and with cold water; with the hand, a washcloth, and a sponge; with or without rubbing, with all possible modern improvements. In a word, the very conception "ablution" is of a wide latitude. Real effective washing is a fine art.

There are various kinds of ablutions. The first and most simple is to wash a child. This is done by dipping the hand into cold water and wash the child; then, skin touches skin or as Priessnitz says, "Life touches life." Taken all in all, children are too restless to like ablutions. The best way is to wash them with a sponge. In special cases, even with two sponges at a time, that the process may be accomplished as quickly as possible.

The washing with the hand has many advantages. The first one is that a pressure is exercised by one human organism on the other; the second is that the humidity to be imparted can be fairly gauged. The temperature of the hand, which is normally 36° to 37° C / 96.8° to 98.6° F, will not change by stroking equally and uniformly.

The washing by hand is recommended in the following cases. In order to induce sleep, the abdomen has to be washed. A basin with cold water is put beside the bed. The hand having dipped into cold water, goes then in circular strokes up the abdomen on the right side and down on the left side. As soon as the hand is dry, it has to be wetted again and the strokes have to be repeated for five or ten minutes. This cold water massage of the abdomen affects the whole nervous system most favorably and brings on sleep. People who are very sensitive and suffer from hyperesthesia would be greatly benefited by such ablutions. The hand which applies them has to be soft and fleshy to avoid unnecessary pain.

The next method is applied to cold feet. Fill a basin with two-thirds of water and one-third of vinegar. Dip the hands into this liquid, rub the feet thoroughly and without wiping them wrap them up in dry linen and then retire. This process undergone for three or four minutes will warm the feet.

Ablutions made with the hand [are preferred] and not with the rag [or washcloth]. This rag has to be of soft, thin linen and to be folded several times. If the rag is rough and hard, it scratches the skin and causes sensations of pain. A rag of old, soft linen, folded together several times will attach itself to the skin. The rag used in the right way preserves the cold, absorbs the warmth, fills the pores with water and soothes the nerves.

Nor must the rag be too wet, it has to be wrung until no water drops off, then it has to be folded, to be taken between thumb and forefinger and rubbed over the body.

If your patient is in bed, it is best to have an assistant who has always the next rag ready so that the whole process may be gone through in as little time as possible. Rapidity is here of the greatest consequence and insures success. When the ablution is finished the patient is not wiped, but a warm shirt is put on and he is lightly covered. All this has to be done in a minute.

The pressure has to be regulated according to the constitution of the patient. Nervous people have to be touched slightly but quickly; corpulent people who lack natural warmth, vitality and buoyancy, whose circulation is slow, have to be washed with a strong pressure that the water permeate the system.

Whenever the ablution has not the expected and soothing effect, the ablution has either been made too slow or too late in the evening. If the skin of a nervous man is irritated too much, the whole nervous system is upset; the patient becomes rather worse than better and so excited that even sleep will flee him. Therefore, nervous people are not to be washed at all in the evening.

The best time for washing is the early morning. If the patient is washed as soon as he is awake and again covered lightly, he will drop into a light sleep which will rest him. Sleep is the best remedy for all ailments.

All nervous people appreciate an ablution in the morning. Even here discriminations have to be made. Some people are so nervous that they prefer a quick flushing to an ablution. This is natural. If the skin of a patient is touched with a rough rag, pains may be caused, but if the skin comes only in contact with a flush of water, the skin is less irritated.

After all, water treatment is an art. One must only be willing to stand it and know how to do it. Each patient has to be treated differently and the skill of the physician reveals itself just in the right discrimination in each particular case.

My various methods in various cases are the following ones. For patients who are out of bed, I have them strip to the waist, then with rag in hand I go up and down with the right arm, touch the chest, take the other arm, pass over the back and shoulder; the abdomen has to be stroked from right to left, according to the position of the bowels.

A patient who is unable to leave the bed I strip to the waist, let him lie quiet and wash the front of the body. Then I raise him, holding him with one arm while I wash his back; then I put on him a clean warm shirt, lay him down and cover him. In the same way, I continue with the lower part of the body if the patient cannot move at all and yet has to be washed. The shirt to be put on is opened up in the back and then easily adjusted around the sick person.

The lighter the cover, the better the effect; not a perspiration but a pleasant warmth has to be brought on.

In these ablutions one may also begin with the legs. In this case, one has to have two separate linen cloths to wrap each leg separately. These are trifles, yet of great importance. In these washes not one part of the human body has to be forgotten; each finger, each toe, and each space between them has to be washed—neither are soles or armpits to be forgotten.

The ablution with the sponge differs from that made with the rag. If you wash with the sponge, the water remains in the sponge instead of permeating the pores. The rag, permeated evenly with water, touches every part of the body regularly and uniformly. Ablutions with sponges are only good for children who are too restless to keep quiet for any length of time.

If a child is sick, I treat the child in the following way: I put the child before me on the floor, have a basin with water and two sponges beside me; with these two sponges I wash the child as quickly as possible.

All ablutions have to be made with cold water; old people may take tepid water. Anemic people ought to add some vinegar to the water. Vinegar will produce warmth. These vinegar additions must not be made too frequently; they are but a tonic to the exhausted organism.

The first and most simple is to wash a child. This is done by dipping the hand into cold water and wash the child; then, skin touches skin or as Priessnitz says, "Life touches life."

The washing with the hand has many advantages. The first one is that a pressure is exercised by one human organism on the other; the second is that the humidity to be imparted can be fairly gauged.

This cold water massage of the abdomen affects the whole nervous system most favorably and brings on sleep.

Nor must the rag be too wet, it has to be wrung until no water drops off, then it has to be folded, to be taken between thumb and forefinger and rubbed over the body.

When the ablution is finished the patient is not wiped, but a warm shirt is put on and he is lightly covered. All this has to be done in a minute.

The pressure has to be regulated according to the constitution of the patient.

Whenever the ablution has not the expected and soothing effect, the ablution has either been made too slow or too late in the evening.

If you wash with the sponge the water remains in the sponge instead of permeating the pores, the rag permeated evenly with water touches every part of the body regularly and uniformly. Ablutions with sponges are only good for children who are too restless to keep quiet for any length of time.

All ablutions have to be made with cold water; old people may take tepid water. Anemic people ought to add some vinegar to the water.

1908

1907 Visit To Germany
Benedict Lust

How Should Kneipp's Treatment Be Taken?
Dr. Bauergmund

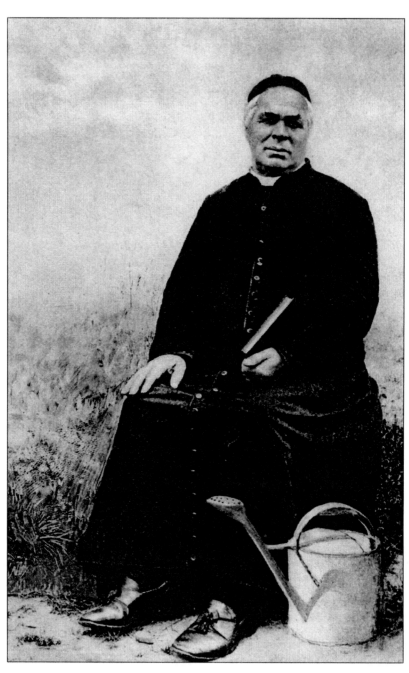

Father Kneipp with his indispensable garden watering can that he used for gushes.

1907 Visit To Germany

by Benedict Lust

The Naturopath and Herald of Health, IX (3), 76. (1908)

O n my visit to Germany the final conclusion was that the best results are accomplished in institutions where no treatments are given and where patients are instructed how to live close to Nature and how to think right.

The health home is a place where people learn how to live. I have found two or three institutions where this is carried on in the full sense of the word. I do not know of any institution in American except the "Yungborn," at Butler, New Jersey, where such an ideal condition exists.

A Naturopath is a teacher, not a physician. The word "doctor" is derived from the Greek and means teacher. This explains why our physicians generally are a failure. They tell you all about diseases but nothing about health. We have to get the idea of diseases out of our minds.

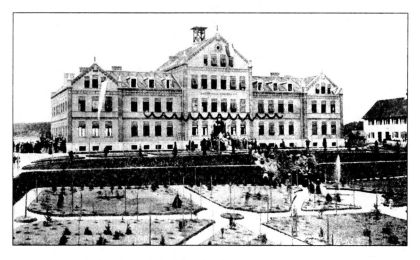

Father Kneipp's building for the treatment of children.

HOW SHOULD KNEIPP'S TREATMENT BE TAKEN?

by Dr. Bauergmund, Wurttemberg

The Naturopath and Herald of Health, IX (3), 69-76. (1908)

FIRST COMMANDMENT
COLD WATER HAS ONLY TO BE APPLIED IF THE BODY IS WARM

In the protoplasm and the cells, the lowest organic beings, we see changes of movement under the influence of cold. The ciliary motions of the ciliated cell at the least sensation of cold proves this fact. The same may be said of the muscle cells and muscular fibers which encircle the blood, this "strange juice" in elastic tissues, in cavities and tubes. Under the influence of cold even these cells draw together; the rising blood is thrown out and the skin becomes pale and bloodless. This only happens if pronounced differences of temperature exist between the water entering from outside and the skin. Suppose the blood were encircled by water, the irritation through the water will be low, even mechanical. The more the temperatures vary, the greater are the effects. If we know that the congestions and contractions of the capillary plexus are in proportion to the irritation, the cold water will be applied in such a way as to bring about this irritation. If the skin is cold and chilly, very little blood is in the capillaries; then the skin is pale and its nerves are not sensitive. What would be the consequence if we would pour cold water on such a skin?

If the non-excitable nerves continue in their insensibility, if the chilliness becomes more intense, if the poverty of the blood remains unchanged, while the inner organs are overloaded with blood causing a sense of repletion, headache and general indisposition also develop into morbid changes of the organs; then the application of water would be fatal.

The effect of cold water on a warm skin would be altogether different. The cold water, the warm blood and the warm tissues are only separated by a thin epidermis. The skin is irritated, the blood begins to circulate, and the vascular network draws together. The irritation passes then also over to the lower blood vessels, and as soon as the feet are put into the cold water the head is relieved and deep breathing is necessary as soon as the respiratory organs experience a sensation of cold.

These effects, the energetic drawing together of the blood vessels and the quick circulation of the blood which is driven to the heart, can only be made possible if the skin is warm. The irritation of the nerves is the greater, the greater the difference of the temperature of the blood circulating in the skin, as well as the water application, not to mention the mechanical influence of the cold water effect. Consequently, the warmer the body and the colder the water, the greater the effect.

But there is a limit; if the water is too cold, no stimulation in the blood vessels but lameness and relaxation would be the consequence.

Such consequences will never happen if the water applied for treatment is never below 45° F / 7° C.

The supposition that people in high fever cannot stand the application of cold water is altogether wrong. Even in the highest perspiration, if only brought on by exercise, as well as in fever heat, cold baths may well be taken. The perspiration must not evaporate, and the undressing should be done quickly. If the heart is highly excited, it is best to wait until it beats normally. Of course, one must protect one's self against draught.

Water being a poor conductor of heat, nevertheless, protects the skin by closing the pores and forming goose bumps whereby the blood is stimulated to greater activity.

If the body is not warm, one should make it warm by exercise. Each contraction of the muscles produces warmth; thus getting warm by the activity of the muscles depends on age, sex, mood and the quantity of blood. Indigestion and nervous indisposition play also here a part. I know a lady who for years has suffered from chills and only by massage and kneading can a reaction be made possible. Others have to be put to bed or to be treated to a warm bath before the cold water can be applied. I repeat, before the cold water can be applied, the body or that part to be treated with water must be warm.

"Well trimmed is well fed," say the hostlers. There is no doubt that currying [grooming] not only cleanses the pores of the horse, but also promotes the evaporation of the skin; the skin will be irritated by rubbing and the assimilation increased. We can realize the same result by irritating the skin by cold water. By the increased circulation of the blood the accumulated superfluous matter in the muscles, and organs will be the sooner removed; new matter will be replaced and fill the organs with vital force.

Second Commandment

Before Each Application Of Cold Water, Wet The Chest And Temples With Water

It is an old custom to wet the forehead, the chest and the temples before taking a bath. This practice has excellent warrant. The internal organs, most affected by the congestion of blood, are in this way prepared for it. By wetting the forehead, throat, chest, temples and head the activity of the blood vessels, lying near these parts will be sufficiently strengthened at the touch of

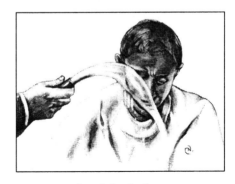

A gush for the face

cold water. In persons of advanced age, the blood vessels, especially those of the brain, become benumbed and calcified. Such vessels deprived of activity can, of course, not stand the pressure of the rush of the blood, and the slightest neglect of this rule might cause apoplexy.

THIRD COMMANDMENT

NO COLD WATER APPLICATION MUST BE MADE IMMEDIATELY AFTER A MEAL

No cold water treatment must ever be applied immediately after a heavy meal. After a meal, the body must digest the food so its activity is required for this process. As animals rest after a meal, men should do likewise. If not, the work, be it mental or physical, cannot be well done. In order to receive the full benefit of a cold water application, the body's full activity must come into play.

FOURTH COMMANDMENT

NO COLD WATER TREATMENT MUST LAST LONGER THAN IS NECESSARY FOR THE REACTION OF THE BLOOD

The object of all cold water applications is to cause a stimulation in the circulation of the blood, and they must last only long enough for this reaction to take place.

A sound box on the ear first whitens and then reddens the ear. The mechanical stimulation of the blood has first caused a bloodless condition and then a return flow of the blood to the auricle. A similar manifestation is noticed when cold water is brought in contact with the warm skin. At the touch of the cold water, the blood in the vessels near the heart as well as that in the centripetal veins, will be forced back, though only for a short time. Soon these vessels enlarge and are again filled with blood; the paleness of the skin will be replaced by redness and the sensation of chilliness by that of comfortable warmth; that is the result of the reaction. This done, our purpose is attained. If after the reaction cold water would again be applied, it would produce injurious results.

It is altogether impossible to say exactly how long an application should last; but certainly not beyond the reaction. This is not visible to the same degree in everybody, especially not in nervous people whose skin scarcely becomes red; it is enough for them if they only become warm.

There are very few people, if any at all, who are not benefited by cold water. They should only be exposed to cold water for a few minutes; and their proper warmth must be produced by exercise. Such individuals have become emaciated and anemic by long illness; they lack blood, and their organs fail to properly perform their functions. As no one individual is like his fellow being, each has to be treated in a different way. Therefore,

I must repeat it, one of the most important things in cold water treatment is to individualize accurately.

The reaction depends always on the degree of cold. The colder the water, the more intense the narrowing of the vessels and the quicker and the stronger the reaction. By pouring water on the patient, a quicker reaction is brought on than by bathing; pouring was Father Kneipp's special method. Though all processes of the cold water treatment must be administered quickly, the cooling of the body should be done slowly. Rapid passages from one condition to another are unnatural and likely to be followed by harmful consequences. The so-called crises which used to be welcomed by physicians as proof of curative effects revealing themselves in lack of appetite, indisposition, headache, and so forth, were only caused by too abrupt, too long or too many applications. The headache in the forehead, usually removed by walking, will altogether be avoided if the process is made by degrees.

Finally, I repeat: Wet yourself only slowly and only long enough to cause a reaction to be felt.

Fifth Commandment

Only The Parts Of The Body Exposed To The Air Should Be Dried

This commandment is a two-edged sword. If correctly followed, it is full of blessing; if not, serious consequences may be expected. I have made many experiments, and have come to the following conclusions. If the body is not dried, more warmth will be developed and appear on the surface, the blood circulates more quickly, and the assimilation is increased. This, of course, can only be effected if the individual dresses quickly. If the cold air touches the wet skin, the moisture will evaporate too quickly, and the cold caused by the evaporation cannot be so easily equalized by the warmth of the body. That is the reason why we recommend the drying of the parts which are exposed to the air. Besides, if the body is not dried, a great deal of exercise must be taken. On the body covered with porous clothing, the water evaporates slowly; the evaporation produces some cold, thereby stimulating the skin and exciting it to continual reaction and attaining better results if the cold is conquered by the warmth by slow degrees. The water-steam between the clothes and the skin affects the whole nervous system like a calming tonic.

Besides, one must bear in mind that by not drying the body it becomes hardened and less sensible to the changes of temperature, climate and season. I beg to quote from the writing of the famous Dubois Reymond:

Protection against cold will be effected by keeping the most sensitive parts of the skin warm; by right clothing; by accustoming the skin to stand cold; by exercise and gymnastics, and by cold washes and baths.

The best results will be attained, if the body is not dried after a wash. By this process the body will become accustomed to more intense and to more prolonged cold. I must still draw attention to one point which is, usually, neglected. The garment, touching the body, must never be thoroughly wet. Many a cold has been caused by a thoroughly wet shirt. Finally, this axiom may be taken for granted: Only the parts exposed to the air should be dried.

SIXTH COMMANDMENT

AFTER THE USE OF THE COLD WATER, EVERYBODY OUGHT TO MAKE HIMSELF WARM, DRY AND COMFORTABLE

German soldiers were once forbidden, on pain of imprisonment, to drink a drop of cold water, either after or during a march. Now at all stations through which troops pass, tubs of water are provided at which the soldiers may quench their thirst, on condition that they continue their march without stopping. Why was this permitted, contrary to the prohibition, given? This question I answer thus:

1) Anyone who stops walking while in perspiration, will catch cold.
2) By a sudden stopping in any movement, the blood will cease to circulate because the transition from the quick pulsation of the heart to rest is too sudden.

Why do I make this comparison? We have seen in the first commandment that by the contact of cold water with the warm body the activity of the latter is roused to a high degree. Through the cold water conditions are created in the human body, analogous to a highly perspiring organism; then, a more rapid assimilation and increased activity and vitality become apparent. If these conditions were stopped, the sudden change might become fatal. Here and there a stagnation of blood would be unavoidable, and disease, though not noticeable in the beginning, would develop.

Cold water makes the skin cool off. If exercise were not taken, the skin would not be warmed and the circulation of the blood, though roused and put in motion, would proceed but slowly. The effect of the reaction would be too short and insufficient, and the more so, as the body has not been dried. As the body cannot throw off the water by evaporation, it begins to feel chilly, and a cold is inevitable.

The reaction and its continuation have to be developed by exercise. The lost warmth will be replaced by increased assimilation and for this purpose the activity of the muscles is imperative. The more exercise is taken, the more the muscles have to work. The flow of blood toward the skin, as begun by the reaction, is continued and kept up by exercise; then the sensation of warmth is not only pleasant to the body, but a proof that the inner organs are not flooded by blood, the respiration is increased and sweat is secreted by the warm skin. If we know that the number of skin glands equals that of one kidney, it will be seen how necessary it is to keep the skin up to the performances of its functions. How long these exercises must be made depends altogether on the constitution of the individual, as well as on the temperature of the air. If this be below 60° F / 16° C, though strong individuals may take exercise out-of-doors, weak ones should do so indoors. If warmth is not brought on by exercise, the patient ought to be put to bed. If this does not produce the desired effect, the patient ought to be rubbed and massaged, until he is warm. Warmth must follow any cold application.

SEVENTH COMMANDMENT
NO EXCESSES

In the second commandment I have already cautioned against too many applications. Once I was called to a man who complained of dullness in one foot. The blue color of the skin proved that the blood in this foot had ceased to circulate and that the used up blue [venous] blood could not flow off. After having examined this patient, I learned that he suffered gout and that he had been advised to put his foot in cold water, which he had done while sitting on the sofa. Meanwhile he had fallen asleep, his foot all the while in cold spring water. No wonder then that his foot was so dull that I feared chronic gangrene might follow.

Excess in all cases is productive of mischief. A horse that is continually spurred on and whipped will become dull and indifferent, while a good horseman will only use his spurs in case of emergency, but manage and control his animal by his equestrian art. A plant too thickly manured will produce fruits scanty and low quality. Every vine-grower knows that too much manure will spoil the vine. If by cold water the skin shall be induced to promote assimilation, rouse vitality in the body, and drive out the impurities, this stimulating process must be kept within certain lines, or more harm than good will be done, and the body will be weakened rather than strengthened. I have seen a man treated to a hip and an upper douche at the same time; this was foolish and even dangerous. Sick, but otherwise strong, people may take three applications a day during the summer and one every day during the winter. Healthy people may take three applications every week. This rule is imperative: each individual has to be treated individually. The real physician understands each individuality at first slight; this understanding has then to be reached by physical and chemical experiments.

Diagnosing is a matter of experience. The man who is able to do this correctly is a good physician. The evil of excess has often caused fatal crises and has brought Hydropathy into evil repute.

Any one-sided treatment produces bad effects. The nursery [laborer] will not manure his trees on one side, but wherever the roots are running out; else the tree would not develop in proportion. It is just the same with the human body. The blood accumulated in the head should be drawn off to the feet. This, of course, must not be done continually or we would have a disturbed instead of a regulated circulation of the blood. As stated before, we must avoid uniform cold water applications. "Individualize and avoid excess," must be our motto.

EIGHTH COMMANDMENT

CLOTHING HAS TO BE LIGHT AND COMFORTABLE AND EVEN IN WINTER NOT TOO WARM

On this subject as on almost any other, the views of the public differ very widely. Clothing must protect man against the detrimental influences of the weather and keep the body warm. The skin, to a certain degree, acts as a reflector of the warmth of the body. If we lose more warmth than we are able to stand, the circulation of the blood recedes and goose bumps are there.

Let us begin with the clothes next to the skin. It is generally believed that wool is the best material, but it is not. Woolen material keeps warm, absorbs humidity, but it hinders the evaporation of the skin, and for this reason it should be totally rejected for underwear; the more so, as its lack of evaporation contradicts the principles of the cold water treatment. Woolen underwear tends to make the skin delicate and for this reason it ought not to be worn.

How about linen? It absorbs but little humidity and soon gives it out again. If linen underwear is of fine texture, it is at once permeated with water and adheres to the skin. Consequently, there is no air between the skin and the clothing. A sensation of cold will be felt, and the individual will feel uncomfortable. Coarse linen, on the contrary, will both absorb and exhale more humidity and is, therefore, to be recommended for use during cold water treatment. The other garments must likewise be porous, that the pores of the skin are in no way impeded. Anyone who wears a rubber coat on wet days has experienced the disagreeable sensation inseparable from the use of this material.

Now a few remarks about the fetters [restrictions] in which the human body or at least certain parts of it is enclosed, which prevent the proper circulation of the blood and can never make amends for the sins of fashion: narrow high collars, tight corsets, the elastic garters and narrow shoes. It is a downright sin to obstruct by force the regular circulation of the blood, to mar the natural form of the body and to disfigure it. Everybody ought to bear in mind that almost on the surface of the throat lie certain vessels which carry the blood from the brain to the heart. A continued pressure on these vessels must to a certain degree check the activity of the brain. Every woman ought to know that too tight a corset impedes the right breathing of the lungs, oppresses the heart, and consequently impairs the blood and disturbs the functions of the organs in the abdomen. Belts oppress considerably the strong vascular cord of the abdomen and make more difficult the work of the digestive organs. Elastic garters impede the circulation of the blood in the feet and often enough cause abscesses or varicose veins with their painful additions. And, finally, a too tight shoe, oppressing the foot with its thousands of glands, is altogether sufficient to increase all these irregularities and inconveniences.

Taken all in all, everybody ought to wear porous clothing, that the evaporation of the skin be not disturbed in any way.

Ninth Commandment

A Successful Water Cure Depends On The Right Kind Of Food And Drink

Hydrotherapy would never have been attended by so many excellent results, if diet had not been one of its chief healing factors. What and how much shall we eat and drink are questions now ventilated in the press day after day. Whether food should be animal or vegetable is a point of long and much dispute.

From a pecuniary point of view a vegetarian diet is to be preferred; but if we consider the nutritious value of the vegetables, their turning to best advantage and their influence on the digestive organs, we have somewhat different results.

The greater part of the combustible material of the human body is albumen, and for its replacing albumen is necessary. By feeding the body, we preserve its material substance, that all its functions may be performed regularly and normally. By the gastric juice the food is brought into such a condition that it may assimilate with the blood. It is beyond doubt that this emulsion (as the metamorphosed chyme is called) may be produced from animal, as well as from vegetable food that one may live exclusively on either one kind or the other. The point in question is, which of these kinds is most wholesome, or if either is to be avoided. An exclusively meat diet does not sufficiently stimulate the digestion, and affects certain digestive glands too much, while exclusively vegetable food makes too great demands on all the digestive organs. Vegetables are to a great extent composed of fibres. Grains and legumes have to be hulled before the kernel can be eaten. This means a good deal of work for the stomach. If we were to live exclusively on vegetables, we should require a large quantity in order to get enough albumen for the building up and keeping our body in due health and well-being. For this reason mixed food is the best; then albumen will be quickly formed, and we also obtain the stimulating effects of vegetable diet.

The proportion between animal and vegetable food depends on the constitution of the individual, age, climate, the manner or rather the art of preparing the food and also, on the quality of the chewing and digestive organs. It is almost impossible to give general rules on this point, either for healthy people or for sick ones.

It is a great mistake to eat too quickly, that means putting too much work on the stomach and the digestive organs. Biting, chewing and soaking the food must be properly done, before it is swallowed. Eating too quickly makes digestion very difficult. Regular times for the meals are of the first importance; the last meal ought to be taken three or four hours before retiring. When eating, one should never go beyond one's appetite; luxurious banquets and gourmandizing cause all the well-known abdominal complaints, with their serious and sometimes fatal consequences.

Opinions differ about water drinking. We all know that water plays an important part in our body. The body of an adult person contains about 65%, that is almost two thirds of water. The water in the human body keeps the blood in circulation, enables it to assimilate food, to combine it with the tissues and to deposit the waste in the glands. The nerves and muscles can only act, if they have a certain amount of water at their disposal. Cramps in the calves of the legs, as they occur in cholera and diarrhea, are caused by too much water being drawn away from the muscles. It is evident, therefore, that the body needs a certain quantity of water. This water is contained in food and in alcoholic drinks, but the natural way of getting it is by drinking it.

Care must be taken by not drinking too much, lest the gastric juices become inefficient. Lack of appetite, pains in the stomach, and indigestion are the natural consequences of doing so. One should drink water whenever one is thirsty; that is, take from time to time a draught of fresh spring water. This stimulates the digestion and is conducive to the general well-being.

I have still a word to say about coffee, tea and alcoholic drinks. I do not exaggerate, when I say that human beings would live on an average two decades longer, if these drinks were taken only in moderation. Experiments have demonstrated that people consuming tea, coffee, and alcoholic drinks, throw off less morbid matter while doing the same work that people who abstain from them. To a certain extent they are so called means of saving. Beyond this limit their poisonous effects become more and more apparent. The sensation of hunger is soon annihilated, and the natural wants are no longer felt in this frenzy. It is an old experience that drunkards, who are more or less in an uninterrupted condition of intoxication, consult a physician when they have pronounced pulmonary phthisis, from which they must have suffered for years, though they state that up to this day they have been in perfect health. By the continued drinking of spirits, the nerves have been excited to such a degree that the drunkard is no more able to notice any weakness; and not until the system is almost on the point of collapse will he turn away from this vice.

Once a minister, who was a walking skeleton, called on me for advice after having tried all kinds of remedies for his dreadful emaciation. He had no special complaint; he only seemed to lack appetite, and nothing abnormal could be found in his organism after the most careful examination. He simply subsisted, however, on coffee and tobacco. His treatment was a very simple one. After his abandonment of coffee and tea his appetite and strength were speedily restored.

I beg to repeat: a moderate consumption of light beer and wine do not interfere with the water treatment; but concentrated liquors, tea and coffee develop poisonous effects because they continually excite the desire for more.

Tenth Commandment

In Any Water Treatment, Rest And Sleep Must Be Given In Due Proportion

By most conscientious experiments, Professor Ranke has demonstrated that the health of the organism is based on the alternation of rest and food, and on greater or less assimilation. There is no doubt that many abdominal diseases are caused by lack of exercise, and others are increased by it or made incurable. The vital powers must be stimulated by vital activity. Continued rest and neglect to use the muscles, not only injures the latter, but slackens the circulation of the blood and injured the whole organism. The assimilation is impaired and a state of weakness and debility is developed. Everybody has experienced the pleasant sensations caused by a quick walk. The respiration and the pulsations of the heart are increased; the circulation of the blood and the assimilation are stimulated, and excretion, as well as the formation of new matter, is accomplished with greater rapidity.

But this increased activity has its limits. Rest is necessary; this is an eternal law on which depends man's health and life. The laws of Nature must be borne in mind by everybody. All living (organic) beings, even the plants, express in some way the desire for rest. This indispensable recreation, this revival of force, is essentially facilitated by a regular division of activity, rest and sleep, especially sleep at night. During a course of water treatment, the patient ought to retire at eight o'clock in the evening, and rise at six o'clock in the morning; then sleeping during the day is not necessary; though weak and anemic persons may rest for an hour or so during the day. Fresh air being a necessity to healthy sleep, the bedroom should be light, airy and spacious; good ventilation is of the first importance. As we need rest and change every day, so we need a full day of rest after several days of toil. The story of the Creation states fully and distinctly that it is the Lord's will that one day of rest should follow six days of toil. The Sabbath rest is as necessary to humanity as food and drink. It is a law of Nature; and all who neglect it will surely have to suffer for their disobedience.

This also applies to the activity and the rest of the mind, and the restriction of the desires and passions. Moderation in satisfying the natural wants is a means of prolonging life. The keeping of this law born within us, but so often neglected and forgotten, is the open secret of prolonging human life.

I would not have exhausted my subject if I failed to add a few words about compresses. Compresses are of great value. If one removes them after they have been used, and noticed the intense development of steam and the penetrating odor, one can understand that very bad evaporations have been thrown out from the body. That this may be done, one has to bear in mind the three following rules:

1) Compresses after having been dipped into cold water must be thoroughly wrung; then they absorb warmth and evaporate more quickly.

2) The piece of flannel put over the compress should lap over one hand-breadth.

3) If no perspiration has been drawn from the body, the compress must be taken off as soon as it is as warm as the skin. In normal cases, this warmth is effected in from one hour to one hour and a half; in cases of fever within a quarter of an hour. If it takes too long a time to warm the compress, it must be removed at once, for it will do no good. Such cases are, however, very rare.

These effects, the energetic drawing together of the blood vessels and the quick circulation of the blood which is driven to the heart, can only be made possible if the skin is warm.

Consequently, the warmer the body and the colder the water the greater the effect.

If the body is not warm one should make it warm by exercise.

No cold water treatment must ever be applied immediately after a heavy meal.

The object of all cold water applications is to cause a stimulation in the circulation of the blood, and they must last only long enough for this reaction to take place.

It is altogether impossible to say exactly how long an application should last; but certainly not beyond the reaction.

As no one individual is like his fellow being, each has to be treated in a different way. Therefore, I must repeat it, one of the most important things in cold water treatment is to individualize accurately.

By pouring water on the patient a quicker reaction is brought on than by bathing; pouring was Father Kneipp's special method.

The so-called crises which used to be welcomed by physicians as proof of curative effects revealing themselves in lack of appetite, indisposition, headache, and so forth, were only caused by too abrupt, too long or too many applications.

If the body is not dried, more warmth will be developed and appear on the surface, the blood circulates more quickly, and the assimilation is increased.

The lost warmth will be replaced by increased assimilation and for this purpose the activity of the muscles is imperative.

Diagnosing is a matter of experience. The man who is able to do this correctly is a good physician. The evil of excess has often caused fatal crises and has brought Hydropathy into evil repute.

"Individualize and avoid excess," must be our motto.

Hydrotherapy would never have been attended by so many excellent results, if diet had not been one of its chief healing factors.

During a course of water treatment the patient ought to retire at eight o'clock in the evening, and rise at six o'clock in the morning; then sleeping during the day is not necessary; though weak and anemic persons may rest for an hour or so during the day.

1909

Is Kneipp's Hydrotherapeutic Treatment Unscientific?
Dr. L. Winternitz

Hydrotherapy
C. E. Judd

Kneipp's Cold Water Douches
Sebastian Kneipp

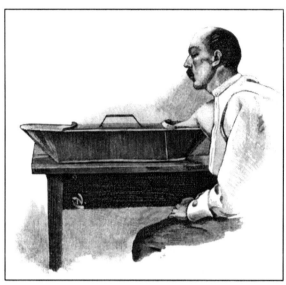

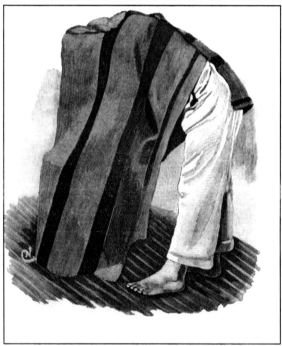

Illustration above: an arm gush. Illustation below: a vapor bath for the head.

IS KNEIPP'S HYDROTHERAPEUTIC TREATMENT UNSCIENTIFIC?

by Dr. L. Winternitz

The Naturopath and Herald of Health, XIV (4), 221-223. (1909)

That this question should stand in need of discussion seems hardly credible, seeing that a number of years has elapsed during which the method of the Pastor of Wörishofen has become known and an established practice. One main argument I could adduce for the scientific justification of Kneipp's curative methods—their success; for it is patent, that the means actually producing a desired effect must be apt means and their scientific justification must be the result of physiological facts, known to everybody who has busied himself with the matter not only empirically, but also with its theoretical aspects.

The problem is not whether water is actually an eminent curative medium, for this question the history of medicine has definitely settled. Hippocrates already knew its excellent effects. During the time of the Roman Cæsars it wielded a predominating influence upon medicine. Throughout the entire Middle Ages and up to our own times, every century has protagonists of the Water Cure to show who successfully battled against the predominating school of medicine. My present object is only to vindicate the scientific rationality of the Kneipp cure as coexistent with the usual methods and to prevail upon my medical colleagues to study the matter without bias.

The first aspect of hydriatic procedures is the thermic one. Kneipp

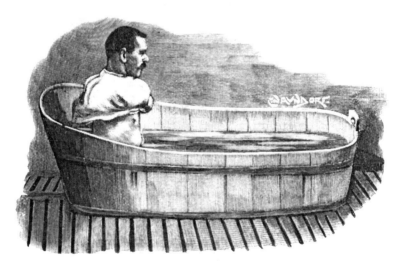

A half bath

has been wrongly accused to operate only with very low degrees of temperature. No one knew better than he how to individualize and to adapt the temperature of his procedures to the individuality, i.e., to the status of vitality of his patient. This stands in no contradiction to his principle that water temperatures of 7.5° to 10° C / 45.5° to 50° F are, in general, the most effective. This principle refers only to individuals with normal reaction, and on this ground he meets in perfect harmony with French Hydropaths. The most eminent French Hydropath, Fleury, knows only water of very low temperature, and his pupils all adopt the same principle. The German Hydropaths operate with more temperate degrees, and blame Kneipp for going too far in using rigid temperatures. They forget that Kneipp requires only five to six seconds for his half bath, while a half bath with tepid water requires several minutes to produce reaction, and demands the mechanical procedure of friction after the bath, if the patient is not to leave it in a shiver. Whereas, the reaction after a Kneipp half bath promptly ensues as soon as the patient has emerged from it. He who has tried both forms of half bath on his own person, will be sure to prefer Kneipp's, on account of the more lasting reaction.

The *apriori* assumption that the unpleasant sensation produced by a tepid half bath is less perceptible than that of a cold one, is erroneous. Experience has proved the contrary; the patient very soon gets used to the cold water and prefers it then under all circumstances to the tepid one. Kneipp's half bath, lasting only a few seconds, will produce the same effect which a tepid half bath (24° to 18 ° C / 75° to 64° F) will produce only after several minutes, and only with the help of a servant to rub the patient during the bath. This procedure of rubbing, which looks so facile to the beholder, is very often done in a perfunctory way, especially when the [masseuse] has been tired out by previous treatments. Thus it happens not infrequently, that the patient leaves the bath pale-skinned and shivering, and warms up under difficulties which the short, cold, half bath of Kneipp doesn't entail. The cold Kneipp treatment has, besides, the big advantage of simplicity. A tub and a few buckets of cold water are all the requirements, which are readily at hand in any household; whereas the tepid bath requires both hot and cold water and besides, an expert [masseuse].

Tepid half baths are, therefore, generally speaking, obtainable only in hydropathic institutions, whereas the Kneipp half bath is ready at hand for everyone, at any hour, day or night.

The opponents of Kneipp's methods insist that they deprive the body of too much warmth. This accusation, too, is wrong.

According to physiological laws, the large vessels of the skin contract after every stimulus of cold and all the more energetically, the stronger the sensation, the colder the water applied has been. After a Kneipp half bath, lasting five to ten seconds only, this spasm of the capillaries persists, after the bather has left the tub. After a while he will feel an agreeable sensation of warmth over the entire surface of his body, the reaction sets in, the contracted skin vessels expand, and the patient is no more in contact with the cold medium.

During the bath, while the main capillaries are narrowly contracted, very little blood can flow into them, and since the whole procedure lasts only a few seconds, the loss of temperature can only be a minimal one.

It is otherwise with the tepid half bath, lasting several minutes, of modern Hydrotherapy. The stimulus of cold is smaller, the contraction of the skin vessels less energetic, more blood circulates in the skin than during a cold bath, and the blood has to yield up more heat to the water. This reduction of heat is heightened by the long stay in the water, and particularly through the rubbing during the bath. The mechanical stimulus of the hand dissolves the spasm of the capillaries, the blood vessels expand during the very process of bathing. Bath and friction are continued, until the skin has become wholly red and replete with blood. In such a status the skin will lose plenty of heat, and it has been actually shown by thermometric measurement that the blood temperature had been reduced several tenths by a tepid bath. It is, therefore, potent in the matter of loss of heat that this last must be bigger after the tepid half bath in vogue with modern Hydrotherapy than after a Kneipp half bath. One great advantage the Kneipp half bath has above all others. The continued use of tepid baths will often produce furuncles [skin reactions], which annoy the patient and retard the natural progress of the cure.

The patient will be be likely to console himself with the thought that these excrescences [healing reactions] are morbid matter leaving the body. They are nothing of the kind. Those furuncles are simply the reaction of maltreated skin vessels against brutal friction. Inflammation of the skin after Kneipp procedures are out of the question.

The opponents of Kneipp think it ridiculous and harmful to don undergarments over a wet body. They imagine such a procedure to be the cause of many colds. But practice proves the contrary. Even in winter, the linen can be put on the wet body without evil after-effects. Even patients suffering from bronchitis may do so, if they only will be careful to comply with this paramount condition: to get heated at once by energetic movement. Without that, colds are inevitable, no matter how carefully the patient has dried his body after the bath. Not to dry the body after the bath has this great advantage: it strengthens and lengthens the reaction.

Through the wet covering a stimulus is exerted upon the nerves of the skin, which effects by way of reflex an expansion of the main capillaries and a strengthening of the blood influx within the periphery to further the evaporation of the damp matter. Those who wear the coarse linen appropriate for the purpose will get dry in winter by a brisk walk of 20 to 30 minutes.

The Kneipp method is furthermore charged with an exaggerated preference for douches, while modern Hydrotherapy insists upon half baths and rubbings.

It might be adduced that the French Hydropaths—who certainly are not open to the charge of unscientific laxity; as their works prove—are also laying stress upon douches as against baths. The douche, with its stronger mechanical stimulus, combined with the stimulus of the temperature of the water applied, elicits a more energetic reflex-action of the nerves controlling motion and secretion, which is the reason why the French prefer the douche.

The Kneipp *Guesse* [gush], however, are preferable to the douches of the French. The French use mostly douches over the entire surface of the body, whereas Kneipp prefers partial douches over the head, thigh, spine or knee. This procedure of Kneipp seems to me physiologically well founded.

The thermo-mechanical stimulus of the douche has a reflex effect upon the entire nervous system which is the stronger, the bigger surface touched by the stimulus. This means that a partial douche will reflect upon the entire nervous system as well as a complete one, with this difference, that the reflex action after a *Theilguss* [part gush] is milder than after a douche over the whole body. It being evidently unwise to resort to the strongest means where milder ones suffice, the partial douche of Kneipp, as a preserver of nerve force, ought to have the preference.

The ratio of blood circulating is also influenced by partial douches. They make the parts so treated richer in blood, which deflects it from other parts suffering from turgidity.

Walking barefoot has been often ridiculed by the ignorant. As a Hydropath, I confess, I would never forgo the extensive use of this procedure. To be sure, the novice must be warned against mistakes. After every barefoot promenade the clad foot must be heated by exercise. Walking barefoot, as means of restoring circulation to the nether limbs [feet], is one of the chief means of curing headaches, giddiness, cold feet and neurasthenia.

In conclusion, I wish to defend Kneipp against the baseless accusation that he uses cold temperatures regardless of individuality. With delicate individuals he proceeds by carefully graded partial washings, leading to more extensive douches and other applications at low temperature.

It is much to be desired that medical circles should treat Kneipp with the same objectivity assumed toward Priessnitz—after several years, to be sure, had demonstrated his efficiency as a healer. As regards myself,

I can't refuse myself to the conviction, that the Kneipp treatment means progress—a fact, which future science will appreciate, as it has appreciated the merits of Priessnitz.

> *Kneipp has been wrongly accused to operate only with very low degrees of temperature. No one knew better than he how to individualize and to adapt the temperature of his procedures to the individuality, i.e., to the status of vitality of his patient.*
>
> *They forget that Kneipp requires only five to six seconds for his half bath, while a half bath with tepid water requires several minutes to produce reaction, and demands the mechanical procedure of friction after the bath, if the patient is not to leave it in a shiver. Whereas the reaction after a Kneipp half bath promptly ensues as soon as the patient has emerged from it.*
>
> *A tub and a few buckets of cold water are all the requirements, which are readily at hand in any household, whereas the tepid bath requires both hot and cold water, and besides, an expert [masseuse].*
>
> *According to physiological laws, the large vessels of the skin contract after every stimulus of cold and all the more energetically, the stronger the sensation, the colder the water applied has been. After a Kneipp half bath, lasting five to ten seconds only, this spasm of the capillaries persists, after the bather has left the tub.*
>
> *Not to dry the body after the bath has this great advantage: it strengthens and lengthens the reaction.*
>
> *The French use mostly douches over the entire surface of the body, whereas Kneipp prefers partial douches over the head, thigh, spine or knee. This procedure of Kneipp seems to me physiologically well founded.*
>
> *Walking barefoot, as means of restoring circulation to the nether limbs [feet], is one of the chief means of curing headaches, giddiness, cold feet and neurasthenia.*

HYDROTHERAPY

by C. E. Judd

The Naturopath and Herald of Health, XIV (7), 411-414. (1909)

The use of water in curing disease has made for itself a large place in drugless methods of healing. Its forms of use have so multiplied that now there are hundreds of variations in its applications. A mere knowledge of all the bandages, compresses, douches, and baths does not suffice. Far better a definite knowledge concerning the most practicable applications, coupled with common sense and good judgment of character and vitality. The simplest methods, varied according to case and circumstances, will work wonders; while complex and 'multitudinous' directions, which are the more likely to be misapplied, often irritate the patient and defeat the very purpose intended.

Neither should one attempt to cure by Hydrotherapy alone, while the patient indulges in unnatural food hastily eaten, lives and works in poor light, or breathes 'second-hand' air.

Good cheer, hopefulness, and implicit faith in Nature should always be remembered and practiced as part of the cure—and no small part either.

Where there is no zeal for health, there is not much chance for recovery. Nothing should be forced, but kindness, patience, inspiration and intuition are needed in a continual supply.

Hydrotherapy's greatest advantage is that we do not, or should not, wait for developments as M.D.'s often do, but may apply at once harmless and helpful measures, often preventing any serious sickness. Yes, not even serious enough to be given a name.

In the following pages, I will attempt to describe only those methods or measures, which from my own point of view, are most valuable, yet simple and applicable to nearly all cases. Still we should not forget that even the simplest remedies are subject to variations. As the alphabet of twenty-six letters forms thousands of words, so the combination of climate, habits, work, recreation, food and clothing form any number of variations in character, person, vitality, and disability in different people. Yet, disease is nothing but the result of perverted use of Nature's gifts—light, air, water, and food—and therefore the return to natural living cures all defects.

I begin to believe that too harsh treatment and too little discrimination in character, nervous conditions, and vitality have often caused too severe crises. No doubt Friedrich Bilz had this in mind when using tempered water, and then gradually reducing it one or two degrees at each bath or douche, until quite cold water was applied without discomfort.*

The average chronic sufferer can, if he will, find health through the constant breathing of pure, fresh air, and the use of the dry friction bath, the "Just" [natural] bath, and the sun and air bath. Of course, these are to be reinforced by a simple moderate diet of foods, which do not require cooking or messing to be palatable. The simpler the regime, the better, providing it accomplishes the purpose.

The dry friction bath, being so often used in connection with water treatment, may justly be included in the realm of Hydrotherapy. It is not valued enough by most people. Alone, or just before the natural bath, or any cold application, it quite fills the 'bill' as an exciter and stimulator of the skin, preparing it for a good reaction in the bath or douche. A good Turkish bath towel, friction glove or soft bristle brushes may be used for rubbing. By trying, one soon finds the best way to rub all parts of the body till warmth is felt from the friction.

The average person finds it most convenient to take a cold bath in the morning. And this is the most natural time for a "Just" or natural bath. Water should be had for the bath four or five inches deep, so that the sexual organs are covered by the cold water when the bather sits down with his knees drawn up. The abdomen, anus and sexual organs are thoroughly rubbed and washed from one to ten minutes, according to season, climate, and person. When these parts of the body are cooled, the water is quickly splashed over the whole body as the finishing touch. The bath may be somewhat varied when circumstances make it more convenient to do so. Exercise should immediately follow or else one should return to bed and stay till warm. Never take this bath or any such water bath within one-half hour before or two hours after eating. A good and also convenient time for a cold air bath is just before retiring for the night. Let the cold fresh air play upon the skin of the entire body, from ten to thirty minutes. Contrary to popular opinion, you will not 'catch cold', but fresh air is an excellent way to cure a cold. Very few there are indeed who dare try it long enough to attain this result. A daily cold air bath would do away with most of the colds and 'grippes' [flu].

A sun and air bath of not too long duration, at first, taken before and after the natural bath, is both a pleasure and a benefit. Out of doors there is not much danger after the skin has become a little hardened. But under glass or within small enclosures, care must be taken to not expose the body too long at one time. Neither has it as good effect as when practiced out of doors.

---

*Friederich Eduard Bilz (1842-1922) wrote a colossal two volume set, *Natural Methods of Healing* (1898) that provided guidance for the early Naturopaths. —Ed.

Before going farther it may be well to note a few of the dangers of water treatment when incorrectly applied.

As all disease consists of more or less fever or inflammation: control of the circulation and reduction of excessive heat are the first things essential. Therefore, to an intensely fevered organ or body, a stimulating [cold] pack or compress, or any stimulating or heating application should not be applied, for less heat is the object, not more. Such treatment should be applied where heat is lacking, while tepid, (lukewarm) or cooling packs but a few degrees lower than the temperature of the body should be placed where fever is highest.

In chronic affections, stimulating treatment is often given direct to that diseased organ or spot. If too much inflamed for that, the soothing or cooling compresses are applied, while the stimulating or warming treatment—douche, pack, or bath—is given to parts, most distant from the inflammation for derivative purpose.

Stimulating packs or compresses are changed or removed, when they become uncomfortable. Soothing or cooling compresses or packs are renewed as soon as warm and repeated, till fever or inflammation is reduced.

Never give a cold or cool bath or pack when the patient is not comfortably warm. Warmth must first be restored by exercise, friction or steam bath. Persons of low vitality or poor blood cannot respond too readily to cold water treatment; hence the treatment should be tempered to suit patient and circumstances.

Gushes applied to any part or whole of body should not be applied with a careless hand, lest the good effect be lost.

Hot baths and compresses are relaxing, and therefore are used to relieve pain and cramps, to induce perspiration, to cleanse, and often to prepare a patient for cold or stimulating treatment. As a rule, all hot water or steam applications should be followed by a cold ablution, wet rubbing or douche, lest the patient be weakened by the relaxing bath. The rotation is generally given as follows: warm application first, stimulating pack or compress second, and cold ablution or wet rubbing last.

A most profitable method of using water is the internal bath, which is neglected by most people and overused by others. By the internal bath, I mean the thoroughly flushing of the whole colon, the water being discharged through a flexible rectal tube, reaching the sigmoid flexure. Thus, the water is applied where most needed, and without ballooning the rectum. During a fast, or in acute disease such as typhoid, diphtheria, appendicitis, etc., its value can hardly be overestimated. But do not by any means depend upon it in the place of the natural bath, exercise, and the natural diet.

Two or four quarts of warm water are used in a full internal bath.

Herbs are sometimes steeped in the water, thus furthering its effects. After the water is ejected from the bowel, one pint to one quart of cold water is introduced, the effect being similar to any other cold bath after a warm bath.

Bilz recommends simple stimulating of the muscles and nerves of the lower bowel by injecting from one-fourth to one full cup of cold water and retaining. I hardly think this is very thorough in cleansing the colon. But it has the advantage of not weakening the patient and can be repeated until feces are moved.

In fevers, the cooling internal bath followed by the introduction of olive oil is a great aid in checking inflammation. Thousands of cases of appendicitis might have been cured by this same method.

For building up vital power and toning the nervous system, Bernarr Macfadden recommends stimulating the nerve centers along the spinal column. I call this a hot towel treatment, combined with exercise. So far, through numerous trials, I have found only good results.

It is best performed by an assistant, although the patient may be able to do it for himself. He should lie face down upon a bed or couch, while the assistant applies the hot towel to whole length of spinal column. The towel is first folded lengthwise four or five inches wide, wrung from very hot water and then laid upon the spine as hot as can be borne. While this is held in place, movements are made, which vigorously exercise the muscles lying close to the spine. Arm and head movements are also made, acting upon cervical and upper dorsal regions. After the back is treated, the towel is applied in similar manner to the abdomen.

One should remember to wring the towel from the boiling hot water two or three times, while exercising the spinal muscles, and also when using the abdominal muscles, which affects the abdominal plexuses. The theory of the treatments is that the rapid circulation of blood, thus induced, supplies extra nourishment to these nerve centres. Better fed nerve centers mean better action of the nervous functions, hence a better control of life's vital processes.

In acute disease, there is necessarily, no great difference in the treatment—the primary essentials being to induce a normal flow of the blood and the activity of the skin and all other eliminative organs. Of course, fresh pure air is always essential and light also.

The following method may be used successfully in nearly all acute diseases; surprising though it may be to the average physician.

First: Absolutely no food allowed, neither liquid nor solid.

Second: Every few minutes while awake, the patient must drink a swallow of water, either hot or cold, according to taste. Lemon may be added to the water if desired, but no sugar.

Third: Once each day give a full hot pack—as hot as can be borne—to be removed after forty to sixty minutes. In fevers, soothing or cooling packs are used instead, and renewed as often as they get warm until fever is reduced.

Fourth: If constipated, give internal bath, using two to four quarts of water. Repeat once in two days, if constipation continues. If taken more often it weakens the patient.

Fifth: After crisis, and not before—that is when normal pulse and normal temperature have returned, give, if desired, one or two glasses of fruit juice, such as orange juice, pineapple juice, or sweet cider.

When able to walk around, one or two glasses of milk may be taken, the amount being increased as strength is gained.

If patient is inclined to walk or exercise, let him. Moderate movements of the body seems to aid the natural functions even in acute disease.

Sun and air baths, as a matter of course, should be made one of the main features of this simple treatment. If handled in this manner, disease fulfills its mission as house cleaner and the patient is left purer in body and brain than he was before. From this no one need infer that disease is necessary for cleansing the body, for it is far better to get and keep so clean that there is no excuse for a sudden and severe house cleaning. Such cleanliness can be gained through the right use of Nature's own light, air, water and food.

A mere knowledge of all the bandages, compresses, douches, and baths does not suffice. Far better a definite knowledge concerning the most practicable applications, coupled with common sense and good judgment of character and vitality.

Yet disease is nothing but the result of perverted use of Nature's gifts—light, air, water, and food—and therefore the return to natural living cures all defects.

The average chronic sufferer can, if he will, find health through the constant breathing of pure, fresh air, and the use of the dry friction bath, the "Just" [natural] bath, and the sun and air bath.

The dry friction bath, being so often used in connection with water treatment, may justly be included in the realm of Hydrotherapy. It is not valued enough by most people. Alone, or just before the natural bath, or any cold application, it quite fills the 'bill' as an exciter and stimulator of the skin, preparing it for a good reaction in the bath or douche.

The average person finds it most convenient to take a cold bath in the morning. And this is the most natural time for a "Just" or natural bath. Water should be had for the bath four or five inches deep, so that the sexual organs are covered by the cold water when the bather sits down with his knees drawn up.

Never take this [natural] bath or any such water bath within one-half hour before or two hours after eating.

As all disease consists of more or less fever or inflammation: control of the circulation and reduction of excessive heat are the first things essential.

Never give a cold or cool bath or pack when the patient is not comfortably warm. Warmth must first be restored by exercise, friction or steam bath.

Hot baths and compresses are relaxing, and therefore are used to relieve pain and cramps; to induce perspiration, to cleanse and often to prepare a patient for cold, or stimulating treatment. As a rule, all hot water or steam applications should be followed by a cold ablution, wet rubbing or douche, lest the patient be weakened by the relaxing bath.

For building up vital power and toning the nervous system, Bernarr Macfadden recommends stimulating of the nerve centers along the spinal column. I call this a hot towel treatment, combined with exercise.

In acute disease, there is necessarily, no great difference in the treatment—the primary essentials being to induce a normal flow of the blood and the activity of the skin and all other eliminative organs.

KNEIPP'S COLD WATER DOUCHES

by Sebastian Kneipp

The Naturopath and Herald of Health, XIV (8), 492-499. (1909)

THE ARM DOUCHE

The arm douche consists in douching the whole arm beginning with the fingers, every one of which must be douched, and continuing up to the shoulder, and the whole process must not take more than a minute. It is generally employed when powerlessness of the arm sets in, caused either by paralysis or any like trouble; or when the arm is very feeble and abnormally cold, or in rheumatism of the arm. In writers' cramp and neuralgia, generally it is a most excellent remedy. It may be taken every day, and in exceptional cases twice a day.

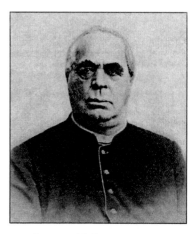

Reverend Sebastian Kneipp
[1821-1897]

THE UPPER DOUCHE

In administering an upper douche one must take into consideration the parts of the body which will be subject to its action. These are the heart, the lungs, the bronchial tubes and the vocal cords. This being so, one must be advised whether the douche is to be weak or strong, or even at first, whether it may be given at all. For example, in case of lung disease it would not be wise to begin with the upper douche, but to substitute for a time washing the upper part of the body morning and evening with cold water and to increase the action by mixing vinegar with the water. I advise the same for one who has palpitation or

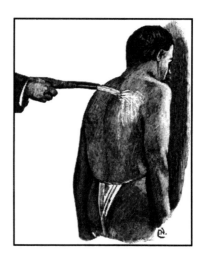

An upper gush using a hose

any other disease of the heart; otherwise it may be safely administered in all cases. A weak upper douche is not much stronger or very different to a washing. Should a few days' trial of the upper washing prove a success, then the upper douche may follow, which will gradually strengthen the patient. This advice must be strictly followed in heart troubles. As this special douche has so much effect upon the organs of the chest it is of the highest importance it should be rightly administered.

It should be applied by beginning from the neck down one-half of the back. The water, which may be given either from a hose or a water can, should spread evenly like a sheet over the back. Whether the water come from can or hose does not really matter, although I personally prefer the can, because with it the stream can be more easily regulated, and increased or diminished, at pleasure. For a weak upper douche one uses an ordinary garden hose containing three or four gallons of water.* For a powerful upper douche, double the quantity. Where the patients have taken several douches and with them have made great progress, three or four hose or cans may be used, and for a very hardy person even six, seven, and eight. If a sick person bears the upper douche well, its power may be gradually increased. If the upper part of the body is weak, one begins gently with the left or right arm, coming gradually from one side to the other with the water till the loins are reached. There is generally at the right or left side of the lower part of the back a point from which the water more easily covers the back, and flows equally, looking as if covered with a sheet.

Before taking an upper douche, the upper part of the body should be quite warm, and as soon as it is over the shirt or chemise must go on as quickly as possible, followed by the remaining articles of clothing without drying the body in the very least. After the body is covered, the neck and hair, if they have become wet, should be made dry, and exercise taken till the whole body has recovered its normal warmth.

The Hip Douche

As the upper douche principally affects the upper part of the body, so the hip douche affects the lower part of it. It is a continuation of the knee douche, and exercises its influence particularly upon the kidneys, the liver and bladder and upon all parts of the abdomen. It regulates the blood in the lower part of the body and has great curative power in case of piles.

The method of administering it is as follows: take either a water can or a hose and begin to pour the water at the back part of the feet and bring it up very slowly and gradually till the knee is reached; then over the hip halfway to the back. With beginners one always commences from the feet, gradually getting the stream higher. One does it in the same way with

---

*To establish the equivalence of three or four gallons of water when using water running from a hose, one must experiment to determine the length of time required. —Ed.

people who suffer from continued cold feet, in order that the blood should rapidly find its way to them, for where the water first falls that part is the soonest warmed. We say emphatically that the douching from below to above must be conducted very slowly. If it is begun at the hip, douche first one and then the other rapidly, and this may be done three or four times. What we said about the upper douche we repeat here, that the water must flow equally over the hip so that it looks as though covered with a sheet of glass. He who gives the douche without method and is content if the water is poured over the hip anyhow will neither douche the hips properly nor procure warmth to the feet.

When four or five douches have been taken from the feet upward there is no harm in beginning from the hip, because the blood is now in better order. Those which strengthen the most are those which are given from the upper part of the hip, the water flowing to the feet.

For the hip douche one uses from six to ten cans or hose full of water, containing about four gallons. For a weak person one can is enough at first, then later two or three, and if the effect of these is good the amount can be increased. If the body is in good condition and able to bear the action of these douches on the abdomen, three or four cans of water may be used, and in cases where special force is required five or six cans or hose. I have sometimes used as many as ten when it has been very desirable to reduce corpulence.

While the knee douche acts beneficially upon part of the abdomen as well as upon the feet, so the hip douche benefits all parts of the abdomen. The hip douche is beyond comparison the best for acting on the kidneys; its effect is not only to strengthen, but to dissolve and disperse. One sees this from the urine, which becomes thick and dark when the kidneys are out of order.

Nor is it less beneficial on the bladder, the liver, and indeed on all parts of the abdomen, the organs of which are in combination with the upper part of the body; therefore, we may say it strengthens the whole body.

A girl suffered so much from headache that she was compelled to keep her bed, and every remedy she applied seemed to increase the suffering. In order to free her from pain, I prescribed a powerful hip douche, the result being that in a short time the headache disappeared and she was able to get a few hours' sleep. Evidently in this case the cause of the headache was stomach trouble, and this being removed by the hip douche she obtained relief.

A man named Jacob suffered intensely from cramps in the feet. I prescribed hip douches, back douches and half baths, and by these he was completely cured, though I think the most effective was the hip douche.

As the hip douche is easy to take and as the abdomen, and indeed, the whole system, can bear it well, it may be taken two, three, or four times a week, according to the strength of the patient.

THE KNEE DOUCHE

As the heading shows, this douche is applied from below to above the knee and is a reinforcement of the foot bath. One begins at the instep, covers the foot and continues the stream upward to above the knee. For weak people it will be enough at first to use one can or hose of water for both knees, while for those who are strong two, three, or four may be poured on.

The more carefully this douche is administered, the more often it may be taken. Like a strong foot bath its special object is to attract the blood to the feet, to increase the normal warmth, and to brace and strengthen the whole body.

Those who suffer constantly from cold feet may take the knee douche frequently, two or three times a week, for example: those who are weak and delicate may use this douche with advantage, as its chief property is to strengthen. It is of great benefit in urinary trouble, diseases of the stomach and kidney, and in removing headaches which are caused by too much blood in the head; and even sore throats are relieved by this douche, because of its power to strengthen and draw blood downward.

It is quite as important here as in other douches how the water is poured over the knee and foot. The water must flow evenly and smoothly down and over the foot. If it be asked, why must it be poured with so much regularity, and why cannot it be thrown onto the body? The answer is that during the time the water is flowing over the body all the warmth which otherwise would evaporate is held back and develops an increased warmth under the water, which combats with the cold pressed in by the water.

Thus, the warmth gains a quicker and surer victory over the cold; or in other words, the reaction will set in sooner; the more regularly and quietly the water is poured, the greater will be the warmth retained. If, on the other hand, the water is carelessly poured on, the chance is there will be no possibility of developing the necessary warmth, and the cold will so gain the mastery that it will be most difficult to get warmth back to the body.

Therefore, I maintain that the more regularly and quietly the water flows over the body, the greater the chance of obtaining and retaining the desirable warmth.

THE BACK DOUCHE

I once saw a cat spring leisurely up into a tree. She did it so easily that one thought it must be her usual way. I believe she did it out of pure

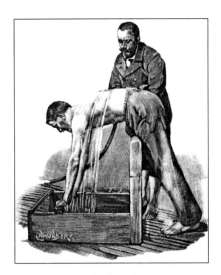

A back gush

pleasure. As she alighted on a branch she settled herself quietly on it, and from her elevated position looked about.

This picture of the cat reminded me of the back douche. The question is, how is it to be given? Exactly as the cat climbed into the tree. She began from below, stuck her claws in right and left and so mounted slowly.

Just so the back douche commences from below and is directed gradually upward till the water flows in a gentle even stream over the shoulders. This last point, as we have remarked, is important in all the douches, but perhaps in none so important as in the back douche.

Many dislike this douche, complaining that it gives them headache and makes them restless. If this be so, there has, without doubt, been some fault in administering it! This is why I prefer a watering can, because the person who applies the douche can do so with a freer hand and guide the flow so that it spreads evenly and broadly over the whole back.

To administer the back douche properly one proceeds as follows: commence from below and on getting to the middle of the back go upward till you get above the shoulder. When the watering can approaches the back it forms a sheet of water which spreads itself over half the back. When the water is poured from the middle of the back upwards, it does not matter which side is first douched, whether right or left, so long as the water flows quietly and uninterruptedly over the whole surface. When both sides have been douched, one can direct the water either up or down the middle of the back—the more quietly and uninterruptedly the water flows over the middle and both sides of the back the better. It is a great fault when the back douche is turned into a spraying douche, and when the stream is poured on to the back from a distance of a quarter or half a yard, or when the water is thrown superficially on the surface, as if it did not matter at all as long as the water fell out of the can on to the back somehow.

A patient complained to me that he could not endure the back douche. It made him so nervous and excitable and gave him so much headache that he could not sleep at night. He begged of me that I would give him this douche myself. I did so, and the next morning he could not speak too highly of the benefit it had been to him.

The chief point to observe is, and I repeat it again and again, to pour the water gently and regularly over the back. If this be not done there can be no good result.

In administering a back douche to a weak and nervous person, one can is enough at first. As the patient gets accustomed to it, two or three may be given containing about four gallons of water, and as the condition of the patient improves, the number of cans may be still further increased to six or seven.

For a long time I continued to give back douches to a bishop. Overall, I gave him ten or twelve cans. This was an exceptional case, and I certainly should not recommend it at any time. He laughed and said I should get tired of applying the douche long before he would get weary of receiving it.

When the patient has taken several of these douches the beginning may be made from above instead of below, because the circulation is regular.

You will scarcely find another douche which will raise and increase the heat as quickly as the back douche. While the water pours over the back, the warmth concentrates itself within and gradually appears on the surface so that in a very short time the patient feels great benefit. Scarcely has he received the douche than a gentle glow is felt on the skin and one knows that there is an increase of warmth. One has seen the same effect from wading in the water. At first, on stepping in, one experiences a cutting cold, followed almost immediately by an agreeable warmth, and just as one puts on a dress directly on coming out of the water without drying the body so one does the moment after taking the back douche.

I know of no douche so generally strengthening as the back douche; its effects are excellent. It is of the greatest service in regulating the circulation of the blood and in dissolving and dispersing obstructions in the blood and secretions. It braces and strengthens the lower part of the body, in that it disperses gases, and works upon the liver and kidneys. Its effect is also very good upon the breast, and indeed upon the whole body, which it warms and strengthens and purifies.

As the effect of this douche is so excellent, people will naturally think they cannot take it too often. My answer is: "All good results come slowly; and the excessive use of a remedy, be it ever so good, is productive of evil." To expect to remove all obstructions of blood or secretions at once is unreasonable, and strength can be reinstated only by degrees.

In some cases, however, the back douche may be given oftener than in others. For example, to a strong, healthy, and too well-fed brewer who wished to reduce his corpulence I prescribed one every other day, and then one every day, and he was pleased with the result. In most cases, however, it must be taken in combination with other douches once or twice a week only, and then for a very short time.

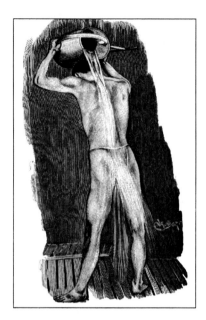

A self-administered full gush or douche

THE FULL DOUCHE

People generally think that the full douche is the most difficult to take of all the douches and the least easy for the body to endure, whereas the opposite is the case.

My great rule is to treat the system gently, and this is why I prescribe all the douches of the shortest duration. The number of small douches are proofs that one need not begin with the full douche—indeed, it is by these that Nature is prepared and braced to take the full douche. This last is to the series what the mantle is to the articles of dress, the completion of the set. One does not take the full douche until the system is prepared for it by first taking the knee douche, the hip douche, the upper douche, the back douche, and the half bath. This douche is merely a higher development of the douches, and almost without exception those who have enjoyed it once desire it again. It is clear that when all parts of the body have been prepared and strengthened, the full douche comes in with the greatest benefit to the whole body. In taking this, as other douches, the body must be thoroughly warm, and unless it be so, on no account must the douche be taken. Indeed, the very best time to take it is in full perspiration.

One begins the full douche from the heels upward to the hips, then over the whole back to the shoulders, over which the water must flow backward and forward, as evenly as possible, over the whole body. Or one may begin at the shoulders, pouring the water first over the back and then over the front of the body. It is quite immaterial whether a hose or a water can be used, the great point being that the water must flow evenly on both sides of the body; and the greater the regularity and gentleness of this process, the more successful will be the effect on the sick man.

In administering a full douche to a hunchback, or a corpulent person, be careful to pour a sufficient amount of water on the enlarged parts. By placing the patient in a somewhat forward position this may be done quite easily, without neglecting the even flow over the whole body. I say again, the more regularly the water flows, so much the more will the body be benefited. It must not be supposed that spraying or wetting the body in all sorts of ways, whether with a hose or a water can, is a full douche.

It must be administered according to the instructions or it is no full douche. When the body has been prepared by other applications for the reception of the full douche, as many as eight or even ten cans of water may be used at one time. For a very weak person one would begin with one or two cans of water, but as his strength increases he will not be content with less than eight or ten and sometimes a patient asks for twelve.

For the robust and those who wish to reduce their corpulency, I have not only used hose and water cans, but large pails, from which the water falls like a cascade. Sometimes, although not necessary, but by desire of the patients, I have given as many as twenty pails. This, however, is an exception and can only be allowed to a strong person who has too fat or too sleepy a body.

I have often administered the full douche in another way. The patient kneels in a large bath and bends slightly forward. A very light full douche is first administered, and then comes the pail, and the water is dashed over the entire body. This is more or less an amusement, but the patient gradually comes to prefer it. Such a douche is the strongest proof of the power of water to strengthen and harden the human body. When an invalid is so far improved as to be able to take a full douche, it is the best indication of renewed life. If in administering this douche to the strong and healthy the utmost care and caution is to be exercised, the necessity for care is double when given to a weak or delicate person.

A consumptive person came to me from Würtzburg, having been given up by all the doctors, and said that if I could give him no hope he would bear his fate and try nothing more. He did not look so very ill and he had at least muscles.

During four weeks he took daily two small douches, then heavier ones; then followed a back douche, very gently given, and then, as a continuation, a short full douche, applied upwards to the shoulders, from which the water fell over the front of the body. This douche did him much good, although he shuddered at first; he was not quite dressed when he exclaimed, "This has done me most good of all!" The application was repeated every two or three days, and he assured me he gained more strength and warmth by this application than by any other. The full douche is no tyrant! It may appear so to the weak or effeminate, but to those who have become by its means strengthened and cured it is the conclusion of the cure.

I never prescribe a remedy that I have not personally tried, so I gave myself the full douche. I took a can of water, held it high with both hands, and turned it over my chest, the water running from spout and top quite evenly over the front of the body. Then I bent the head forward, and taking a second can poured it from my neck over the back, first on one shoulder and then on another, and continued the process till I have used four cans.

The full douche is often given to children. It is applied simply from the heels upwards to the shoulders, from which points the water flows over the whole body, the front receiving as much water as the back. At first one can of water is sufficient for the whole body; then two, one for each side. Children like this douche quite as much as adults do. After having other douches they like the full one best of all, which is a proof that they gain health and strength by it.

The full douche is generally used in combination with other applications once or twice a week. Where a general strengthening of the body is required, it may be given three times a week. It must not be given to nervous or weak children quite so often, once or twice a week being sufficient.

The name full douche is very appropriate, for its effects are general and complete. Its special work is to increase the normal warmth of the body, strengthen the whole system and regulate the circulation of the blood.

As to the time of taking this douche it is immaterial; it can be taken in the early morning or before the midday meal; if in the afternoon it will be better to let two hours pass by after the meal. In the winter it will be better to take before and not after four, in the summer not after six o'clock.

In taking the full douche it is better not to wet the head, especially if the hair is thick and long, for fear of neuralgia and headaches. If, however, the temperature is warm and the hair neither thick nor heavy, there will be no danger; but it must be rubbed thoroughly dry or harm may come of it.

THE LIGHTNING DOUCHE

Looking at the Parish Church of Wörishofen today, one would scarcely credit it the deplorable condition it was in when I first took charge of the Parish. The walls were wet and stained, even up to the roof, and looked as though they had stood partly in water and collected all the mud and dirt round about. They were not only wet through but thoroughly rotten, and if one leaned against them one displaced the plaster.

In order to remove the decay and prevent the dampness from extending, I sent for six masons to investigate and remove the rottenness of the walls, even if they had to penetrate to the stone. So they went to work with their picks, and the rotten plaster fell like rain on the floor. This being fully done, the inner walls were found to be sound and dry. They had evidently had three layers of plaster on them, none of which had been dry. The church was not well ventilated, and during the service it was crowded with people and full of a hazy mist that settled in the walls.

When the masons had exposed the walls, we had a thin plaster laid on, made of the best materials, and today they are perfectly free of damp and there is no lack of fresh air or proper ventilation in the church.

This picture of my church represents to my mind the conditions of a man who carries about with him fifty or sixty pounds of flesh without being able to get rid of it; and the result is a weariness and a hindrance to him. And yet this burden can easily be taken away.

There came to me one day a gentleman who weighed three hundred and fifty pounds. He told me he greatly desired to be free of some of this heavy burden. I applied to him all the douches—the hip, the back, the half bath, and the full douche, and being by this time quite accustomed to the water I gave him the lightning douche. This worked upon the man exactly as the mason's pick had acted upon the walls of my church.

To give the lightning douche correctly, one begins at the heel of the right foot and works slowly upwards till the whole of the back is douched, and this process is repeated for the front of the body. In the meantime a comfortable heat is developed and the sick person is so relieved that he says "I feel new born." If you wish to know something of the effect of the lightning douche go and look at a burning building. In order to quench the flames a hose is directed to them and with such force that the burning wall is sometimes thrown in and the fire is smothered.

In the same way through a hose the water is directed like lightning over the body, beginning either from above or below. This lightning-like stream, although it takes good strong hold, is by no means painful, but as one can see, it drives out everything from the system that is superfluous or harmful. It reminds one of beating a coat or carpet with a stick; the dust is all driven out, but the coat and the carpet remain intact.

In giving the lightning douche the distance of the hose from the patient is from three to five yards, according to the force desired for the jet, and the application may last from three to eight minutes. First a full sharp douche is given, then the finger is placed across the opening so that the stream is broken and a rapid spray dashes against the body like a rainstorm against a window. The opening of the hose should be only large enough to hold a lead pencil, and that the system may be treated as gently as possible the stream should not be too strong. The effects of the lightning douche are as follows: increased warmth, improved appearance, lighter breathing, better appetite, free expectoration, an unusual amount of and deposit in the urine, at which last symptom many are needlessly alarmed.

According to the condition of the patient the lightning douche may be applied every second day, every day, or even twice a day.

I am radically opposed to massage, which has been introduced by the allopathic practitioners. Many patients have come to me complaining not only of pains but of injuries resulting from it. The pressure, rubbing, and squeezing may very easily burst the vessels and liberate the blood from the smaller veins, producing serious disturbances. A patient came to me with more than fifty ulcers produced by inflammation of the blood and secretions, the result of a course of massage. In its stead, I recommend with a good conscience the lightning douche, and affirm that it will not only replace but surpass the former in good effects. This douche hammers and beats upon the body, removing everything which is not made fast.

Everyone knows that the body of the corpulent person is porous and spongy, and it is equally clear that the porous matter can easily be dispersed. The cold water draws all the dispersed matter together and causes it to escape either by perspiration or through the urine. It is precisely those who are corpulent who have weak organs. Too much blood is formed, and this leaves a deposit in the system just as a thick smoke leaves a deposit of soot in the chimney through which it passes. A proof that this is so, is the heavy breathing and gait and the tendency to be easily fatigued. A double or triple layer is formed in the inside like the plaster on the walls of my church and must be got rid of.

An Austrian official lost seventy-three pounds after a somewhat long course of treatment. When he first came, he could scarcely breathe, he was in low spirits and could with difficulty drag his weight about. The lightning douche relieved him of these troubles—he looked fresh, healthy and young; his breathing became easy, he could walk without fatigue and resumed his official duties which he had been about to give up. He had previously tried many remedies and the doctors had prescribed rigid dieting, which came hard upon him, and although the amount of nourishment he took was reduced, it did not reduce his size and weight.

He looked quite extraordinary in his clothes, and when one day he showed me his trousers I jokingly remarked that really in the need of dwellings nowadays he could allow a tailor a lodging in them.

I advised him strongly not to change anything in his way of living, which I knew to be temperate. His corpulence was due to a too great formation of blood, which built up a porous spongy mass, and also to his vocation, which conduced to obstructions in the system.

It is because a sudden and entire change of diet has often an injurious effect upon the system that I am distinctly opposed to it.

Just as in the world there is nothing good that does not meet with more or less opposition, so with the lightning douche, the working of which has been falsely judged and in heart disease has been declared dangerous.

Even my own physician objected to this douche as dangerous in this disease. I maintained the contrary opinion, always supposing it to be given in the proper way.

But when a man will not believe in a remedy, be he Thomas or a Doctor, he will not accept it. We made many trials of the lightning douche; we counted the pulse of the patient before, during and after the douche and then came the surprise. The result of this so-called torture was in my favor, and even the unbelieving doctors were convinced.

A young priest who, on account of disease of the heart (*insufficientia valvula mitralis*), could not advance in his profession, and took lightning douches. The first day, before taking the douche, his pulse was 108—after it, it was not more than 80.

The doctors thought that some mistake had been made and still would not believe in its power. The next day another lightning douche was administered to the young man. Previous to his taking it the pulse was 120—afterwards it was 88.

He himself felt extremely well and unexcited and declared: "There is nothing the matter with me; I have not felt so well and comfortable for years."

(Extracts from Kneipp's book *My Will, a Legacy for the Healthy and the Sick*. Price, 85 cents. For sale by the Kneipp Store, 133 E. 59th Street, New York.)

[The arm douche] is generally employed when powerlessness of the arm sets in, caused either by paralysis or any like trouble; or when the arm is very feeble and abnormally cold, or in rheumatism of the arm. In writers' cramp and neuralgia generally it is a most excellent remedy. It may be taken every day, and in exceptional cases twice a day.

The water, which may be given either from a hose or a water can, should spread evenly like a sheet over the back.

With beginners one always commences from the feet, gradually getting the stream higher—one does it in the same way with people who suffer from continued cold feet, in order that the blood should rapidly find its way to them, for where the water first falls that part is the soonest warmed.

What we said about the upper douche we repeat here, that the water must flow equally over the hip so that it looks as though covered with a sheet of glass.

While the knee douche acts beneficially upon part of the abdomen, as well as upon the feet, so the hip douche benefits all parts of the abdomen. The hip douche is beyond comparison the best for acting on the kidneys; its effect is not only to strengthen, but to dissolve and disperse.

Those who suffer constantly from cold feet may take the knee douche frequently, two or three times a week, for example: those who are weak and delicate may use this douche with advantage, as its chief property is to strengthen.

Many dislike this [the back] douche, complaining that it gives them headache and makes them restless. If this be so, there has, without doubt, been some fault in administering it! This is why I prefer a watering can, because the person who applies the douche can do so with a freer hand and guide the flow so that it spreads evenly and broadly over the whole back.

My great rule is to treat the system gently, and this is why I prescribe all the douches of the shortest duration.

One does not take the full douche until the system is prepared for it by first taking the knee douche, the hip douche, the upper douche, the back douche, and the half bath.

The full douche is often given to children. It is applied simply from the heels upwards to the shoulders, from which points the water flows over the whole body, the front receiving as much water as the back. At first one can of water is sufficient for the whole body; then two, one for each side.

The name full douche is very appropriate, for its effects are general and complete. Its special work is to increase the normal warmth of the body, strengthen the whole system and regulate the circulation of the blood.

1910

The Treatment Of Acute Diseases
Benedict Lust

—·—

The Water Cure In Gay Paris
Robert Biéri, N.D.

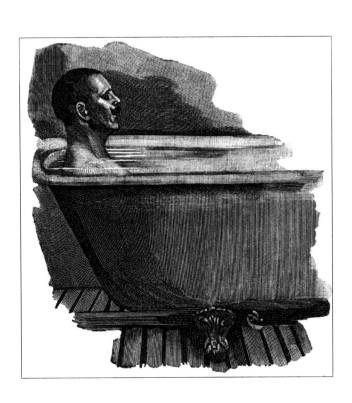

The Treatment Of Acute Diseases

by Benedict Lust

The Naturopath and Herald of Health, XV (2), 85-86. (1910)

Whatever the acute conditions may be—a simple cold, measles, typhoid fever or smallpox—the following treatments applied singly, combined or alternating, in accordance with individual conditions, will always be in order.

The Cold Bath

Cold baths or when the patient is too weak to leave his bed, cold sponge baths, repeated whenever indicated by the rise of temperature, are very beneficial for reducing temperature, relieving congestion and for stimulating elimination through the skin. Care, however, must be taken not to lower the temperature too much by the coldness or duration of the application.

Do not forget that we can suppress a fever or inflammation just as easily by cold water or ice bags as by drugs; we never, under any circumstances, use ice bags or ice water, but only water of natural temperature, as it comes from well or hydrant.

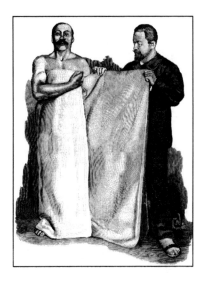

The first layer of the wet sheet wrap or pack is a wet sheet.

Never, by means of cold baths, ablutions, sponges, wet packs, etc., suppress the fever temperature but merely lower it below the danger point. For instance, if the fever has a tendency to rise to 104° F/40° C or more, we never lower it below 101° or 102° F / 38° or 39° C. If the fever runs at a lower temperature, or if the temperature is abnormal, that is, below the regular body temperature, then the packs are made more warming and are left on the body longer before changing. Never lose sight of the fact that fever itself is a healing, cleansing process.

Whole Body Pack

Spread out on a bed one or more blankets. Cover the top blanket with a linen sheet dipped into cold water and wrung out moderately, then

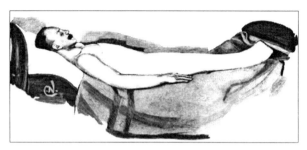

The second layer is the dry blankets

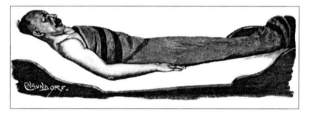

The blankets are wrapped snuggly and quickly to prevent air exposure

let the patient lie down on the wet sheet (the neck above the sheet) and tuck the wet sheet snugly around him, covering every part of the body, including the parts between the arms and body, and between the legs. Then wrap the dry blankets, one by one, tightly around the wet sheet and secure them with safety pins.

The patient stays in this whole body pack from one-half to two hours, according to his power of reaction and endurance. All packs must be adjusted in such a manner that the patient becomes warm within a few minutes. When the pack is taken off, follow with cold bath or towel rub, or if the patient cannot leave the bed, sponge the body, part by part, with cold water. Cover the parts as soon as sponged in order to prevent chilling.

Short Body Packs

The short body pack is applied in a similar manner. One, two or more layers of cold wet linen or muslin are wrapped around the body from under the armpits to the thighs or knees. This wet pack is surrounded by one or more layers of dry flannel, woolen or linen bandages.

Similar wet packs or bandages may be applied to the legs, arms, and throat or to any other part of the body.

The amount of wet linen and dry flannel covering is to be governed by the height of the temperature, the strength of the patient, and the main object of the application.

1) To lower high temperature.

2) To raise the temperature when sub-normal.

3) To promote elimination.

If the object is to lower high temperature, one, two or three layers of wet linens may be wrapped around the body, only loosely, covered by flannel, woolen or linen wrappers in order to protect the bed from becoming wet. For this last purpose, it is also well to spread an oilcloth sheet over the mattress. The packs must be removed as soon as they become hot or dry.

For the purpose is to raise subnormal body temperatures and to promote elimination, less linen and less woolen blankets are used. In cases of exceptionally stubborn constipation, an injection of a few ounces of warm olive oil may be given. Allow this to remain 15 minutes in order to soften the contents of the rectum. Follow with a warm water injection.

Cold baths or when the patient is too weak to leave his bed, cold sponge baths, repeated whenever indicated by the rise of temperature, are very beneficial for reducing temperature, relieving congestion and for stimulating elimination through the skin.

Do not forget that we can suppress a fever or inflammation just as easily by cold water or ice bags as by drugs; we never, under any circumstances, use ice bags or ice water, but only water of natural temperature, as it comes from well or hydrant.

Never, by means of cold baths, ablutions, sponges, wet packs, etc., suppress the fever temperature but merely lower it below the danger point. For instance, if the fever has a tendency to rise to 104° F / 40° C or more, we never lower it below 101° or 102° F / 38° or 39° C.

The patient stays in this whole body pack from one-half to two hours, according to his power of reaction and endurance. All packs must be adjusted in such a manner that the patient becomes warm within a few minutes.

The amount of wet linen and dry flannel covering is to be governed by the height of the temperature, the strength of the patient, and the main object of the application.

The Water Cure In Gay Paris

by Robert Biéri, N.D.

The Naturopath and Herald of Health, XV (9), 517-521. (1910)

Impressions Of A Live Wire Naturopath In The French Metropolis

It is difficult to understand why the notion has gained ground with Americans that the Parisian has no "goût" for serious matters. Of course, the idea has limits, and no intelligent person in the entire United States would dispute that Paris is not a centre for great learning, science and culture. Still, the dominating belief is that the French are very gay, the Parisian frivolous, and that they would much prefer to die than to imitate, say, the Germans.

As a rule, they are more imitated than any nation in the world, because they are clever and original. When, however, the bugle call sounds for humanity's sake, to cure the sick, to feed the poor, and console the distressed, then the gay Parisian hurries home from the boulevards and rushes to the spot where his services are required.

It is then immaterial to him to use anything at all, as long as it serves his purpose, and because the French have their pose, and because the French have their hearts in the right spot, they have wisely followed the Germans in the Water Cure and have improved it.

Here are observations made by Dr. Beni-Barde, practicing Hydropathy for the last fifty years in Paris. I am quite enthusiastic in presenting to our readers this splendid treatise on Hydrotherapy.

A master mind like Dr. Beni-Barde hates to give us anything but what would prove useful to our science and to suffering humanity. One need only read ten minutes in his works, to realize that there is an authority whose keen philosophical insight, whose learning is exceeded only by his love for his suffering fellow-man.

He has great sympathy for every physician who is discouraged and urges us to the conviction that, after all, medicine and therapeutics for science's sake are worthless; that our profession derives its splendor and glory from the fact that above all else, it is humanitarian in character.

Cold Douche

Action and Reaction

Cold and hot water, used separately or combined with one another in well-defined proportions, are the principal factors of the hydrotherapic method. In addition to these, there are also processes for the production of heat and perspiration, vapor baths, which are extremely serviceable auxiliaries.

Cold water, which may be utilized in the form of ablutions, affusions, compresses or abdominal bandages, or which may be applied by the aid of moist cloths, and especially by the douche, occupies the predominant place in this method.

The cold douche exerts on all parts of the organism a physical and dynamical action.

The first is generally due to the simple contact of the cold water with the external or internal integuments. The second has its origin in an impression set up at the surface of the body. This impression is transported by the sensory nerves to their nervous centres, which they leave again immediately after having been transformed, and regain by the aid of the motor nerves the regions in which they originated, inducing along their whole course dynamogenic or inhibitory reflex actions, which concern all the organs encountered enroute, and particularly the generative cells. In fact, the effects of the cold douche begin in a sensory impression and end in an organic reparation. Such is the direct action which cold water, employed more especially in the form of the douche, exerts on the organism.

Immediately after its application the skin is chilled, the superficial blood vessels contract and the blood is driven into the deeper regions of the body, which momentarily undergo a lowering of temperature. At the same time the nerves receive a strong shock. But the nervous system, promptly recovering from its surprise, mobilizes all the forces of the organism which stand under its control. It arrests the movement of concentration of the blood, increases the chemical combinations which produce the animal heat and arouses the activity of all the functions. Under its influence the blood returns to the skin, to which it gives a red tint that brings it a part of the heat which it has gained in its course.

The sequence of all these phenomenon constitutes the reaction, which is rightly considered as the indirect action of cold Hydrotherapy. The reaction of the circulatory system, the thermal and nervous reactions are closely interconnected, but they are all obedient to the nervous system, which has the power of regulating them when they are incorrect or defective.

This triple reaction should always occur after all applications made methodically. There are, however, some cases in which the reactionary phenomena must be attenuated or even annihilated.

But in any case it may be said that the direct action is the work of the doctor and the indirect action is the work of the patient. This latter action is the response to the attack which the patient has undergone.

WARM DOUCHE

Its Properties
Range of Applications

I shall now proceed to deal with the services which may be rendered by warm water in applications of Hydrotherapy.

The warm douche has stimulating and heat producing properties, which enable the patient fittingly to support the effects of the cold water and to render them more beneficial. The preparatory or acclimatizing douche is the one which is best adapted to this special case.

Apart from its special action, the warm douche, when combined with cold water, allows the constitution of the Scotch douche with all the gradations which it should have in the succession of cold and warm water, the alternating douche, the temperate douche made expressly sedative and which may also be hypotensive, the more or less lukewarm douches in which the degree of temperature, adapted to each morbid individuality, may be found instantaneously or by means of a well calculated progression. Such mixed douches can only be administered with the special hydro mixing apparatus which is known by my name. They are essentially beneficial to patients who present at the same time the signs of both excitation and distress or of perversion of the nervous system.

EFFECTS OF HYDRO-THERMAL TREATMENTS

Sedative Effects
Special or Mixed Effects
Anti-Thermal, Anti-Phlogistic [anti-inflammatory] and
Hemostatic Effects
Calorific-Sudorific Effects

With the agents which I have just indicated, Hydrotherapy may render every service that can be reasonably expected from it.

It produces stimulating, tonic and reconstructive or simply perturbative effects. These are produced by refrigerant applications and especially by the cold douche, which should be of brief duration and sufficiently energetic. Such applications are suitable for all those who are victims of debility and who want to develop tone and energy.

Hydrotherapy may also be credited with sedative effects, which are called into play to calm disorders engendered by an immoderate nervous agitation. These effects may be produced by means of baths or partial baths at an agreeable temperature, by certain moist bandages and especially by the temperate douches, lasting fairly long (from three to five minutes), with very gentle percussion and fed by water which is neither hot nor cold.

Hydrotherapy produces special or mixed effects which are obtained with douches, the temperature of which should be made to vary during the course of the same application. They are utilized in the case of patients overcome by an excessive nervous agitation and prostration.

I must also refer to the revulsive, derivative and analgesic effects for which recourse is generally had to warm douches, vapor baths and especially to Scotch douches,* in which it should always be possible to make cold water succeed warm, sometimes with a rapid, sometimes with a progressive transition. They are called into play to dissipate congestions, to effect the requisite flux and reflux of the blood and to soothe pains seated in comparatively accessible regions of the body.

Hydrotherapy likewise exerts resolving or alternative effects, which are used with advantage in affections of the nutritive system, in auto-intoxications and in certain benign nutritive changes. Such effects are obtained with the cold douche, the warm douche, the Scotch douche and particularly with the alternating douche, which consists of a series of cold and warm douches, succeeding one another very rapidly and separated by very brief intervals.

There must also be noted the anti-thermal, anti-phlogistic [or anti-inflammatory] and at times hemostatic effects of this method of treatment. They are induced by cold applications, in which there is no percussion, notably by immersions, moist compresses, damp cloths, more or less continuous irrigations.

Recourse is had to them in the majority of traumatic accidents, in some morbid conditions of inflammatory nature, and in certain febrile diseases, such as typhoid and scarlet fever.

Lastly, I must mention the calorific or sudorific effects, which are always serviceable to patients who have need of warmth or of benefiting by a more or less copious perspiration. To obtain these results the various sudation methods, the warm douche sufficiently prolonged, are employed. These agents render very great services to patients who are victims of a great algidity complicated by incessant shivering or of an auto-infection.

To all these therapeutic effects may be added those produced by water taken internally. It contributes to modifying the composition and the pressure of the blood. It stimulates the movement of the histological elements, furnishes the cells with a liquid medium which favors their nutritive changes, opens the channels of absorption and serves as a support to the secretory organs by aiding them to prepare and to accomplish the expulsion of the residues which are imprisoned in the mesh of their tissues.

Such is the succinct summary of the therapeutic effects of Hydrotherapy. It is requisite before making an appeal to their aid to know to

---

*The Scotch douche gradually increases and decreases temperatures, alternating from hot to cold during the douche. —Ed.

what ailments they should be applied. Accordingly it is necessary for me to define the indications and contraindications of Hydrotherapy.

CLINICAL ASPECTS

Water Treatment in Diagnosis
Individual Specialization
Pulmonary Disease and Typhoid Fever

Formerly, when the doctor had at his disposal only the agents of sudation and exclusively cold applications, the study of this clinical question was rather complex. But nowadays, owing to the introduction of warm water into hydrotherapic installations, what I call a trial douche with varying temperature may be applied to patients whose temperament is unknown. When it is manipulated with discernment it may furnish the doctor with most valuable information. By this means the contraindications have been better defined and considerably reduced, but it is indispensable to refer "en bloc" to those that remain.

Hydrotherapy must be remorselessly prescribed in serious or incurable organic affections and even in functional ailments occurring in subjects who have not the strength to support a too intense stimulation or too accentuated a depression.

In certain eruptive fevers and pulmonary complaints, Hydrotherapy is most valuable.

Against contagious fevers, the hydrotherapic interventions that can be made are moist bandages, more or less cold affusions and baths, always regulated by the various complications that may be seen to arise. These applications are suitable for typhoid patients when the animal heat is elevated and the beating of the heart and pulse is accelerated. They are equally useful for combating the principal symptoms which accompany ataroadynamia [sic].

In typhoid fever the use of the bath may be renewed several times during the same day. Its duration should not exceed ten minutes. On the other hand, the refrigerant applications should be renounced if the patient is extremely feeble and if his heart reveals frequent weakness. They must not be employed in cases where serious hemorrhage or danger of intestinal perforation is observed.

I will now briefly study the various morbid conditions by bringing into relief the particular processes which are suitable to each of them and by leaving in the shade the agents which ought not to be used. In other words, I will say what should and what should not be done.

In order to realize this programme, I have no need to make a didactic exposition of the diseases which may be treated by Hydrotherapy and of those which do not require intervention. I prefer to cite some examples in which I shall define the indications which may aid the practitioner to extend to a large number of invalids the benefits of the hydrotherapic treatment which he will institute and conduct.

I may at once turn my attention to the most striking pathological facts, without studying them in the sequence required in writing a methodically classified book.

THE TREATMENT OF CHLORO-ANEMIA*
Fortifying Enfeebled Organism
The Patient's Animal Heat
Complications

First, take the case of a young chloro-anemic patient who is recommended hydrotherapic treatment to reconstitute her accidentally enfeebled organism. A cold douche of brief duration is administered, which immediately induces a spontaneous and regular action. The use of this douche should be continued. It will lead to a cure.

A second example is a case in which the reactionary phenomena are excessive and almost always followed by great lassitude. In this instance, a less cold douche should be given, and it should last slightly longer.

In the third case, that of a patient who is never warm before or after the douche, a fairly brief preparatory Scotch douche should be given, taking care not to turn on the cold water too suddenly. At the same time all the maneuvers which are known to be capable of elevating the animal heat should be employed. They will aid the patient to benefit by the douche.

I will assume that the doctor is called upon to treat a chloro-anemic patient who evidently needs a cold douche to restore her manifestly enfeebled powers. Unfortunately, it is found that she belongs to the gouty race, whose nerves, muscles, joints and viscera are frequently the seat of intolerable pains. In such a case, which is often met with, some doctors would hesitate to prescribe hydrotherapic treatment. This reserve would be quite intelligible had the practitioner only a cold douche at this disposal, but nowadays when douches of all temperatures may be administered, it is no longer necessary to recommend abstention.

Should such a young chloro-anemic subject, liable to gout, be plunged into a cold bath or be given at the outset a very cold douche, the treatment would be detestable. It might easily induce or revive pains which are always only too ready to manifest themselves. The course of treatment must be commenced with warm douches, which are progressively cooled.

---

*The word "chloro-anemia" refers to a common diagnosis for weakness accompanied by digestive disorders, greenish complexion, lack of appetite, constipation and vomiting in young girls and women. —*Ed.*

Exclusively cold applications will not be made use of until the patient is guaranteed against the recurrence of gouty pains by a daily training methodically pursued. By taking these precautions the patient will be freed from her sufferings, and success will be attained at the same time in giving a healthy vigor to all the functions of her organism.

In the category of chloro-anemic patients are found many persons liable to functional derangements, which may be easily modified by cold douches or by douches at an agreeable temperature. Here are some other examples, furnished by anemic or simply debilitated subjects. Some present symptoms of great nervous weakness, going almost to the limit of cerebral torpor. The douche in the form of a vertical shower, of brief duration and moderately energetic, will do them a great deal of good.

Others who have a constitution almost analogous to the former are subject to sanguineal stasis in the upper parts of the body and complain of being troubled by a very painful nervous excitation. A vertical shower bath is not suitable for them. They must be given a gentle, adjustable douche, of very brief duration and at an agreeable temperature, which may be progressively cooled. The douche will be first directed gently over the upper parts of the body and afterward with greater force over the lower limbs.

The douche in which the water is used at variable temperatures is suitable for some asthmatic subjects, and to patients attached or menaced by an irritation of the air passages, by a perturbation of the cardiac functions or by arteriosclerosis in its first stages.

The latter indications lead me to denote the services which Hydrotherapy may render in diseases of the chest, the heart and the vascular system.

THE TREATMENT OF ASTHMA

Asthma when it occurs in the form of nervous asthma and of the seasonal asthma which is known as hay fever, may happily be modified by hydrotherapic applications. The following is the treatment I prefer. An adjustable and agreeable warm douche is very rapidly administered by spreading it over the whole extent of the cutaneous surface for about a minute. The jet is then directed with greater force on the lower limbs, which may be given a more or less cold sprinkling according to the susceptibilities of the patient.

A similar treatment may be instituted in the case of phthisic [tuberculosis] patients who are obstinately held in the clutches of the first stage of the ailment. Only in this case, the douche must be very short and less cold at the end of the operation.

Venous Circulation

In diseases of the venous system, Hydrotherapy may render service. A douche suitably chilled very beneficially modifies the varices disseminated in the limbs. In the presence of inflammation of the veins, all hydrotherapic practices must be abandoned.

Later, hydrotherapic treatments may be employed to facilitate the circulation of the blood, to tonify the venous tissues, to soothe the pain and get rid of the infiltrated matter; but this must be on the express condition that there is no doubt whatever about the existence of any clot. In this case, a brief and very light, chilled douche will produce the best results.

The reaction of the circulatory system, the thermal and nervous reactions are closely interconnected, but they are all obedient to the nervous system, which has the power of regulating them when they are incorrect or defective.

I must also refer to the revulsive, derivative and analgesic effects for which recourse is generally had to warm douches, vapor baths and especially to Scotch douches, in which it should always be possible to make cold water succeed warm, sometimes with a rapid, sometimes with a progressive transition.

Hydrotherapy must be remorselessly prescribed in serious or incurable organic affections and even in functional ailments occurring in subjects who have not the strength to support a too intense stimulation or too accentuated a depression.

On the other hand, the refrigerant applications should be renounced if the patient is extremely feeble and if his heart reveals frequent weakness. They must not be employed in cases where serious hemorrhage or danger of intestinal perforation is observed.

Should such a young chloro-anemic subject, liable to gout, be plunged into a cold bath or be given at the outset a very cold douche, the treatment would be detestable.

1911

SYSTEMATIC BATHING, A PRESERVATIVE OF HEALTH
JOHN LUEPKE, M.D.

WATER CURE, WATER APPLICATIONS
LOUISA LUST

VINEGAR
M. HABEL

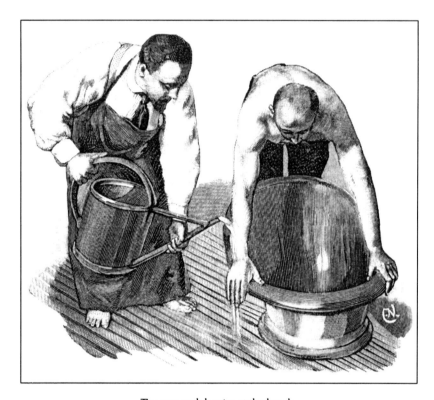

The arm gush begins at the hands.

Systematic Bathing, A Preservative Of Health

by John Luepke, M.D.

The Naturopath and Herald of Health, XVI (2), 103-104. (1911)

The necessity of systematic bathing to preserve health and strengthen the body was already recognized among the most ancient civilized nations. For this purpose bathing houses were also built in the Middle Ages for public use in winter as well as in summer. Later on, the culture of the body became neglected. Only in modern times has the idea of an extended application of water become popular; people of intellect begin to employ this natural therapy as one of the best means to regain health and preserve it.

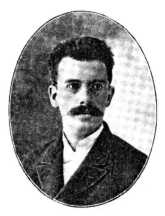

John F. G. Luepke, M.D., S.D.

If we consider the effect of water at different temperatures on the human body, aside from its combination with soap for the sake of cleanliness, we must acknowledge the importance of systematic bathing as a special protection against disease.

Man's physical welfare depends greatly upon his power of adapting himself to all climatic changes. This must be done by getting accustomed to heat and cold beginning in younger days, and gradually advancing throughout life. Yet this general rule cannot be applied to everybody. One must individualize. Delicate children, the aged and convalescents must be treated with special care and precaution, for imprudent cold bathing often has very grave effects. Pernicious anemia, nervous troubles, irritability, loss of appetite, chronic indigestion and intestinal derangements are some of such serious sequellae or consequences.

If children, barely recovered from measles, or adults from pneumonia were subjected to a harsh cold water treatment, only a serious outcome could be expected. All cold water procedures must be adapted to the constitution of the individual, his or her age, vitality, surroundings, etc.

Anemia and other chronic derangements—if they should appear after the use of cold water on the debilitated—are not due to the art of Hydrotherapy, but to its wrong and irrational application. Therefore, no such treatment should be attempted without previously consulting an experienced physician.

In order to get the child accustomed to sudden changes of the atmosphere, it is wise to give baths of varying temperatures, followed by short cooler sponge baths, but never by douches, as they irritate the nerves. The procedures should always be very short. They will be of greatest benefit in the morning right after rising, when the body is warm and well rested, the room properly ventilated and an early hour of rising. They invigorate body and soul and strengthen the whole nervous system, help to regulate the temperature of the body and last, but not least, cultivate and preserve health and beauty.

Cold water applications must be avoided at night; here the body is exhausted, and energy and superfluous animal heat are consumed. Furthermore, the fear which some children and even adults have of cold water increases irritability and causes loss of appetite, indigestion, insomnia, anemia, muscular atrophy, etc.

The same general rules hold good for adults, if they want to protect themselves against catching cold, which may happen in damp weather. 80° F/27° C is a good temperature of the water to begin with, gradually decreasing it. Besides cold water baths, light air baths accompanied by manual friction are of great value. Both produce an energetic contraction of the pores and thereby protect the body against cold. They also regulate cardiac action, deepen respiration, increase metabolism, stimulate the appetite and absorption, and thereby prevent certain diseases of the circulatory, respiratory and digestive apparatus to develop.

Lukewarm baths are also of priceless value. They promote the cutaneous circulation of the blood and give the skin its peculiar luster, its incompatible softness and flexibility. They improve the emunctory function of the skin to excrete from the body, as the kidneys do, such obnoxious matters, which will—should they remain in the system—cause autointoxication and death.

Moderately hot baths of short duration prevent skin diseases and have a soothing effect in nervousness, atony, neurasthenia, irritability, convulsions, etc. The same benefits may apply to warm packs, especially in insomniacs. In such ailments, Hydrotherapy shows the best results.

But without going into further detail into the modes of application of water in sickness, which must remain with the physician, systematic bathing *per se*, if properly understood, will train people to give good attention to the body and to develop an ethical sense for purity, cleanliness and self-preservation.

If we consider the effect of water at different temperatures on the human body, aside from its combination with soap for the sake of cleanliness, we must acknowledge the importance of systematic bathing as a special protection against disease.

Anemia and other chronic derangements—if they should appear after the use of cold water on the debilitated—are not due to the art of Hydrotherapy, but to its wrong and irrational application.

Cold water applications must be avoided at night; here the body is exhausted, energy and superfluous animal heat are consumed.

80° F/27° C is a good temperature of the water to begin with, gradually decreasing it. Besides cold water baths, light air baths accompanied by manual friction are of great value.

WATER CURE, WATER APPLICATIONS

by Louisa Lust

The Naturopath and Herald of Health, XVI (4), 231, 233. (1911)

Water, air, food and exercise are considered necessities for good health by all intelligent reformers.

Water, air and exercise can be obtained freely. Still, only a few comprehend the value of water in health or sickness. In fact, if all people understood how to use water, its value of cooling, cleansing, invigorating and sustained life, one-half of all the afflictions from disease would be removed and the other half banished as soon as all the people understood how and when to eat, how to breathe and the necessity of daily exercise.

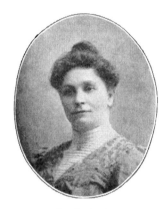

Louisa Lust
[1864-1925]

To quote Liebig, the great chemist: "Greater organic changes transpire in the human system under six months' active water treatment than in three year's ordinary action of nature."

We all recognize the comfort and pleasure experienced from cleanliness and order in all places and conditions of life. If the masses could be taught right living, how and what to eat and drink, how to dress, and how to strictly conform to hygienic laws, there would undoubtedly be less necessity for bathing. As society is now constituted, bathing is a necessity for the best physiological conditions. Obstructions or impeded circulation, internal and external congestion are common, everyday experiences, to be met with in the best-ordered homes.

There is no better treatment for acute or chronic disease than the steam bath—for pneumonia, la grippe [flu], a severe cold, or any clogged condition. This bath is a safe and sure remedy and will accomplish a good deal. The object sought in this bath is to open the pores and cause perspiration, which will relax the system, remove congestive and clogged conditions of the blood and the vital organs.

Herbs are used for nerve baths and are very beneficial. Sage, hay flower, bark of oak, pine needle, fenugreek, yarrow, etc., may be used. They form an agreeable medication. A bath prepared with any of these herbs may last from ten to fifteen minutes. The water in the tub should be as hot as the patient can bear it. The bath should always conclude with a cool ablution, so as to close the pores and prevent cold. The patient should be out of doors most of the day.

Another most valuable water treatment is the wet sheet pack, to loosen up waste matter. A warm pack is the best, but when fever rages, use it cold. The bed should be in a quiet, well-ventilated sunny room. Cover the mattress with a rubber sheet, place two to three woolen blankets on the rubber sheet and an ordinary bedsheet on top of the blankets, as well as a hot water bottle for the feet. After wringing the cold or hot water out of the linen sheets, which must be done in the bathtub, so as to avoid its dripping in the bed, place the sheet smoothly upon the blanket. The patient, disrobed, is assisted to the middle of the wet sheet, the arms resting at the side of the body. The sheet is then wrapped smoothly and rapidly around the body and closely around the neck. Each blanket should be quickly wrapped in a like manner around the patient, taking pains to tuck them well about the neck and feet in particular. One hour is sufficient to remain in such pack.

If a patient goes to sleep, do not disturb him. If patient is uneasy and restless, remove the pack before the hour is up. Two water packs are advisable each day, morning and evening, until the fever is removed.

For scarlet fever, measles, bilious and intermittent fever, the water pack in connection with drinking lemonade or spring water, to keep the head cool and feet warm is the safest method. Entire fasting until the fever is removed and then a fruit diet for a few weeks ought to be taken up.

A thorough airing of the bed and blankets after each pack, and washing of the sheet is one of the requirements. Always keep the air of the sickroom as pure as the outdoor air. To neglect ventilation means to invite sickness and death.

Fever inflammation and deep-seated disease is drawn to the surface and absorbed in the pack. After the pack is removed, the body is washed all over with cool water.

By understanding the object of this important treatment, the necessity for airing and sunning the clothing and bedroom becomes apparent.

For acute and chronic disease, to reduce abnormal heat of the body, to correct morbid secretions and aid in restoring healthy ones, to cleanse the circulating system and soothe and quiet overworked nerves, water packs are excellent. Fasting and not feasting is all important in acute attacks. The Water Cure is quite often misrepresented by so-called healers and practitioners and they object to packs and other Nature Cure methods, because there is too much work. Too much work, indeed—in Nature Cure methods, too much work to restore life with safe, natural methods and remedies. It is less work to bow, smile and *talk* health, or write out prescriptions and await the results. The only qualification being in this case, a diploma.

HEAD AND THROAT COMPRESSES

For hoarseness or sore throat use a piece of soft, old linen or towel, doubled, or four thicknesses, wring cold water out of it, apply and cover throat with a piece of flannel.

For severe cases of croup, diphtheria, snow compresses are to be preferred; they must be renewed every five minutes.

ABDOMINAL COMPRESSES

These are most excellent for bladder, kidney, uterus and many other diseases.

Sunlight, pure air and water are Nature's important healing factors and remedies. There is no deception or fraud attached to them. Try them, and you will not be disappointed.

—*Yungborn*, Butler, New Jersey

If the masses could be taught right living, how and what to eat and drink, how to dress, and how to strictly conform to hygienic laws, there would undoubtedly be less necessity for bathing.

There is no better treatment for acute or chronic disease than the steam bath—for pneumonia, la grippe [flu], a severe cold, or any clogged condition.

Herbs are used for nerve baths and are very beneficial. Sage, hay flower, bark of oak, pine needle, fenugreek, yarrow, etc., may be used.

Always keep the air of the sickroom as pure as the outdoor air. To neglect ventilation means to invite sickness and death.

For acute and chronic disease, to reduce abnormal heat of the body, to correct morbid secretions and aid in restoring healthy ones, to cleanse the circulating system and soothe and quiet overworked nerves, water packs are excellent.

The Water Cure is quite often misrepresented by so-called healers and practitioners and they object to packs and other Nature Cure methods, because there is too much work.

Vinegar

by M. Habel

The Naturopath and Herald of Health, XVI (5), 294-295. (1911)

Vinegar plays quite an important role in the household of Nature. It is used for seasoning many dishes, as a means to prevent putrefaction and to macerate the meat till it becomes tender; for the manufacture and fixation of dyestuffs, and finally also in the medical arts. Popular medicine as well as the medical science make use of vinegar, and Sebastian Kneipp also has not failed to make it serve his cures.

To rightly comprehend the efficacy of vinegar, it is necessary to know its nature, i.e., its essential physical and chemical qualities. Vinegar is a composition of an organic kind, for it can evolve only out of organic, of grown materials. It is formed by a special kind of fermentation, the sour fermentation, and by dry distillation.

The usual way of making vinegar is the so-called sour fermentation. If liquids that contain alcohol are exposed to the air, they take oxygen at a temperature of 30° to 35° C/86° to 95° F, by which process alcohol becomes vinegar. It is well known that the fermentation of the vinegar is being accelerated by adding a little white film or some vinegar. The exciter of the oxidation, a certain microscopic fungus (*Mycoderma aceti*), which usually is drawn into from the air by accident, is hereby added directly. The dry distillation is, in general, the heating of organic stuffs with the seclusion of air. There is also in the dry distillation vinegar to be found among the many products of decomposition, the so-called wood vinegar.

In our household there can, according to Kneipp, a good vinegar be produced out of apple parings, fallen fruits, honey, the scorched stinging nettle, leaves of the blackberry and elderberry, out of beer or wine. An earthen glass vessel is filled two-thirds with the cut up fruits or something else, water is poured over it, acetous ferment is added, and then paper is tied about the vessel in which some holes have been made. It must stand now near a warm stove. In three to eight weeks the best vinegar has been obtained. It is ready as soon as it has cleared off, i. e., has become perfectly bright.

Acetous ferment can, according to Kneipp, be made in a simple way. Take a crust of black bread, let it become very dry, dip it in good vinegar and let it soak in as much as possible. Dip it in thrice and let it dry as often. This acid is then put in the pot of vinegar.

Vinegar is a mixture of two to five percent of acetic acid and water which mostly contains also some aromatic stuffs, evolving from the mother substance.

Acetous acid, methylcarbonic acid, $C_2H_4O_2$ is C_2H_3OOH is a colorless liquid of a sour taste and smell, which affects our skin, corroding it; is easily mixed with water and alcohol; dissolves various stuffs, camphor, gums and etheric oils, and enters into chemical combinations with oxides, hydroxides and carbonates, and forms thus the acetous salts, acetates which are partly used in medicine, partly in the trades. We consider here only the qualities and effects of the vinegar itself and not of its combinations, because this alone is also known everywhere and is easily accessible.

First of all the sharp smell is physiologically effective, which we also mentioned first, and which is a quality of the vinegar, which at first attacks our senses. Strong, sharp smells excite our consciousness by affecting the nerves of our nose. Vinegar, therefore, has been used and is still used when the consciousness becomes weak or has disappeared entirely, i.e., in cases of fainting fits.

The spare volatility, which the vinegar contains, the evaporation, is also used for medical purposes. A fluid which evaporates from the skin, extracts some warmth of the skin and causes a local irritation which is the stronger, the quicker the evaporation sets in. As vinegar is more volatile than water at the same temperature, it can under certain conditions when water is used be applied to increase the effect.

The thermic irritation is heightened also by a chemical one. The vinegar can impregnate the horny part of our skin; it is dissolving the skin in a corrosive manner.

If, therefore, we want more to make use of the cooling quality of the vinegar, the vinegar must be mixed with cold water, as is done with the vinegar washings, vinegar compresses, clay bandages, etc. of Kneipp. If a corrosion is wanted, for example, to remove warts or corns, the acetous acid must be used in its totally waterless form, which is called the ice vinegar because at 17° C/63° F, it congeals to icy crystals.

The dissolving power of the vinegar is used to make different extracts—for example, the hair water made of the stinging nettle.

A remedy which is so strong and variously used, like vinegar, can also do harm if improperly used. It must not be forgotten that the vinegar dissolves copper chemically and produces with its help the poisonous copper rust. Salad must be prepared with wooden spoons, fruits and vegetables must never be boiled in copper vessels. We must not ourselves corrode spots on our skin by acetic acid, but let a physician do it. The immediate use of the vinegar injures the stomach and is also hindering the formation of the blood and therefore injurious.

The smell of vinegar is disagreeable mostly to nervous persons because it excites and irritates too much their sensitive nerves. Who can bear in daytime a compress of vinegar cannot always bear it at night, etc. If vinegar, therefore, though it seems to be so harmless and is quite familiar with us, is used as a remedy, the condition of the patient must be considered carefully. Laymen, therefore, should use it with great caution.

In our household there can, according to Kneipp, a good vinegar be produced out of apple parings, fallen fruits, honey, the scorched stinging nettle, leaves of the blackberry and elderberry, out of beer or wine.

Acetous ferment can, according to Kneipp, be made in a simple way. Take a crust of black bread, let it become very dry, dip it in good vinegar and let it soak in as much as possible. Dip it in thrice and let it dry as often.

As vinegar is more volatile than water at the same temperature, it can under certain conditions when water is used be applied to increase the effect.

If, therefore, we want more to make use of the cooling quality of the vinegar, the vinegar must be mixed with cold water, as is done with the vinegar washings, vinegar compresses, clay bandages, etc. of Kneipp.

The dissolving power of the vinegar is used to make different extracts—for example, the hair water made of the stinging nettle.

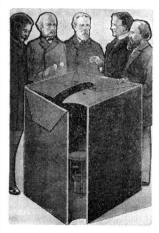
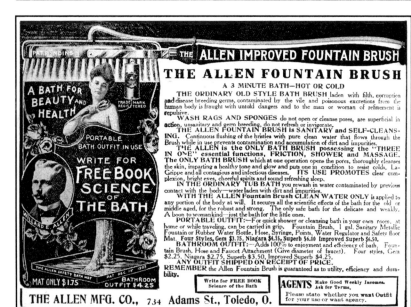
So many products for the bath

1912

AM UNKNOWN, INEXPENSIVE AND YET EFFECTIVE SWEAT BATH

F. J. BUTTGENBACH

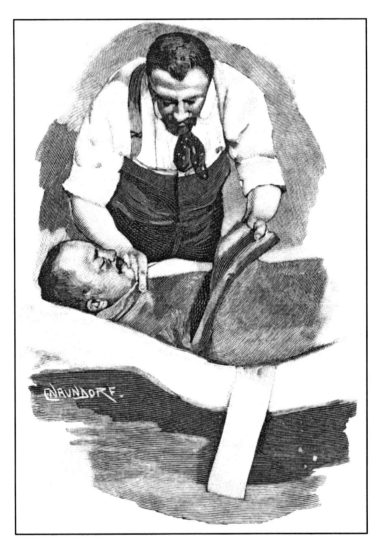

The most attention given in the application of a wet sheet wrap is the careful and tight closure of the blanket around the neck and feet.

An Unknown, Inexpensive And Yet Effective Sweat Bath

by F. J. Buttgenbach

The Naturopath and Herald of Health, XVII (8), 522-523. (1912)

Everybody ought to take a sweat bath once in a while; included are laborers and farmers who are apt to sweat much. If they knew how to handle themselves after such a procedure, they would be benefited physically by it, but generally they don't know, they gain a little financially and lose on the other end. To sit down, light a cigarette or take another chew of tobacco while resting a little while will not do it. The perspiration will be reabsorbed by the body (which is scientifically called auto-intoxication, self-poisoning) closes the pores and so sickness and ailments of every kind appear. Those unfortunates, who, on account of their financial and social standing, think they can afford to have someone else sweat for them, are still worse off. Of course, they enjoy their automobile and carriage ride very much, but deprive themselves of the exercise of a brisk, healthful walk and besides they swallow the dust of the roads. They ought to take two, three or more sweat baths every so often.

It is not necessary to take a sweat bath in an expensive bath cabinet or go for this purpose to a steam bath house; it can be done cheaper and at least just, or even more, effective. For those who cannot afford to have one of the above mentioned sweat baths—the others need not read this— I will in the following suggest, describe and recommend an unknown, inexpensive, safe and still powerful sweat bath.

Secure some of that fresh mown grass from lawns or back yards (take out the thistle leaves, briars and sticks, of course); the other greens are all good, and fill it into sacks so it will get quickly self-heated. While this process is going on, make a box about ten to twelve inches deep and as long and wide as necessary for the respective person to lie comfortable in, just as big as the coffin should be in which some time hence, the earthly remains of this person will be taken to the cemetery. So much is sure that if that person will use this bath frequently and henceforth live correctly, the supposed lumber for the real coffin will grow in the woods for a while yet.

If the grass is now hot enough to suit you, put a layer six to eight inches in the box, undress yourself and wash the whole body with water mixed with good cider vinegar (about one-half pint of cold water and one-half teacup of vinegar); then lie down in the box, cover yourself up to the neck with the grass, and call somebody else to cover your arms insulated from the body, tight and good. If you are sweating lively, drink lots of cold water—city, well or rain water, uncooked—never mind those microbes; they are harmless little scavengers. I laugh at the whole microbe and bacillus theory—what others think, talk and fear about are none of my business. I did and do my own thinking. Remember the more cold water you drink while sweating, the more you will sweat. The more you sweat, the more of that morbid matter (what ails you) will come out of your system, and the more of this morbid matter you lose, the better you will feel after the bath. The better you feel, the better you will think, act and live on this earth, and so according to this life your future life will be shaped.

Everything has its consequences: *Ergo bibamus aquam puram, frigidamsatis;* that means in English: "Therefore let us drink plenty of pure, cold water." After you have thus sweated ten, twenty or thirty minutes (the longer the better), jump right away in a bathtub filled with cold water, roll around, stay in it for about a half a minute, jump out and rub your whole body with your dry bare hands. In case you deem your hands not good enough for this and where you cannot reach, take a piece of a clean, old, rough gunnysack. I used for years a piece of an old fishnet, soaked it in water, put on some river bottom sand and so scrubbed my back thoroughly, pulling the sandy old fishnet right and left, up and down. When the skin is getting dry, rub it with the palm of your hand hard in short strokes in every direction until the real dirt comes to the surface and rolls off. Wet the palms again, and rub again, repeat this till your skin glows like fire, then the dirt is out. Remember, the morbid matter, impurities, waste matter or whatever it is called—I call it dirt for short—and it is this that is in and below your skin that causes your ailments and troubles. After your skin is dry, take a strong solution of salt water, rub it with your bare hands thoroughly over the whole body. This saves a trip to the ocean and is just as good as a swim in the ocean.

The salt water on the skin generates positive electricity and magnetism. Those who have neither box nor bathtub can have the same results if they put the grass bed in one corner of the room, and take a pail full of water; any clean old rag or stocking will answer the purpose. With sufficient will power and some gumption, one can accomplish a whole lot! The main thing is to see that it is done, and done correctly and quickly. Don't get scared about the cold water. Cold water, since the creation of the world, has never harmed anybody if applied and used right. It has always a strengthening and vivifying effect, while hot baths, if not [finished] by a short cold bath or at least by a cold ablution are weakening and are if repeated the cause of an enervated and effeminated system.

If anyone suffers with rheumatism, cancer, or any other deviltry, or is liable to have the blues, or the hay fever again, or is all the time ailing with bad colds, etc., I recommend them to take sweat baths frequently; that will settle the quarrel. It will restore the original color of gray hair—caused by nothing else but by impurities of the blood. The saying: "Gray hair is a sign of wisdom and must be honored" is alright, but the shade of this kind of gray is different from that which we see now a days; it is ash-gray, while the sign of whitish or yellow-gray is something that rather should be pitied.

Now parents, an appeal to you: your children, little ones, and big ones, perhaps, enjoy at present good health, but you know, maybe by experience, observation or hearsay, how quickly and how suddenly such conditions can change. If you use the opportunity, while at hand to take first yourself the above sweat bath to get acquainted with the procedure and then put the children, one after the other, in the sweat box and let them soak thoroughly, and treat them besides with proper food, drink and clothing, you will see the end of the year 1912 without being bothered by diphtheria, scarlet fever, typhoid fever, etc., for all these deviltries cannot afflict you or your children if the blood is clean.

I don't doubt a good many who read this article will laugh about it, or doubt my assertions, but if those doubting Thomas's or scoffers would give it one trial, I would not risk a wager of four cents that they wouldn't try it again and again. Certainly they cannot overdo it, because this and correct breathing exercise cannot be overdone.

This bath is a clean bath in comparison with a mud bath in which waterdogs, lizards, bugs, wiggle tails, snakes and numberless other creeping creatures live, but poor suffering mankind has often to use the latter.

—Eugene, Oregon

Secure some of that fresh mown grass from lawns or back yards (take out the thistle leaves, briars and sticks, of course), the other greens are all good, and fill it into sacks so it will get quickly self-heated.

If the grass is now hot enough to suit you, put a layer six to eight inches in the box, undress yourself and wash the whole body with water mixed with good cider vinegar (about one-half pint of cold water and one-half teacup of vinegar), then lay down in the box, cover yourself up to the neck with the grass, call somebody else to cover your arms (insulated from the body, tight and good.

After you have thus sweated ten, twenty or thirty minutes (the longer the better) jump right away in a bathtub filled with cold water, roll around, stay in it for about a half a minute, jump out and rub your whole body with your dry bare hands.

After your skin is dry, take a strong solution of salt water, rub it with your bare hands thoroughly over the whole body.

Cold water, since the creation of the world, has never harmed anybody if applied and used right.

1913

THE PRIESSNITZ OR ABDOMINAL BANDAGE

WET SOCKS

BENEDICT LUST, N.D.

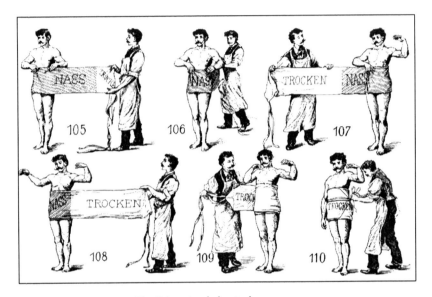

The Priessnitz abdominal compress

THE PRIESSNITZ OR ABDOMINAL BANDAGE
by Benedict Lust, N.D.

The Naturopath and Herald of Health, XVIII (9), 617-618. (1913)

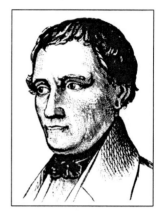

Vincent Priessnitz
[1799-1851]

This bandage has been called a "universal remedy". There is almost no disease, acute or chronic, in which this simple treatment cannot find application and it has become, so to say, the starting point of Naturopathy. As all diseases have their origin in the abdomen more or less, the abdominal bandage, therefore, is the first remedy commonly applied and the first relief to the patient and many times the only treatment necessary. Very few people realize what a great healing effect is produced by this simple old-time Priessnitz bandage and not to wait till the doctor is called.

We will, therefore, take the opportunity to recollect to our readers the physiological effects of this bandage and what is necessary to know in using it. See also Bilz', *Natural Method of Healing*, pages 1678-1685.

Each complete bandage consists of two parts, a wet one and a dry one, or an internal one and an external one. The internal bandage should be about seven or eight inches wide and long enough to reach around the whole abdomen, double on the front, and that means the two ends form a double cover on the stomach part and single on the back. The dry or external part must be about 10 to 12 inches wide in order to cover the wet or internal one thoroughly. The best material for the internal bandage is raw silk; if not within reach, crash linen or any old linen table cloth, bed sheet or towel may be used. For the cover, thick flannel or a piece of a woolen blanket is practical. The internal bandage must be dipped in cold water and wrung thoroughly to avoid wetting of the cover bandage, which would retard the reaction.

It must be borne in mind that the Priessnitz bandage cannot be applied when the patient is feeling chilly. If this is the case, the patient must first be warmed entirely, which can be done by a steam bath, or a hot bath, or a hot foot bath, or by resting in bed with hot water bottles applied to the feet and calves, or if the patient is able, by a brisk walk or exercises; also through a vigorous rubbing of the whole body with warm cloths or with alcohol, warm oil, etc.

The bandage must be put on airtight, but not too tight, as the patient may feel uncomfortable. If the bandage is too loose, the steam escapes and the body feels chilly and a reaction cannot take place. If the bandage becomes too warm and the patient in consequence restless, the bandage must be removed and renewed and this must eventually be repeated several times till he falls asleep. The sleep must not be interrupted no matter how long it lasts. After awakening, the bandage is to be taken off and a short cool sponge bath round the abdomen is to be given, after which the patient may remain in bed for a short time yet till perfectly dry, or in case he wants to get up, the abdomen must be rubbed carefully till dry.

Let us recapitulate now in short words what has to be observed:

1. The whole body must be warm.
2. The wet cloth must be wrung thoroughly.
3. The wet bandage must be applied cold directly to the skin.
4. The bandage must be well-fitting and not too loose.
5. The bandage must be removed when irritating or after having become dry.
6. When falling asleep, sleep must not be disturbed.
7. A cool sponge bath and dry rubbing of the parts which were bandaged must follow the removal of the abdominal pack.

The physiological effects of the Priessnitz bandage are like those of any wet sheet packing. As soon as the cold wet cloth comes in contact with the skin a contraction of the cutaneous blood vessels takes place, the result of which is a flowing back of the blood in the inner body. This condition lasts, however, only for a very short time and quickly a reaction answers in the form of a rushing of the blood toward and in the skin, which produces now a dilation of the blood vessels, and the apparent short low tide at first is followed by a long-lasting high tide of arterial blood.

This tide of blood causes as a natural consequence a high moist temperature below the woolen cover, but the water of the internal bandage, evaporating slowly through the cover, produces on the other hand a slow sinking of the temperature. And on this alternating process of refrigeration, rushing of blood to the inner body and hence back to the skin, heating temperature and evaporation depends the physiological effect of all wet packing.

During this process all the morbid and foreign substances in gaseous and liquid form are eliminated through the dilated blood vessels and pores of the skin and are finally absorbed by the wet cloth, while on the other hand the rich provision of arterial blood causes a better nutrition of the cells.

As all diseases have their origin in the abdomen more or less, the abdominal bandage, therefore, is the first remedy commonly applied and the first relief to the patient and many times the only treatment necessary.

The internal bandage should be about seven or eight inches wide and long enough to reach around the whole abdomen, double on the front, and that means the two ends form a double cover on the stomach part and single on the back.

The bandage must be put on airtight, but not too tight, as the patient may feel uncomfortable. If the bandage is too loose, the steam escapes and the body feels chilly and a reaction cannot take place.

If the bandage becomes too warm and the patient in consequence restless, the bandage must be removed and renewed and this must eventually be repeated several times till he falls asleep. The sleep must not be interrupted no matter how long it lasts.

As soon as the cold wet cloth comes in contact with the skin a contraction of the cutaneous blood vessels takes place, the result of which is a flowing back of the blood in the inner body.

During this process all the morbid and foreign substances in gaseous and liquid form are eliminated through the dilated blood vessels and pores of the skin and are finally absorbed by the wet cloth, while on the other hand the rich provision of arterial blood causes a better nutrition of the cells.

WET SOCKS

by Benedict Lust, N.D.

The Naturopath and Herald of Health, XVIII (11), 770. (1913)

Here are some rules to be observed in the use of wet socks:

1. Take thin linen socks or stockings and put them in fresh water; twist them and put them on if possible in the evening, when going to bed, taking care, however, that the feet be first very warm.* Over them put on thick, dry woolen socks or stockings, which must be longer than the thin ones of about one inch in order that the wet socks be completely covered by the other ones. If this should not give a steady warmth to the feet, it will be necessary to cover them with another warm cloth. Care should be taken that the feet become warm at once and stays so, for otherwise, the treatment instead of bringing the desired results will cause displeasing effects.

2. In the case in which the socks, after having become warm through the heat of the body, should become cold again, this will prove that the feet were not well covered and to avoid a cold the best thing is the take them off right away and to try over again, being more careful the second time.

3. If one does not find any trouble with them, the best thing is to keep the wet socks overnight. But this should not be at the cost of sleep and if the patient has not rest through [wearing] them or if his feet should become too warm, the advisable thing to do is to take them off. To reach any result they ought to be kept on, however, at least a couple of hours and only with very hot feet (in case of high fever) they ought to be changed after a shorter time, every half-hour, for instance.

4. Select if possible white linen socks in order that no dangerous color might affect the body. Colored socks however can be used, if they have already been washed or if one is sure that their color is not of a dangerous nature.

5. There are cases in which instead of thin linen socks, thick ones are more advisable, cases where it is better not to twist them too much and this in order to keep more water in its pores. Sometimes instead of cold water, warm water ought to be used; instead of

---

*Possessing cold feet did not rule out cold water application to the feet by Sebastian Kneipp. In fact, cold wet socks and walking in cold water were the very means to restore natural warmth to chronic cold feet.—*Ed.*

plain water, water with vinegar (half water, half vinegar or two thirds water and one third vinegar) or water with salt. But only a naturopathic doctor could tell this and the patient should not change the general prescription without competent advice.

6. In some cases wet socks are used for the hands.

7. The socks must be kept a much longer time than bandages on the abdomen for they do not become warm as quick as those bandages.

8. The great utility of this remedy is in the fact that by attracting the blood circulation towards the feet, these become warm and head and chest are relieved of an excess of circulation. Chronic cold feet will by and by become warmer and excessive perspiration of the feet will stop. In case of fever, a very considerable decrease of temperature will soon be noticed.

9. To reach the best results on should not depend only on this remedy but use it together with other naturopathic agencies, advised by the special case of the patient.

Care should be taken that the feet become warm at once and stays so, for otherwise, the treatment instead of bringing the desired results will cause displeasing effects.

The socks must be kept a much longer time than bandages on the abdomen for they do not become warm as quick as those bandages.

The great utility of this remedy is in the fact that by attracting the blood circulation towards the feet, these become warm and head and chest are relieved of an excess of circulation.

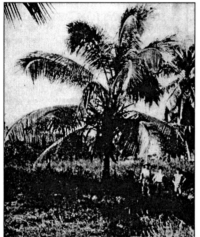
By 1913, Louisa and Benedict Lust moved at full throttle to promote their second
Yungborn located at Tangerine, Florida.

1914

HYDROTHERAPY OR WATER CURE
Dr. Carl Schultz

Dr. Carl Schultz championed Naturopathy in California

Hydrotherapy Or Water Cure*

by Dr. Carl Schultz

The Naturopath and Herald of Health, XIX (6), 345-349. (1914)

One of the many therapeutic agencies of the naturopathic school is Hydrotherapy. I claim it is the most important one, for the following reasons:

First: Water can be had for the asking in almost any place.

Second: It is the most effective of all natural therapeutic agencies.

Third: It can be used in one form or another, in the broadest sense of the word, in all ailments and diseases, without exception.

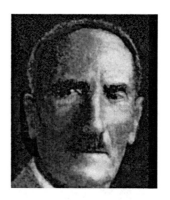

Dr. Carl Schultz

Of course, Hydrotherapy is not a *cure all*. It often has to be used in connection with other natural remedies, and must be used with common sense. This is one reason why it has become so popular with the laity, especially in Germany, while it is not popular with physicians.

The reasons why Hydrotherapy is not practiced by all physicians are several, mostly selfish ones. I am sorry to add that many naturopathic physicians have abandoned Hydrotherapy. Sometimes the physician has not money enough, or thinks he has not money enough to equip his treatment rooms with the suitable arrangements and appliances. Expensive equipment is not necessary. Father Kneipp for many years used a common sprinkling can with the sprinkler taken off and a wash tub. An ordinary bathtub, a wash tub, a sprinkling can, and a lounge or massage table, blankets and sheets will suffice in many cases, and have served me well for many years. Fine equipment does not make a physician.

Another reason for not practicing Hydrotherapy is that a majority of physicians think it beneath their dignity to use water. As if anything that will help a patient could be beneath the dignity of any physician, no matter what his name or school may be. What the leading physicians of the continent of Europe think of Hydrotherapy is shown by the fact that it is not only taught in every university, but in most of them special independent chairs of Hydrotherapy have been established. I am sorry that this

---

*Carl Schultz wrote two other articles in this series on Hydrotherapy that can be found in *Principles Of Naturopathic Medicine* (2014) pp. 262-274. —*Ed.*

is not the case in America, where even trained nurses have very little or no training in the use of water. Often I have found it necessary not only to instruct the nurse in the practical use of water but also have had to do most of the water treatment myself. All nurses seem to know is how to administer drugs, give hypodermics and take the pulse and temperature; that is, unless one has a nurse who has been trained in a naturopathic institute, or in one of the Battle Creek Sanitariums.

The founders, or rather the rediscoverers of Hydrotherapy (for Hydrotherapy is as old as history), were men from every walk of life, educated and uneducated. Singular to say, among them was not one regular physician. I do not mean to say that the medical profession did not finally accept Hydrotherapy, as they did other natural therapeutic measures. Of course, as naturopathic physicians you are more or less acquainted with the history of Hydrotherapy. Therefore, it would be a waste of time to go into a detailed history. I must, however, make reference to Professor Wilhelm Winternitz, of Vienna, who, in my opinion, has done more to make Hydrotherapy acceptable to the profession than any other writer. His books and writings have convinced the profession that Hydrotherapy was a most powerful healing agent in the hands of a well-trained and honest physician. What Father Kneipp did for the people, Winternitz has done for the profession.

Father Kneipp, whose books have been translated into thirty-two languages, has surely done more than any man to popularize the Water Cure. Many a physician has sat at his feet and has learned from him the first principles of Hydrotherapy. I mention this because it seems to be the tendency of many of the profession to belittle the work of this great master. "Honor to whom honor is due."

Some physicians have endeavored to restrict the use of the term "Hydrotherapy" to the employment of cold water alone. This is a mistake that could only be made by those who have not studied this subject thoroughly. Hydrotherapy includes the application of water in any form, from the solid and fluid to vapor; from ice to steam, internally and externally.

I will not here go into a discussion of internal treatment by water, but take for my subject its thermal and mechanical action upon the cutaneous surfaces of the body. In order to understand this we must study:

1. The anatomical construction and physiology of the skin from a hydriatric standpoint.
2. The physical properties of water, which render it capable of producing these effects.

As important as the intimate knowledge of this subject is to the

Hydrotherapist, the time is too short for me to enter into this subject thoroughly.

The skin has three functions to perform:

1. It is an organ of sense.
2. It is an organ of excretion.
3. It is a heat regulator.

This third function is the most important function of the skin, when considered in connection with Hydrotherapy. Those portions of the skin which contain the blood and nerve supplies interest us most. I hold that a more careful and elaborate study of these structures than is usually made by Hydrotherapists would be of great benefit to them.

I will discuss first the tissue of the skin. The skin comprises a large variety of the tissue elements in a complicated arrangement, directly or indirectly connected with the functions of all other parts of the body. The epidermis, or outer layer, acts as a protection to the more delicate and sensitive structures underneath. The dermis, or true skin, is made up of two fairly distinct layers, the pars papillaris, upon which the epithelium rests and the pars reticularis beneath, the former lying next to the panniculus adiposis.

The knob-like projections of the papillary layer are of two types. Those containing blood vessels (vascular papillae), and those containing nerve endings (tactile papillae). Both layers of the dermis consist of the reticulum, composed of bundles of connective tissue, surrounded by elastic fibers. For the most part, the fibrous bundles lie parallel to the skin surface. Those fibres nearer to the surface are finer and more densely packed, producing a felt-like texture, while those of the deeper layers nearer the subcutaneous fat, are coarser and more loosely arranged. Smooth muscle fibres are intimately associated with elastic fibres. The two together constitute one of the most important anatomic arrangements of the skin.

In many parts of the skin the muscle fibres are formed like a network, contracting diagonally. The muscular tissue exists mostly as the erectors pilorum, disposed in bundles in connection with the hair follicles, and lying in an oblique direction through the thickness of the skin. These muscle bundles are surrounded and traversed by elastic fibres, so that they are enclosed in a dense network of elastic tissue, threads of which serve as tendons to connect the ends of the muscular fasciuclus to the connective tissue bundles of the corium, or deep layer of the skin.

I now turn to the functions of the skin. First, as an organ of sense. Professor Roehrig has well said that next to sight, the sense of touch is the most important of all the senses. This brings us to the nervous system of the skin. The nerves of the skin are: the secretory, the vasomotor and the temperature [receptors].   Dr. Baruch in, *Principle and Practice of Hydro-therapy*, says:

> The anatomical distribution of the nerves throughout the skin
> and their connection with the central nervous system are so per-
> fect and complete that not the finest pinpoint may penetrate its
> uppermost layer without calling into action all those agencies by
> which the human organism protects itself.

The cutaneous nerve endings guard most of the functions of the
human body. They are constantly exposed to irritation by heat and cold,
which they convey to the vasomotor, respiratory and cardiac centers and
to the muscles, in order to arouse in them by reflex action such a degree of
innervation as may be required to ward off any damaging influence that
may approach from without.

The nerve endings which fulfill this important function are the tactile
corpuscles and pacinian bodies, club-shape terminals which compose the
sense of touch. The latter is composed, according to Goldschneider, of
a large number of specific sensations, each of which is brought about by
separate nerves. There is a system of nervous sensation spread through
the skin, not arranged in any recognizable manner, which seems to enable
us to "feel our skin". While the pressure nerves give information of those
objects which touch us from without, the nerves of sensation are the carriers or conveyors of the so-called general sense. Temperature sensations
are divided into positive or sensations of heat, and negative or sensations
of cold, according to whether the temperature of the object is higher or
lower than that of the body. Inasmuch as the temperature of the skin is
constantly subjected to fluctuations, it is clear that a sharp distinction
between these conceptions is not easily made. Temperature impression is
intensified by the number of nerve endings receiving it, and by the greater
or lesser thickness of the epidermis, which is a poor conductor of heat.

To sum up, we have in the nerve apparatus of the skin, facilities for
perceiving pain, temperature and space, all the intricate functions of an
organ of sensation.

I will now turn to the second function of the skin, that of excretion.
The skin is important as an organ of excretion has been recognized since
the time of Galen. Suppression of the perspiration is a menace to health.
The extensive glandular structure of the skin discharges an enormous
amount of water. Carbonic acid also is exhaled through the skin, and
even urea, the latter more frequently and copiously in cases where the kidneys are not in good working order. In various other diseases, especially
in diseases of the lungs and heart, in which other physiological functions
of these organs are diminished, the exhalation of carbonic acid by cutaneous excretion is usually increased. You will have witnessed in severe cases

of asthma, the profuse perspiration of the patient. In such cases the walls of the cutaneous vessels are dilated, more water, aqueous vapor, and carbonic acid are excreted, and the difficulty of breathing is relieved. Also, when the heart's action is depressed, the lumina of the cutaneous vessels become distended, affording some compensatory action to tide the patient over immediate danger. The clammy sweat, so characteristic of cardiac inadequacy, is a commonly observed clinical phenomenon.

Now we come to the third phase, the skin as a heat regulator. This is the most important function of the skin in connection with Hydrotherapy. It depends to a great extent upon the two functions previously referred to. The maintenance of the body's temperature is of great importance to the human organism and the contribution of the skin to this process is indispensable. It is a physiological fact that the standard of the body temperature depends upon the maintenance of an equilibrium between heat production and heat loss. Heat is produced by the combustion of non-nitrogenous substances, chiefly in the muscles, and that heat is given off by perspiration and radiation from the cutaneous surface. When heat loss exceeds production, the temperature is lowered until the processes of life are interrupted, and life ceases.

We come now to the physical properties of water. First, these are the capacity for gathering, absorbing and conducting heat and cold. Water possesses a remarkable capacity for absorbing heat without being itself much raised in temperature, and giving off heat without losing materially in temperature. The amount of heat sufficient to raise the temperature of two pounds of oil of turpentine, eight pounds of iron, or thirty-five pounds of mercury to thirty-four degrees, will raise one pound of water only to the same degree.

The temperature conducting capacity of water is twenty-seven times greater than that of air. Water conveys to the skin much stronger thermic impressions than air, a fact easily discovered in exchanging a room with a temperature of 70° F/21° C for a bath at the same temperature.

Second, the flexibility of water. The enormous physical changes which water is capable of exerting as the result of different temperatures enlarges its value as a flexible thermic agent. At 32° F/0° C, water solidifies; at 212° F/100° C it becomes elastic, increasing seventeen hundred times in volume. In the form of ice, it possesses valuable thermic properties which are impossible in other forms.

In the form of steam, it is again a most useful agent. The application of water has a wide range by our ability to apply it at any temperature. A temperature of from 34° to 120° F/1° to 49° C renders water a most flexible therapeutic agent. I use here not the common terms, hot and cold water, because they do not express absolute accuracy. People differ in regards to toleration of heat and cold; what seems warm to one person is very hot to another, and what seems to be cool to one, is cold to another. Therefore, it is more satisfactory to define yourself to degrees. The following table will illustrate the relation of common names as to degrees:

Very hot	104° F and above/40° C and above
Hot	100° to 104° F/38° to 40° C
Warm	92° to 100° F/33° to 38° C
Neutral	94° to 97° F/34°to 36° C
Tepid	80° to 92° F/27° to 33° C
Cool	70° to 80° F/21° to 27° C
Cold	55° to 70° F/13° to 21° C
Very cold	32° to 54° F/0° to 12° C

I say here that I do not approve of the ice bag; in fact I never use the ice upon the cutaneous surface contrary to widespread custom. My reasons are good ones and are endorsed by such authorities as Prof. Baruch, Prof. Winternitz, and others.

If you remember, I said that water had great absorbing power, and that is the reason I do not advocate ice, because ice has not this power. My opinion is that like in any other cases, convenience plays a large part in using ice instead of water. It is so easy to lay the ice bag upon the parts which suffer, because ice keeps cool so long, but water will have to be renewed ten times in the same period that one application of ice would require. The ice does not reduce the inflammation as a cold water application will do. Ice acts as a local anesthetic and therefore, should never be used in cases of appendicitis, pneumonia, peritonitis and even not in cases of fever.

The third physical property of the water is the perfect control of the fluidity. We may change the size, form and character of the stream and direct it to any or all portions of the body and by this limiting the local and general effects with nicety and precision. The various hydriatric procedures, full bath, half bath, sitz bath, spinal douche, upper and lower douche, chest and knee douche, etc., etc., devise their technique and application from this property of water.

The capacity of water as influenced by different degrees of pressure gives it the power to produce mechanical effects upon the nerve and blood supply of the skin, which form one of the most interesting and least appreciated elements of Hydrotherapy. By proper mechanical contrivances, water may be applied almost without pressure, as by a sponge, or by pouring from a vessel, which is just above the level of the cutaneous surface; it may flow from a height with great force, or may be driven upon the skin by compressed air, or applied by a rubber hose with or without a nozzle from a shorter or longer distance.

Here again we find a range of action which enables the physician to produce varied effects, adapted to the therapeutic indications which may present themselves.

In order to show what effect water has in disease, we must show its action in health. I quote here from Simon Baruch:

The action of thermic and mechanical application of water, either cold or hot, is that of irritants to the peripheral sensory nerves.

1. Irritation may be conveyed to some portions of the central nervous system, and thence reflected by motor fibres to the various parts which we desire to influence.

2. Changes of the total enervation of the parts which we desire to influence.

3. May be produced by effects upon the ganglionic centres, which exist in the nerve supply of the vessels, and which perform the function of nerve centres within their immediate sphere without depending upon reflex impulses from the brain or spinal cord. The effect of these nerve irritants depends, like that upon the extent of surface receiving their impact, upon the susceptibility of the entire organism or of the point of application, and also upon the suddenness of the impact. The thermic and mechanical action of water upon the circulation, respiration, temperature, tissue change and secretions, forms the basis of all those notable results which Hydrotherapy has obtained.

[Water] can be used in one form or another, in the broadest sense of the word, in all ailments and diseases, without exception.

I am sorry to add that many naturopathic physicians have abandoned Hydrotherapy. Sometimes the physician has not money enough, or thinks he has not money enough to equip his treatment rooms with the suitable arrangements and appliances. Expensive equipment is not necessary.

Hydrotherapy includes the application of water in any form, from the solid and fluid to vapor; from ice to steam, internally and externally.

Water possesses a remarkable capacity for absorbing heat without being itself much raised in temperature, and giving off heat without losing materially in temperature.

The temperature conducting capacity of water is twenty-seven times greater than that of air. Water conveys to the skin much stronger thermic impressions than air, a fact easily discovered in exchanging a room with a temperature of 70° F/21° C for a bath at the same temperature.

The enormous physical changes which water is capable of exerting as the result of different temperatures enlarges its value as a flexible thermic agent. At 32° F/0° C, water solidifies; at 212° F / 100° C it becomes elastic, increasing seventeen hundred times in volume.

People differ in regards to toleration of heat and cold; what seems warm to one person is very hot to another, and what seems to be cool to one, is cold to another.

If you remember, I said that water had great absorbing power, and that is the reason I do not advocate ice, because ice has not this power.

1915

SITZ BATHS
Dr. Carl Strueh

MAGNESIA SULPHATE OR EPSOM SALTS BATH
Benedict Lust, N.D.

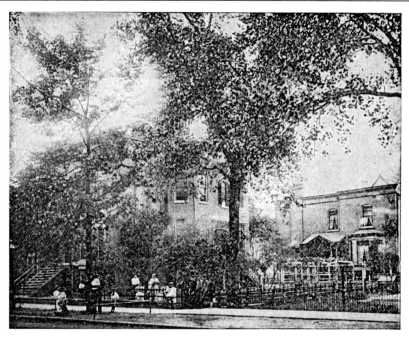

Trained as a medical doctor in Zürich, Dr. Carl Strueh established a practice at 464 Belden Avenue in Chicago. Quickly disillusioned with drug treatments, Strueh became an avid Hydrotherapist and would be one of Benedict Lust's supporters. He placed advertisements in Lust's publications from its inception.

Sitz Baths

by Dr. Carl Strueh

The Naturopath and Herald of Health, XX (4), 215. (1915)

Sitz baths are one of the most important forms of the Water Cure. More has been written about them than about any other water application. Priessnitz, the Father of the Water Cure, already used them extensively at his famous watering place at Freiberg in Silesia, more than a hundred years ago.

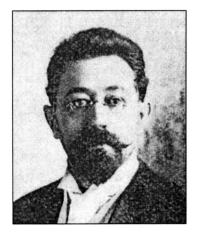

Carl Strueh, M.D.

Special bathtubs are usually used in giving sitz baths; however, an ordinary wash tub can be made to serve the purpose. As a rule, the sitz bath tubs are made of tin or porcelain. The latter are, however, quite expensive. The best and most practical sitz bath tubs are those which have running water connections, as much water can be added as is desired. These tubs can be so adjusted that the appropriate quantity of water can enter and leave the tub at the same time. For some purposes it is advisable to have special spraying attachments, such as circular spray, perineal spray, etc.

As regards the temperature of the water used, we differentiate among cold, lukewarm, warm and hot sitz baths. Cold sitz baths, having the power of abstracting heat from the body, are especially beneficial in inflammatory and feverish diseases.

People afflicted with arteriosclerosis (hardening of the blood vessels) must be cautious about taking cold sitz baths, as a sudden rush of blood to the head may result in apoplexy, i.e. the bursting of a blood vessel in the head. For this reason it is best even by healthy people to place a cold compress on the head while taking a cold sitz bath. Cold sitz baths are advisable for weak intestines, chronic constipation, scanty menstruation, sexual weakness, torpid liver, congestions to the head or lungs, etc.

They are, as a rule, of short duration. In cases of inflammatory conditions of the liver, spleen, intestines, certain kinds of diarrhea, however, cold sitz baths of longer duration are more effective.

Warm and also hot sitz baths must always be from 20 to 30 minutes in order to accomplish their purpose. They are a splendid means of relieving abdominal pains caused by various conditions, such as gallstones, intestinal afflictions, difficult menstruation, etc. They are also helpful in certain cases of nervousness and sleeplessness.

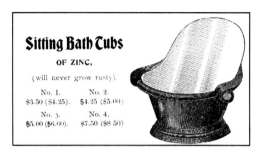

Lukewarm sitz baths which should last from 5-15 minutes and have a temperature of about 68° F/20° C, often work wonders for women being afflicted with headaches and nervousness due to an oversupply of blood to the brain. They are also used successfully for hemorrhoids, sluggish digestion and for weak intestines and sexual organs.

Outdoor exercise should always be taken after a cold or lukewarm sitz bath, otherwise the desired reaction will not take place.

A special form of the sitz bath is the so-called immersion bath which is very beneficial in afflictions of the bowels and in women's diseases. These baths should be taken eight or ten times within twenty-four hours, each immersion requiring only a minute. The water used for these baths must, however, not be too cold.

Priessnitz, the Father of the Water Cure, already used [sitz baths] extensively at his famous watering place at Freiberg in Silesia, more than a hundred years ago.

Cold sitz baths are advisable for weak intestines, chronic constipation, scanty menstruation, sexual weakness, torpid liver, congestions to the head or lungs, etc.

Warm and also hot sitz baths must always be from 20 to 30 minutes in order to accomplish their purpose. They are a splendid means of relieving abdominal pains caused by various conditions, such as gallstones, intestinal afflictions, difficult menstruation, etc.

A special form of the sitz bath is the so-called immersion bath which is very beneficial in afflictions of the bowels and in women's diseases. These baths should be taken eight or ten times within twenty-four hours, each immersion requiring only a minute. The water used for these baths must, however, not be too cold.

Magnesia Sulphate Or Epsom Salts Bath*

by Benedict Lust

The Naturopath and Herald of Health, XX (7). (1915)

No element or compound known to science will so quickly, surely, and readily dissolve uric acid and neutralize all poisons in the blood and tissues of the body as magnesia sulphate or Epsom salts. This bath may be given as a sponge bath, or in a tub with the usual quantity of water. If a patient is not able to get in tub properly, the sponge bath may be given him with the usual quantity, say a gallon for this, with about a teacup full of the salts to this quantity of water, or about an ounce of salts to each pint of water. To relieve rheumatic conditions and dissolve poisons in the body or in the blood and tissues of the body, spend fifteen to thirty minutes several times a day for a day or two, and then about two a day, after a while only one will answer. Recovery from rheumatism using Epsom salts will be very rapid.

The full tub bath is the best of all when it can be given. In this use from three to five pounds of the Epsom salts, according to the capacity of the tub. Let the patient remain in the bath from ten to twenty minutes, or even thirty minutes sometimes, with the water warm. After being [in the Epsom salt bath] for about five minutes, the skin will become somewhat slimy in feeling, as if the poisonous substances had been drawn out by the action of the salts, which is indeed the case. Then rub the body under the water with a coarse sponge. After five or six minutes repeat this rubbing. Take from fifteen to thirty minutes in all for the tub bath.

In giving this bath to chronic rheumatics we have sometimes observed the water to become so foul from the soaked out toxins that the odor in the room became so offensive that windows in the room had to be opened. Sometimes we have let the water run out of the tub, and fresh water run in again, with a new supply of salts, which in turn would also become quite filthy. Next day the water would become less filthy.

The full tub bath may be repeated several times during the first days, and less frequently as the treatment advances. Once a day will answer in most cases, and when more advanced with the work, every other day will suffice. It is a most powerful aid in all rheumatic troubles, paralysis, locomotor ataxia, etc.

Never use soap of any kind in giving Epsom salt baths, as one counteracts the other. You will find it the very best for yourself as a health guard, as it is the best bath ever given for anything. Take it as your regular bath a few times, and you will never want any other. Bed time is always

---

*This article was found among advertisements and letters in the July, 1915 issue. —*Ed.*

a good period for the bath for yourself, but it may be taken at any other hour of the day.

You will find Epsom salts very cheap if purchased in quantity. Before the present war began, the price was less than two cents per pound, but is somewhat higher now. It is the most cleansing, purifying, and invigorating bath ever given.

No element or compound known to science will so quickly, surely, and readily dissolve uric acid and neutralize all poisons in the blood and tissues of the body as magnesia sulphate or Epsom salts.

To relieve rheumatic conditions and dissolve poisons in the body or in the blood and tissues of the body, spend fifteen to thirty minutes several times a day for a day or two, and then about two a day, after a while only one will answer.

In this [full tub] use from three to five pounds of the Epsom salts, according to the capacity of the tub. Let the patient remain in this from ten to twenty minutes, or even thirty minutes sometimes, with the water warm.

In giving this bath to chronic rheumatics we have sometimes observed the water to become so foul from the soaked out toxins that the odor in the room became so offensive that windows in the room had to be opened.

Never use soap of any kind in giving Epsom salt baths, as one counteracts the other.

1916

Sitz Baths
Joseph A. Hoegen, N.D.

The Nauheim Bath
Simon Baruch, M.D.

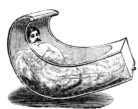
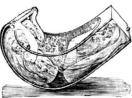
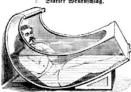
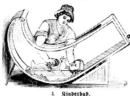
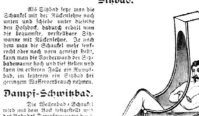
Oh, this is my dream sitz bath tub. This ad appeared in the German issues of *Amerikanischen Kneipp Blätter* in 1900. —Ed.

Hydrotherapy Department

Address all communications for this department to its editor
JOS. A. HOEGEN, N.D., 334 Alexander Avenue, New York

SITZ BATHS

by Joseph A. Hoegen, N.D.

Herald of Health and Naturopath, XXI (7), 468-469. (1916)

The sitz bath is something that should be in every home where health is valued. It is one of the most useful and the oldest of water procedures. A tub is so arranged that the patient can sit down in it while bathing, leaving the feet outside and placed in a smaller vessel during the application. The sitz bath is given cold, tepid, or warm, as the condition requires. The lower part of the hips, abdomen and upper part of the thighs are immersed in the sitz bath. It should be large enough to permit a thorough rubbing and kneading of the diseased parts.

THE COLD SITZ BATH

The cold sitz bath is given at a temperature from 55° to 65° F/13° to 18° C, and while some keep their patients in the tub as long as 15 minutes, I believe from my experience, that one to two minutes is sufficient in all cases when the water is used cold. It is an excellent tonic in cases of relaxed tissues of the pelvis, in debility of the urinary genital organs in piles, prolapsus of the rectum, and constipation. It produces active dilatation of the vessels of the lower abdomen, increasing the blood supply through these parts. It is a good bath for those suffering from congestion of the brain, congestion of the prostate, in gleet and in the atonic forms of seminal weakness. It should not be used where there is acute inflammation of the pelvic or abdominal viscera, in sciatica, in acute cases of pulmonary congestion, neither in painful conditions of the bladder or genital organs, as in cystitis, ovaritis, colitis, appendicitis, and peritonitis, in neuralgia of the ovaries, bladder, testicles, and is decidedly harmful in spermatorrhea or frequent losses. I always use a hot foot bath in connection with the cold sitz bath. Rubbing the whole surface while the patient is in the cold sitz bath is a powerful means of stimulating cerebral activity.

THE TEPID SITZ BATH

The tepid sitz bath is given at a temperature of from 80° to 90° F/27° to 32° C and the duration may be from 20 minutes to one hour. It has a

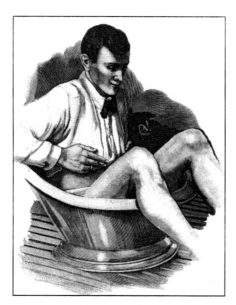

The cold sitz bath

calming, quieting effect upon the viscera of the pelvis and lower abdomen, and there is really no condition in which this bath may not be given. It is especially useful in cases of nervous irritability, bladder catarrh, neuralgia of the fallopian tubes or the testicles, pruritus of the anus and vulva, and in excessive sensitiveness of the urethra and ejaculatory ducts, also in all cases of pelvic disease, where on account of pain or inflammatory conditions, cold applications would be harmful.

THE HOT SITZ BATH

The hot sitz bath is an effective remedial adjunct in menstrual suppression and painful menstruation, gravel, spasmodic and acute inflammatory affections generally. The temperature is from 105° to 115° F/41° to 46° C, and the duration from three to ten minutes. The foot bath taken with it, may be of the same temperature. The hot sitz bath is a most powerful measure of relieving pain. It is excellent in cases of vaginismus, uterine colic and in all painful conditions of a non-inflammatory character, where the viscera of the pelvis and lower abdomen are involved. It is certainly one of the most useful measures that can be employed for the various neuralgias of the genito-urinary organs of which women and also men suffer so much. To get a good effect, the hot sitz bath should be followed by a cold application, but very short. The cost of a sitz bath is so reasonable, that no family should be without one.

A tub is so arranged, that the patient can sit down in it while bathing, leaving the feet outside, and placed in a smaller vessel during the application.

The cold sitz bath is given at a temperature from 55° to 65°F/ 13° to 18° C, and while some keep their patients in the tub as long as 15 minutes, I believe from my experience, that one to two minutes is sufficient in all cases when the water is used cold.

[The cold sitz bath] produces active dilatation of the vessels of the lower abdomen, increasing the blood supply through these parts. It is a good bath for those suffering from congestion of the brain, congestion of the prostate, in gleet and in the atonic forms of seminal weakness.

I always use a hot foot bath in connection with the cold sitz bath. Rubbing the whole surface while the patient is in the cold sitz bath is a powerful means of stimulating cerebral activity.

It has a calming, quieting effect upon the viscera of the pelvis and lower abdomen, and there is really no condition in which this bath may not be given.

The hot sitz bath is an effective remedial adjunct in menstrual suppression and painful menstruation, gravel, spasmodic and acute inflammatory affections generally.

THE NAUHEIM BATH*

by Dr. Simon Baruch, M.D.

Herald of Health and Naturopath, XXI (8), 532-536. (1916)

Dr. Simon Baruch, M.D., writes in the *N.Y. Journal of Medicine* that his reasons for presenting the Nauheim Method as a subject for discussion are:

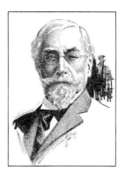

Dr. Simon Baruch
(1840-1921)

First—The success of this method of managing cardiac diseases has been established, during the most enlightened period of the history of medicine, not by the statements of patients, which are often unreliable, but by observations of specialists, who have demonstrated their confidence by continuing to send their patients to this mecca of heart cases.

Second—The mineral springs of Saratoga and certain California springs furnish the most important component of the waters that have made Nauheim famous, viz., carbonic acid gas, and require the addition only of certain salines to be equal to those of Nauheim.

Third—I have been painfully surprised to discover that the large proportion of baths ordered as Nauheim baths are given with simple carbonic acid water from a cylinder of gas or artificially produced by mixing a definite solution of bicarbonate of soda with either muriatic acid or sulphite of sodium cakes, or formic acid. The salines are either omitted or a few pounds of salt, or a natural brine or sea water, or as in one institution, sodium chloride and bicarbonate of soda, which actually counteracts the desired irritating action of the salt, misrepresenting them.

Fourth—It is my aim to obviate this unfortunate substitution, which may be due to the prevailing lack of agreement upon the rationale of the Nauheim method, by offering an explanation of the action of certain elements of the latter, which, though novel, has a rational basis.

Fifth—My warrant for venturing upon this subject may be found in the historical fact that the method consists, as is well known, of the application of baths, in which the patient is submerged entirely, excepting the head, in water, containing carbonic acid gas and certain salines, chief among which are the chloride of calcium and sodium, which in concentrated form would produce a decided hyperemia. These baths are given

---

*Nauheim, a town in Germany, became famous in the 19th century for its mineral waters containing carbon dioxide. Carbon dioxide baths continue to be used throughout the world today for cardiovascular diseases and many other complaints. —*Ed.*

methodically, according to the indications of each case and the effect of each bath, and they are accompanied or followed by certain passive or resisting movements, which offer a systematic but mild exercise of the principal voluntary muscles of the body. Success of the Nauheim method depends upon faithfully following the method.

Artificial CO_2 Bath

In 1896 I brought from Germany the Sandow tablets, consisting of cakes of sodium sulphite and a package of bicarbonate of soda, for the artificial preparation of carbonic acid baths, which I gave to Mr. H. A. Cassebeer, who prepared the Cassebeer Nauheim Baths. The Triton preparation resembles the latter.

In 1902, I visited the Virchow Hospital at Berlin. Here Dr. Laqeur used the ZEO bath, which consists of a solution of formic acid and a package of bicarbonate of soda. From experiments in the Vanderbilt Clinic, I ascertained its advantages, not being corrosive and more quickly prepared. The CO_2 bubbles were more abundant and the consequent hyperemia of the skin more pronounced.

These preparations had never been used in this country before as far as I know.

In 1896, I visited Nauheim for the first time and since then I have made two visits, the last being in 1913. It has been my good fortune to come in contact with Drs. Heineman, Groedel, Schott and Honan, during these visits. The Nauheim method has passed through a gradual evolution, in regard to its theory and practice. I desire to emphasize that the entire series is a methodical training of the insufficient heart to enable it to resist definite attacks made upon the cutaneous periphery, by baths and exercises, alternating with rest. Indeed, we have here the same principle which I have frequently dwelt upon in the application of water in health and disease, viz., that water below the temperature of the skin produces an effect upon the blood vessels and nerves of the skin, which I have termed "neuro-vascular training", by means of which the heart and central nervous system are raised in functional efficiency, so that the organs supplied by them are restored to normal activity, which has been disturbed by toxic agencies, or by products of abnormal tissue change, due to faulty modes of living.

In the most recent publication of Professor J. M. Groedel, this veteran of Nauheim confirms my view, when he writes, "We have it in our power to put into action the excitations which drive the heart to higher activity, by gradual approach. We may stimulate the heart to a greater or lesser degree, within definite limits, through the intensity of the thermic excitation, namely, low temperature of the water."

Formerly the Nauheim doctors began the series with baths of indifferent temperature, about 34° C/93.2° F, with small saline and carbonic acid content. This was followed slowly by a gradual decrease of the bath temperature, until 30° C/86° F, while at the same time the saline and carbonic acid content was increased and the duration of the bath raised from eight or ten minutes to fifteen or twenty minutes, giving at first the bath two days in succession, or every second, third or fourth day. Recently this course has been abandoned for a more individualized scheme, which is based upon the actual effect of each bath, or small series of baths, upon the patient and the type or character of the cardiac insufficiency.

In Nauheim, no treatment is administered for the higher grades of circulatory insufficiency in persons, who, for instance, when at rest or under the slightest movement suffer from dyspnea, or who present large dropsical effusions. I have in mind a case of the former type, in which I advised against a journey to Nauheim, but was not sustained by an eminent specialist, who had advised him to consult me about the Nauheim trip, although I had endeavored to neutralize his obstinacy by telling him that he would return in a coffin. He arrived in Nauheim, but was advised not to remain longer than necessary to recuperate from the journey. He did arrive home in a coffin, dying one day before the ship arrived.

It was the merit of Beneke to retain cases that were promising and to discourage others from remaining in the vain hope of recovery. His successors, though not so rigid, have followed this course, with the result that Nauheim has established a reputation for the amelioration and cure of heart disease. Let me counsel colleagues practicing in Saratoga to follow Beneke's example.

RATIONALE OF THE NAUHEIM BATH

This may be divided into two essential elements, (a) effect of the carbon dioxide, (b) of the salines.

ACTION OF THE CARBON DIOXIDE

From experience on my own person, together with observations made upon many other individuals in Bad Nauheim and in Saratoga Springs, the following are the notable objective and subjective effects:

On entering a bath, with Hathorn No. 1 water, at 90° F/32° C, my first impression was one of decided coolness, with contraction of the scrotum. This coldness disappears as soon as bubbles of CO_2 gas begin to accumulate upon the skin. A prickling sensation begins, sometimes painful, on touching, in the scrotum, which feels as if covered by a very thin layer of dry varnish. If these bubbles are disturbed on large surfaces, coolness is again felt quickly, however, replaced by warmth, so soon as the gas bubbles again are seen on the skin. The skin shows decided hyperemia wherever it is in contact with the gas bubbles. Decided warmth is felt, together with a sense of comfort and *bien aise*, that is not felt when plain cold water produces reaction redness. In fact, the latter only reaches similar intensity of redness but never the same intensity of warmth, after very cold procedures, in vigorous subjects. Certain it is that I have never seen a patient in the condition which is met in the majority of cardiac cases, that could bear a cold procedure with plain water of sufficiently low temperature to produce a hyperemia equal to that which the most depreciated cardiac case can be trained up to bear with the CO_2 bath.

LOCAL ACTION OF CO_2 WATER

The hyperemia, which is invariably manifested when the individual lies in a CO_2 bath, by redness of the skin, cannot be due to reflex action, through the vasomotor system, because it is confined only to the parts expose to the CO_2 water. A careful study of the experiments and observations made by others confirm my conviction that the hyperemia is due to a specific mechanic-chemical irritation by the CO_2 gas. (Oxygen bubbles in the Ozet Bath do not produce hyperemia.)

Ottfried Miller and his school have demonstrated by painstaking observations, the absence of decided vasomotor action, because of absence of resistance at the periphery. There is no plethysmographic volume increase in the arm made red and hyperemic by CO_2.* This has been successfully refuted by Arthur Hurschfelt of Brieger's Clinic, who shows that Miller's plethysmograph rested partly in the bath water. Nevertheless, both agree upon the most important fact that the peripheral arteries are contracted slightly. May this not be due to the constringing action of the absorbed CO_2 upon their muscular coats, which come in direct contact with the gas? More of this later on. The almost invariable slowing of the pulse and its somewhat heightened tension, find in this theory a more rational explanation.

Another undeniable effect of the CO_2 upon the skin is a heightening of cutaneous sensibility, which has been referred to. I regard this phenomenon as explaining the intensifying effect of CO_2 on temperature sensation, whether below or above the point of indifference, which averages in a plain water bath for ambulant patients about 33° C/91.4 F and 35° C/95 F in persons warmed by lying in bed previous to coming in contact with plain water. O. Miller states that this neutral point is (in the CO_2 bath for ambulant patients) about 34° C/93.2° F. Despite the fact that the skin feels a sensation of warmth, the action of the CO_2 bath is equivalent to that of water of lower temperature in its influence upon

---

*Carbon dioxide causes vasodilation and those taking these cool CO_2 baths have a sensation of warmth, a result of increased blood flow. —*Ed.*

the vaso-motor system (Miller). The first time I had occasion to utilize this singular fact was in a desperate case of typhoid fever, I saw with Dr. Joseph Fraenkel, of New York, several years ago. The doctor had been advised by two eminent consultants against using a cold bath and to rely upon alcoholic stimulants to rescue the patient from desperate toxemia, which blunted all reflexes. Believing that it was imperative to arouse the reflexes by refreshment with cold water and fearing to advise the Brand bath, a tubbing in water at 80° F/27° C was advised, with Cassbeer's Nauheim salts, to add a chemical to the thermic and mechanical peripheral excitation. Though there was not the slightest visible response to the cold water and none even to an affusion at 50° F/10° C, her pulse improved in tension and frequency and she slept for three hours after the first bath and awoke from an unconscious state of several days' duration, during the fourth four hourly bath, the pulse improving after each one. ("*Ueber Reaction nach kalten Prozeduren*", *Congress fuer Naturforscher und Aertzte in Karlsbad*, 1902)

This experience was repeated in other consultations, so that in typhoid fever I no longer hesitate to order certain cold baths, from which I formerly refrained in depreciated cases when fortified by CO_2 gas. My experiments have demonstrated the enhancement of sensibility in the peripheral nerves by CO_2 baths, so that the clinical fact above mentioned is accounted for and we are able to deduce from them a phase of therapeutic action of CO_2 baths in cardiac insufficiency that has been hitherto obscure.

The bubbles of CO_2 gas which envelop the body as it were in a network, isolate the portions so protected against extremes of temperatures, so that the beneficial results referred to above are attained. Temperatures that would be obnoxious, either above or below tolerance, are borne with comparative comfort when the water contains CO_2 bubbles.

The systematic effect from absorption of CO_2 is more important in my estimation than is generally believed. Indeed absorption of CO_2 gas is the positive fact undisputed by all authorities. Ottfried Miller and his aids mention it, but do not appear to realize its importance. (*Sammlung Klinischer Vortraege*, No. 711-14, 1915)

The absorption of CO_2 through the skin and its activation of respiration has been indisputably established by the valuable investigations in Von Mering's Clinic at Erlangen by H. Winternitz (*Deutches Archiv. F. Klin. Medizin*, Bd. 72) who regards this action as specific in CO_2, being absent in other cutaneous irritants and he affirms an increase of absorption in the presence of salt solutions. This is a neglected but important fact, which explains what hitherto has been obscure, as I shall show.

In commenting upon my new rationale of the Nauheim Bath, Professor Groedel protests that there is already a fatal increase of CO_2 in many cardiac cases. In rebuttal, I would point to the fact that we deduce from animal experiments with toxic doses of drugs, our most valued therapeutic results from safer doses of the poisons. Moreover, the cyanosis present in extreme cardiac failure is due more to the absence of oxygen than to accumulated CO_2. That CO_2 circulating in the blood in excess stimulates the respiratory center is a well-known physiological fact; an increase of 2 percent causing a tenfold energy of respiratory activity in health. (Burton-Opitz) Starling (*Lancet, 1915*) gave CO_2 the first place as the hormone or chemical regulator of respiration. Therapeutically this enhancement of respiratory activity becomes of immense import, in that it must influence favorably the entire intrathoracic circulation, more especially the venous flow. The right heart is unloaded and the diastole production of edemas and retention of toxins from faulty tissue change, give the bedside clinician most anxiety and but too often close the scene. I am disposed to regard this action of the absorbed CO_2 as most important in temporarily restoring lost cardiac equilibrium. That judicious adaptation of the bath to each individual case is required is evident. It is remarkable that other clinicians do not lay more stress upon this demonstrated action of CO_2.

Distribution of blood as manifested by blood pressure, pulse frequency, volume and tension, has been a bone of contention among investigators, Ottfried Miller and other laboratory reporters claim some increase of blood pressure, while Groede, Jacob and others who practice with natural CO_2 baths, do not find increase of blood pressure to any extent. Nevertheless, all report almost invariably an improvement in the pulse, evidencing bettered cardiac conditions. My own observation, made with Saratoga waters published in the last summer of the *N.Y. Medical Journal* confirms their view.

This difference in the observations of equally reliable clinicians may be explained as follows: The action of water, air and CO_2 gas upon the skin is determined by the temperature conducting capacity of these agents. Air and CO_2 gas differ materially in capacity of absorbing temperatures (cold and heat) and water absorbs temperature with far greater rapidity than either. The point at which the skin is indifferent to water, air or CO_2, as ascertained by changes of blood pressure is 34° to 35° C/93° to 95° F for plain water, and it is lower for atmospheric air, in ordinary humidity, 20° to 25° C/68° to 77° C and for CO_2 gas it is still lower, viz.: 13.5° to 14° C/56.3° to 57.2° F. According to Senator and Frankenheimer (*Therapie der Gegenwart*, 1904) air, water and CO_2 gas differ still more positively in conductivity or capacity for transmitting temperature to objects. Taking the conductivity of air to be 100 that of CO_2 gas is inferior (almost one-half) to that of air, and almost infinitesimal when compared to water (1 to 54). Therefore, CO_2 conducts its own temperature, so slowly to the skin that it must be warmed by the temperature of the water, long before the skin can be affected by it. For example, if the temperature of the water at 90° F / 32° C is conveyed to the skin in one-tenth of a second, the CO_2 temperature would require 540 seconds (nine minutes) to reach the skin, were it not held in the water. This being the case, the water, which absorbs temperature readily, is endowed with the temperature indifference of CO_2 but slightly. The water temperature always dominates, because of its great conductivity, both in the low and high temperature baths. This confirms the results of my clinical observation. (*Principles and Practice of Hydrotherapy*, Wm. Wood & Co., Third Edition, p. 51)

In my estimation, a potent influence upon the circulation has been overlooked by all observers, viz.: the direct stimulation of the heart muscle by absorbed CO_2. We have experimental warrant for such cardiac stimulation in the fact that animals poisoned by CO_2 die with the heart in systolic contraction.

The success of this method of managing cardiac diseases has been established, during the most enlightened period of the history of medicine, not by the statements of patients, which are often unreliable, but by observations of specialists, who have demonstrated their confidence by continuing to send their patients to this mecca of heart cases.

Indeed, we have here the same principle which I have to frequently dwelt upon in the application of water in health and disease, viz., that water below the temperature of the skin produces an effect upon the blood vessels and nerves of the skin, which I have termed "neuro-vascular training," by means of which the heart and central nervous system are raised in functional efficiency, so that the organs supplied by them are restored to normal activity, which has been disturbed by toxic agencies, or by products of abnormal tissue change, due to faulty modes of living.

Formerly the Nauheim doctors began the series with baths of indifferent temperature, about 34° C/93.2° F, with small saline and carbonic acid content. This was followed slowly by a gradual decrease of the bath temperature, until 30° C/86° F, while at the same time the saline and carbonic acid content was increased and the duration of the bath raised from eight or ten minutes to fifteen or twenty minutes, giving at first the bath two days in succession, or every second, third or fourth day.

In Nauheim, no treatment is administered for the higher grades of circulatory insufficiency in persons, who, for instance, when at rest or under the slightest movement suffer from dyspnea, or who present large dropsical effusions.

The skin shows decided hyperemia wherever it is in contact with the gas bubbles. Decided warmth is felt, together with a sense of comfort and bien aise, *that is not felt when plain cold water produces reaction redness.*

A careful study of the experiments and observations made by others confirm my conviction that the hyperemia is due to a specific mechanic-chemical irritation by the CO_2 gas.

My experiments have demonstrated the enhancement of sensibility in the peripheral nerves by CO_2 baths, so that the clinical fact above mentioned is accounted for and we are able to deduce from them a phase of therapeutic action of CO_2 baths in cardiac insufficiency that has been hitherto obscure.

Moreover the cyanosis present in extreme cardiac failure is due more to the absence of oxygen than to accumulated CO_2.

That CO_2 circulating in the blood in excess stimulates the respiratory center is a well-known physiological fact; an increase of 2 percent causing a tenfold energy of respiratory activity in health.

Starling (Lancet, 1915) gave CO_2 the first place as the hormone or chemical regulator of respiration. Therapeutically this enhancement of respiratory activity becomes of immense import, in that it must influence favorably the entire intrathoracic circulation, more especially the venous flow.

It is remarkable that other clinicians do not lay more stress upon this demonstrated action of CO_2.

1917

HYDROTHERAPY
JOSEPH A. HOEGEN, N.D.

MY REMEDIAL AGENTS
LOUIS KUHNE

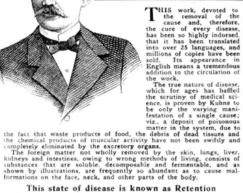
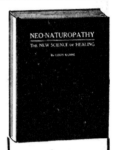
In 1917, Benedict Lust translated Louis Kuhne's book, *The New Science of Healing*, and republished it with a new title, *Neo-Naturopathy, the New Science of Healing.*

HydrotherapyDepartment

Address all communications for this department to its editor

JOS. A. HOEGEN, N.D., 334 Alexander Avenue, New York

HYDROTHERAPY

by Joseph A. Hoegen, N.D.

Herald of Health and Naturopath, XXII (5), 311-316. (1917)

Hydrotherapy! Greatest of all healing factors! Most beneficial system of treatment for human ills! And how much still abused, and how little understood! Many systems of healing have sprung up in late years. Many with much good. Where is there one to compare with the Water Cure? Where is one that produces such wonderful results, leaving no harmful after-effects, provided the treatment is applied in the proper manner?

If I were to choose among all systems of drugless healing, having studied nearly all, and knowing what results I can get, I would select the Water Cure as the most beneficial of all.

Great indeed is the value of a thorough knowledge of this science. I call it science, because it is proven to be an exact science, properly applied. I have time over and again impressed in my lectures and writings, the absolute necessity of knowing how to apply this science.

Every physician, no matter what other good system he may use, must use water to get best results, and I am profoundly sorry that there are many schools, who during their whole term of instruction, do not touch the subject of Hydrotherapy. Our medical schools go over it slightly, but do not impress upon the student sufficiently as to the great value of this simple remedy.

Water is, without any doubt, the oldest and most ancient method of treating disease. Several centuries before Christ, there are records of it being used and prescribed by Chinese physician, who then already used the wrapping up in linen sheets, similar to our pack. Water was always used in the treatment of disease by the ancient Hebrews, Greeks and Egyptians, and it is still used by them up to present day. The cold bath has been in use in Japan nearly 1,000 years. Even old Hippocrates, the famous Greek physician, born 460 B.C., and called "Father of Medicine," had an excellent knowledge of the physiological properties of water, which he employed in the treatment of fevers, ulcers, hemorrhage, and various other ills.

In Europe, Hydrotherapy is not new, and Father Kneipp, the great Bavarian water apostle, simply reviewed some of the crude methods that were used by English peasants almost two centuries ago.

In this country, in the 17th century, we had Dr. Benjamin Rush, who was very successful, and achieved wonderful results with the Water Cure for the treatment of rheumatism, gout, measles and yellow fever.

Within the last century, great and gifted men have taken up the Nature Cure method, principally the Water Cure. These men are Priessnitz, Schroth, Graham, Rausse, Kneipp, Kuhne, Just, Rikli, and many others. Priessnitz was one of the first to organize the use of water into a system, for which he deserves great credit. Winternitz, of Vienna, did much in bringing and establishing Hydrotherapy upon a sound and scientific basis.

As I said in the beginning, this wonderful agent, water, demands a thorough and practical knowledge of physiology. It will yield bad results in the hands of one not experienced in its use. One of the reasons why many physicians are still against recommending the use of water in treating disease, is that there are too many who are inexperienced in giving this treatment.

Too many Hydropaths apply one and the same treatment for nearly all patients, which is a dangerous procedure. No two cases are alike, and the full blooded patient surely does not need the same treatment that an anemic patient would require. A good Naturopath, as a rule, is a good Hydropath, because he has studied all the fundamentals necessary to enable him to apply water in diseased conditions of the body in the proper manner.

Water applied to the body should have the purpose of aiding the body to bring back and restore sick parts to health, and also to bring back proper functions to the organs which are working imperfectly, or it should make abnormal conditions normal. Water is a great and powerful means of restoring normal functions to the body.

An impaired circulation, due to lack of oxygen and muscular activity, cannot be cured by Hydrotherapy alone. Neither will cases of dissipation, overwork, improper partaking of food, etc., respond to Hydrotherapy alone. Unless the patient gives up the causes of his ailments, Hydrotherapy or any other therapy will not be of much use.

We use water, in giving treatments, ranging from very cold to very hot, from 32° to 104° F/0° to 40° C and over, all applications made suitable to the condition of the patient. Cold applications, as a rule, are always of short duration, thereby hastening the reaction.

In using water, we get an action and a reaction. The latter gives the important effect which we need. When we try to relieve pain by the use of hot water, of course we do not look for a reaction. Always adjust and suit the water to the body, not the body to the water, otherwise instead of increasing your patient's vitality, you decrease it. It would be folly to give a cold bath to a person who had been working hard, and was tired and sleepy. While it may make him feel very spry for the moment, it would draw too much on his reserve force, acting like exercise, causing the body to generate more energy, which in reality is only stored up during sleep.

The results we wish to obtain in Hydrotherapy depend almost entirely on the bodily temperature of the patient, and the mode of treatment employed. Also upon the length of time or the duration of the application, its suddenness, and the sensibility of the patient. That is where the true Hydropath must show his knowledge of this science, in order to get the proper results. I will give a few of the most common water applications used.

THE FULL BATH OR HIGH BATH

The high bath is used chiefly in cases of neurasthenia, hysteria, various nerve pains; also in cases of sleeplessness, etc. This is a tub bath, in which the patient is seated, and the water should reach above the shoulders. The patient usually remains in this bath from 15 to 20 minutes, and the temperature should be from 95° to 100° F/35° to 38° C. After the bath, the patient may have someone rub him down gently.

THE COLD FULL BATH

The cold full bath, in which the patient lies down, should not be given more than one minute, and the shortest duration is about 3 seconds. This short immersion, as a rule, is the best. Active movements should be engaged in, so that there is sufficient warmth to cause the skin to become reddened. The circulation and respiration are stimulated, and the cutaneous vessels become dilated. These cold baths are used chiefly when metabolism is retarded, and also where excretory activity is to be greatly increased, as in obesity, syphilis, scrofulosis, in chronic metallic poisoning, and whenever general stimulation is desired. It is given at a temperature of from 40° to 60° F/4° to 16° C, and on account of it being powerfully sedative, is employed for its tonic effects. If the vital powers are low, or the individual remains in it too long, the reaction is slow, and its effects injurious. While it is highly invigorating to robust persons, those who have a low standard of vitality should be cautious in its employment.

THE WARM FULL BATH

The warm full bath, given at a temperature varying from 92° to 98° F/33° to 37° C, is always agreeable and refreshing. It is used for equalizing the circulation, softening the skin, and removing impurities. It moderates pain, and soothes the whole system without weakening or debilitating. It is an efficient agent in many chronic diseases, convulsions, spasmodic affections of the bowels, rheumatism, and derangement of the genitourinary organs. In this bath, one may remain 25 to 30 minutes. It is always preferable to take a cool rub-down after getting out, in order to increase skin activity and promote circulation.

The Half Bath

The half bath is used often, but should be used still more. Patient sits in the water, which must reach the level of the umbilicus. This is a bath that all well persons should take for strengthening the abdomen and the lower organs. If these baths were used more, we would have less cases of piles, colic, hysteria, prolapses of the rectum, etc. The duration of the bath should not be more than one-half to two minutes. While in the water, rub the abdomen well, and have someone give good, vigorous friction on back and shoulders. This is very beneficial. Of course, these treatments must all be used with care, especially in diseased conditions. For instance, in typhoid fever, it would be a dangerous procedure to manipulate the abdomen, although excellent otherwise. Have the temperature from 84° F/28° C down as low as 68° F/20° C. Used in this manner, half baths constitute a good, general, stimulating, refreshing measure. In diseases of the spinal cord these baths should always be given a little warmer, about 85° F/29° C to 90° F / 32° C.

The Tepid Bath

The tepid bath is used for cleansing the body, and is given at a temperature of from 85° to 92° F/29° to 33° C. It is prescribed in fevers and inflammatory affections for its cooling effects. The temperature should always be regulated according to the vitality of the patient, and the bath may be repeated two or three times a day. It removes superfluous heat, and keeps the skin in a condition favorable for excretion.

The Shower Bath

The shower bath produces a shock to the nervous system by coming in contact with skin. Streams of cold water fall upon the neck, shoulders, and the body of the patient, who stands beneath the hose or shower. When the patient is full-blooded, feeble or nervous, or when some internal organ is diseased, the cold shower bath should not be employed. In plain debility, not accompanied by inflammation or symptoms of internal congestion, its use is beneficial. The most delicate persons can endure this procedure, if the force of the shower is moderated, and tepid water used. The usual means for inducing a good reaction, namely friction and exercise, should be employed.

THE SPONGE BATH

A sponge bath may be used extensively in acute or chronic diseases. It consists in a general or local application of water at any desired temperature. In acute diseases it is applied at a temperature agreeable to the patient. It is a pleasant mode of treatment, and may be repeated as often as necessary. It is well, in many cases, to take one part of the body at a time, then quickly drying it, thus avoiding exposure to cold. Excessive animal heat is thereby removed, the capillaries are relaxed, the circulation is equalized, and comfort and sleep are produced.

THE SALT RUB OR GLOW

A salt glow is splendid for patients not too ill, and is without a peer in its effects upon the skin and complexion. With all its virtues, it is the simplest measures, and can be taken very easily at home. Put a few pounds of coarse salt, the coarsest you can get, in an earthen jar, and pour enough water on it to produce a sort of slush, but not enough to dissolve the salt. This should be taken up in handfuls, and rubbed briskly over the entire person. Any one in ordinary health can do it for himself very easily. It is a tonic for feeble patients, who have little blood circulation, or where the skin is inactive. It is also good in cases of Bright's disease and diabetes. It should never be used in cases of eczema or skin diseases. Rub one part of the body after another, and use friction movements, but not too much pressure. After the application use shower or spray to remove any salt on the body. Then rub and dry quickly.

THE FOOT BATH

A foot bath is frequently used as a means of causing diaphoresis in colds, attacks of acute diseases, and also to draw the blood from the head or some internal organ. It is a powerful auxiliary in the treatment of those chronic diseases in which inflammation, congestion and a feeble circulation are prominent symptoms.

THE ALTERNATE FOOT BATH

An alternate foot bath is used by placing both feet in hot water for two to three minutes, then in cold water for half a minute. Then back into the hot, and then the cold, repeating the procedure a number of times. This alternate foot bath is excellent in chilblains, cold and sweating feet.

THE HOT FOOT BATH

The hot foot bath should be 104° to 120° F/40° to 49° C, beginning with about 102° F/39° C, and gradually increasing until 120° F/49° C is reached. The duration is from five minutes to half an hour, and the feet should be completely under water. I believe it is the bath most used. It is excellent in cases of sprained ankle, neuralgia and gout and may be made two to three times daily. This bath is also given to a patient when in the cold sitz bath.

THE COLD FOOT BATH

A cold foot bath is given from 45° to 55° F/7° to 13° C from one to five minutes duration, and is not quite as useful as the hot foot bath, but produces reflex, revulsion and other effects. Always have feet previously warmed; then place in tub, in which the water is three to four inches deep. Use friction on the feet while in the bath by rubbing the feet together. In cases of cerebral congestion, use the bath very short, in fact, all cold applications should always be used quick and short.

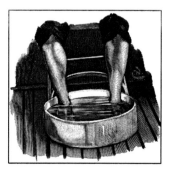

Cold foot bath

THE LEG BATH

The leg bath requires a deeper tub and more water, and its uses are about the same as the foot bath. It is recommended in the treatment of insomnia, pulmonary congestion, painful menstruation, suppressed menses, and ovarian congestion, in which conditions the hot leg bath are used.

THE SITZ BATH

A sitz bath is something that should be in every home where health is valued. It is one of the most useful of water procedures. A tub is so arranged that the patient can sit down in it while bathing, leaving the feet outside and placed in a smaller vessel during the application. The sitz bath is given cold, tepid or warm, as the condition requires. The lower part of the hips, abdomen and upper part of the thighs are immersed in the sitz bath. It should be large enough to permit a thorough rubbing and kneading of the diseased parts.

THE COLD SITZ BATH

The cold sitz bath is given at a temperature from 55° to 65° F/13° to 18° C, and while some keep their patients in the tub as long as 15 minutes, I believe in my experience that one to two minutes is quite enough, when the water is used cold. It is an excellent tonic in cases of relaxed tissues of the pelvis, in debility of the urinary genital organs, in piles, prolapses of the rectum, and constipation. It produces active dilation of the vessels of the lower abdomen, increasing the blood supply through these parts. It is an excellent bath for those suffering from congestion of the brain, congestion of the prostate, in gleet, and in the atonic forms of seminal weakness. It should not be used where there is acute inflammation of the pelvic or abdominal viscera, in sciatica, in acute cases of pulmonary congestion, neither in painful conditions of the bladder or genital organs, as in cystitis, ovaritis, colitis, appendicitis, peritonitis, neuralgia of the ovaries, bladder, testicles, and is decidedly harmful in spermatorrhea or frequent losses. I always use a hot foot bath in connection with the cold sitz bath. Rubbing the whole surface while the patient is in the cold sitz bath is a powerful means of stimulating cerebral activity.

The Tepid Sitz Bath

The tepid sitz bath is given at a temperature from 80° to 90° F/27° to 32° C and the duration is usually from 20 to 30 minutes. It has calming, quieting effect upon the viscera of the pelvis and lower abdomen, and there is really no condition in which this bath may not be given. It is especially useful in cases of nervous irritability, bladder catarrh, neuralgia of the fallopian tubes or the testicles, pruritus of the anus and vulva, and in excessive sensitiveness of the urethra; also in all cases of pelvic diseases where, on account of pain or inflammatory conditions, cold applications would be harmful.

The Hot Sitz Bath

The hot sitz bath is an effective remedial adjunct in menstrual suppression and pain menstruation, gravel [kidney stones], spasmodic and acute inflammatory affections generally. The temperature is from 105° to 115° F/41° to 46° C, and the duration from three to ten minutes. The foot bath taken with it may be of the same temperature. The hot sitz bath is a most powerful measure of relieving pain. It is excellent in cases of vaginismus, uterine colic, and in all cases of a non-inflammatory character where the viscera of the pelvis and lower abdomen is involved. It is certainly one of the most useful measures that can be employed for the various neuralgias of the genitourinary organs, from which women and men suffer so much. To get a good effect, the hot sitz bath should be followed by a cold application, but very short. The cost of a sitz bath is so reasonable, compared with the unlimited good derived from its use that no family should be without it.

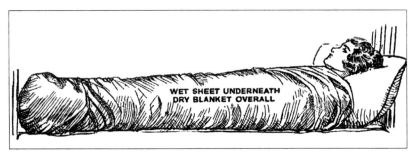

The wet sheet pack

THE WET SHEET PACK

The wet sheet pack is the most powerful and best blood cleanser known. It is without a peer, wherever feverish conditions exist. Spread upon the bed sheet, wring it out, not too tight, in cold water, and spread out smoothly on the woolen blanket. Have patient lie down on this wet sheet, arms extended, then wrap him closely and tightly and as quickly as possible. Each arm may be covered in this manner by the wet sheet, or may be covered separately by wet towels in the same manner as with the sheet. Then cover well with blankets and comforters, making sure that there is no place unwrapped. After the first shock of the chill is over, the pack is very soothing, pleasant and refreshing, and proof that the pack has a beneficial and quieting effecting upon the whole nervous system is, that nearly every patient falls asleep while in it.

The ordinary time for a patient to remain in a pack is about an hour; however, if the patient is in a feeble condition, a half hour is sufficient. After the pack, I usually give a warm bath, with gradual cooling, followed by massage. It is surprising to see how a pack like this throws off impurities from the body, by examining the sheet after the patient is taken out of it. It is one of the most efficient measures in fevers, breaking up cold, grippe, insomnia, and a valuable remedy in most chronic diseases, helping to remove the causes which depress bodily functions.

THE NAUHEIM BATH

A Nauheim bath consists of a salt water bath, properly carbonated. The body of the patient is covered with minute bubbles of carbonic acid gas that form rapidly on the immersed surface, and when disturbed, are quickly replaced by new ones. The effervescing, carbonated bath produces a sensation of warmth to the skin, caused by the prickling of the gas bubbles, and the body of the patient resumes a healthy red color, due to the distension of the cutaneous capillaries. The pulse becomes full and strong, the heart beat is regular, and the breathing easier and more composed. Metabolism is increased by the improved circulation, which means improved cell nutrition, greater cell activity throughout the body, and thus the toxic products of circulatory stagnation are quickly eliminated.

I generally begin the baths with a temperature of 95° F/35° C, keeping the patient in the bath from eight to ten minutes, believing that a short immersion stimulates and a long one depresses. The next day the bath is reduced one degree, and then for two or three days the bath is omitted. The temperature is gradually reduced to 78° F/26° C, not over a degree at a time, and the duration of the bath is gradually prolonged, until nearly half hour is reached. Care should be taken to have the patient completely immersed up to the neck. A series of baths consists of about twenty, and sometimes more are given. No exertion should be made by the patient in preparing for the bath or in leaving it.

A rest for half an hour is essential after the bath, and no massage or exercise is advisable immediately after the bath, but may precede it.

The Nauheim bath is indicated and of great value in cases of compensatory heart failure, dilatation in consequence of overexertion, diseases of the heart muscle, heart neurosis, nutritive disturbances, fatty degeneration, valvular deficiency, disorders of the pericardium, arteriosclerosis, etc. The favorable action of the baths on the nervous system has caused their successful application in hysteria and all kinds of nervous derangements, sciatica, neurosis of the sensory nerves, neuralgia of all kinds, especially of traumatic and rheumatic origin, neuritis, motor neurosis, peripheral paralysis, tabes, myelitis and neurasthenia.

There are many and numerous other water applications, and I have just mentioned a few to show what a wonderful remedial agent we have in so simple a thing as water.

If I were to choose between all systems of drugless healing, having studied nearly all, and knowing what results I can get, I would select the Water Cure as the most beneficial of all.

Every physician, no matter what other good system he may use, must use water to get best results, and I am profoundly sorry that there are many schools, who during their whole term of instruction, do not touch the subject of Hydrotherapy.

Water is, without any doubt, the oldest and most ancient method of treating disease. Several centuries before Christ, there are records of it being used and prescribed by Chinese physician, who then already used the wrapping up in linen sheets, similar to our pack.

Priessnitz was one of the first to organize the use of water into a system, for which he deserves great credit. Winternitz, of Vienna, did much in bringing and establishing Hydrotherapy upon a sound and scientific basis.

In using water, we get an action and a reaction. The latter gives the important effect which we need. When we try to relieve pain by the use of hot water, of course we do not look for a reaction.

The high bath is used chiefly in cases of neurasthenia, hysteria, various nerve pains; also in cases of sleeplessness, etc.

The cold full bath, in which the patient lies down, should not be given more than one minute, and the shortest duration is about 3 seconds. This short immersion, as a rule, is the best.

If [half] baths were used more, we would have less cases of piles, colic, hysteria, prolapses of the rectum, etc. The duration of the bath should not be more than one-half to two minutes.

A salt glow is splendid for patients not too ill, and is without a peer in its effects upon the skin and complexion.

A foot bath is frequently used as a means of causing diaphoresis in colds, attacks of acute diseases, and also to draw the blood from the head or some internal organ.

The hot sitz bath is a most powerful measure of relieving pain.

The wet sheet pack is the most powerful and best blood cleanser known. It is without a peer, wherever feverish conditions exist.

The Nauheim bath is indicated and of great value in cases of compensatory heart failure, dilatation in consequence of overexertion, diseases of the heart muscle, heart neurosis, nutritive disturbances, fatty degeneration, valvular deficiency, disorders of the pericardium, arteriosclerosis, etc.

My Remedial Agents

by Louis Kuhne

Herald of Health and Naturopath, XXII (6), 359-368. (1917)

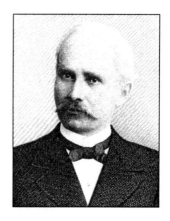

Louis Kuhne (1835-1901)

After having had a description of a number of illnesses and their cause, it will be necessary to become acquainted with the means of curing the various diseases with which mankind is afflicted. Here, again, we must expect to find unity of cure, for the very reason that all forms of disease have one common origin.

First of all come steam baths, of which several forms may be applied. The steam bath is the most reliable means there is of restoring the skin to regular action. And this is an indispensable condition for all those who desire to maintain their health, as well as for those who wish to become healthy.

The Whole Steam Bath

For a long time I endeavored to find a really simple and practical apparatus suited for general family use, and also for cases of serious illness. I was led finally to construct my own folding steam bathing apparatus. This appliance, when folded together, takes up no more room than an ordinary chair and can be set up by anyone.

The only things required in using this apparatus are a large blanket, a few pots and one of my hip baths, or a washtub. A particular advantage of this apparatus is that either the whole body, or only particular parts, can be submitted to the action of the steam, just as desired.

Having set up the apparatus in the manner shown in Figure 1, boil some water in three or four pots on an ordinary fire. Or, better still, employ my specially constructed steam pots with alcohol heaters and water compartments. Three of these steam pots are required for a full steam bath. They render all special assistance unnecessary.

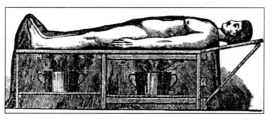

Figure 1

If ordinary pots are used, it is better for the sake of convenience not to fill them quite full. As soon as the water boils, let the patient lie down, quite unclothed, upon the apparatus, preferably upon his back at first. He should then cover himself up with a woolen blanket, letting it hang down loosely on either side, far enough to prevent any steam escaping. It is well, at first, to cover up the head too with the blanket. Another person, lifting the blanket a little, places the pots under the bench. The heat can be regulated as required by lifting the covers of the pots more or less, thus allowing more or less steam to escape. In the case of adults, two or three pots should be used; for children, one will suffice. One pot should be kept boiling on the fire as a reserve. The first pot—in the case of little children, the only one—should be placed in the front compartment under the small of the back, the second under the feet, and the third when required, somewhat further up than the first, under the back.

As soon as the supply of steam begins to diminish (after about ten minutes), put the reserve pot from the range in place of the first, and set the latter on the fire. As a rule, the pot under the feet does not need to be renewed. When my special steam pots with alcohol heating are used, these directions, of course, do not apply. All changing of the pots is then obviated, as is explained in the full and clearly worded instructions always supplied with the apparatus.

In from ten to fifteen minutes the patient may turn over, in order that the heat may better reach the chest and abdomen. Should perspiration not have broken out already, it will now do so most profusely, the head and feet beginning to perspire simultaneously. In the case of children, a renewal of the pots of water is often unnecessary. Persons who do not perspire readily, should keep the head covered; this will not be found to be so disagreeable as may at first be imagined.

The perspiration may be kept up for a quarter or half an hour, as desired, and the pots renewed or not, at will. Those parts of the body which are especially encumbered with fermenting matter, perspire with difficulty and the patient himself will experience the desire for greater heat at such places. His request should always be complied with, for this is the very way in which such successful cures are effected by means of these steam baths.

Weak persons and such as are seriously ill, more especially nervous patients, should never take steam baths. For such, the most effective cure is attained by the use of friction sitz and hip baths, which act derivatively in conjunction with sun baths. Persons who naturally perspire easily, can sometimes dispense with steam baths altogether. More than two steam baths weekly should be taken only if specially prescribed.

On leaving the steam bath, a friction hip bath at 68° to 81°F/20° to 27° C should be taken in order to cool down the body. The manner of taking the friction hip bath is described in detail on page 411, the apparatus being shown in Figure 4. At the commencement or conclusion of the bath, however, in addition to the abdomen, all the remainder of the body (chest, arms, legs, feet, head and neck) should be very quickly washed over, so that they likewise may be cleansed and cooled down. The warmer the body, the less it feels the cold. On perspiring, there is no excitation, but only the skin becomes thoroughly warm. There is no reason to fear the effects of such a bath. Steel, when brought to white heat in the fire, must be plunged into cold water in order to obtain the requisite temper. Similarly the human body after the steam bath, on being cooled down becomes strong and hardy.

After the friction hip bath, it is necessary that the bather should again be warmed, so as to induce slight perspiration. Strong patients can attain this warmth by exercise in the open air, especially in the sun. Weaker persons (though such must be very careful in taking steam baths at all) should be well covered up in bed, the window being left open a little.

Steam is produced immediately when water reaches 212° F/100° C produced in the pots, and therefore is exactly the same as that developed in steam boilers. The only difference is as regards the amount of steam developed; and one trial will convince anyone that the pots are quite sufficient for the purpose.

Where neither my steam bathing apparatus nor a cane-seated bench are available for use, an ordinary cane-seated chair can serve the purpose as a substitute. The patient seats himself upon it and is completely covered up with the blanket. Under the chair is placed, as described above, a pot of boiling water, while the feet are placed over a second pot half full of boiling water, across the top of which two strips of wood have been laid.

My steam bathing apparatus has the great advantage, however, as already pointed out, that the steam can also be applied only to particular parts of the body, if desired.

Abdominal Steam Bath

Bathing for the abdomen, which is especially adapted for use in obstinate abdominal complaints and in cases of chlorosis, menstrual disturbances and other female diseases, is shown in Figure 2. The manner of applying it is clear from the illustration. Only one pot need be used at a time, being renewed as the patient may desire.

As the remaining parts of the body also become warmed, the whole abdomen must be cooled down just as after the steam bath. In fact, the entire procedure in both cases is the same. In many cases, especially in diseases of women, it is well, after the steam bath,

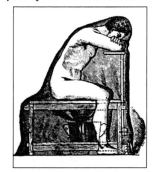

Figure 2

to take a friction sitz bath. This or the friction hip bath must be continued so long until a feeling of coolness commences to be felt. When carefully carried out, these steam baths have a surprising effect.

NECK AND HEAD STEAM BATH

A steam bath for the neck and head is shown by Figure 3. The vessel

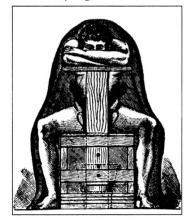

is set on a board laid upon the bench and the head and neck steamed until they perspire profusely. When per-spiration begins, any pain will always cease; this is peculiarly noticeable in the case of toothache. The head and chest, if warm, must be quickly washed over with cold water and a friction hip or sitz bath then taken at once. Should the pains return after a time, whole steam baths (particu-lar attention being given to thorough steaming of the abdomen) and neck steam baths may be taken alternate-ly.

Figure 3

These partial steam baths are of high importance, and afford remarkably quick relief, e.g. in troubles of the ears, eyes, nose and throat, and particularly in toothache, and the treat-ment of boils and carbuncles.

Partial steam baths can also be given, though not so conveniently, without my special apparatus. The abdominal steam bath can be taken on an ordinary cane-seated chair. For the head steam bath, a kitchen bench may be used, the pot being set upon it and a chair placed in front to serve as a rest for the arms.

THE SUN BATH

The method of taking sun baths, which of course can only be done on very warm, sunny days, is as follows. The patient lies down, lightly dressed, on a spot well sheltered from the wind, and preferably on a mat. Shoes and stockings must be taken off, and women and girls must not wear a corset. Head and face should be protected from the rays of the sun, which is best effected by means of a large green leaf, such as rhubarb leaf, or by a number of small leaves. The naked abdomen must also be protected in the same manner by a leaf, or where not at hand, by a wet cloth.

A sun bath should last from half an hour to one and a half hours.Patients who do not perspire easily, can lie still longer, provided they do not feel too tired. On very hot days the bath should not be continued too long.

Those who at first get a headache, or feel dizzy on taking a sun bath should let the first baths be of short duration. This particularly applies to patients who either do not perspire at all, or only with the greatest difficulty.

After the sun bath, a cooling friction hip bath, or friction sitz bath, as shown in illustrations, should be taken to carry off the morbid matter which has been loosened. Patients who do not easily recover their warmth after the cold friction hip or sitz bath, should sit again in the sun, the head being protected, or they may take a walk in the sun. This applies particularly to patients who are seriously ill, and to delicate persons. Indeed, for such, the sun bath is frequently altogether too vigorous a remedy and should not be used at the commencement of the cure.

The best time for taking sun baths is from 10 a.m. to 3 p.m. They may, if desired, be taken just after the mid-day meal, but it is better to wait half an hour, or an hour, since digestion demands bodily warmth, and the cooling baths following the sun baths would cause too great a diminution in the heat of the body.

Partial Sun Baths

I have made use of partial sun baths with the best results in cases where there is a deposit of nodules, for open sores, induration, tumors and internal growths, painful places of all kinds, etc. The partial sun bath is taken in the same manner as the whole sun bath, except that in addition, that particular part of the body which is to receive the partial sun bath, is bared and protected against the sun by one or more green leaves.

Concerning sun baths in general, it may be remarked that with water and diet, the sun is the most important remedial agent we have; and there is no other way in which we can attain a like effect. In chronic cases, especially, there is no other such effective, and at the same time, mild remedial agent as the sun bath for exciting and expelling foreign matter. A comparison will make this clear to the reader. It is well known that if soiled linen is laid in the sun, the dirt dries in all the more. But if we put the linen alternately in sun and water, the sun extracts the impurities more or less, and thus renders the wash cleaner: it bleaches it.

The existence of all living beings on the earth depends upon the alternate action of sun, water, air and earth. Plants and trees can only thrive if they can get sun, water, air and earth; as soon as these factors of life are partly or wholly withdrawn, the plant or tree becomes stunted or fades. It is just the same with all other life, and therefore, also with man

Unfortunately, most people avoid sun and water far more than is good.

The body becomes effeminated and a disposition to disease is the result. A healthy person can bear the heat of the sun without bad effect. A diseased or sickly person, on the contrary, avoids it instinctively, because it causes a feeling of uneasiness. The rapid movement of morbid matter in the body, brought about by the sun, naturally causes headache, giddiness, lassitude and heaviness if the secretory organs are still too weak. These symptoms, however, are a sure indication that foreign matter is being dispersed. The sun bath alone, without the subsequent water bath, would never enable us to attain the desired result. The water has the effect of raising the vitality of the body to increase, which must be our first aim. Plants also, only thrive under the alternate action of sun and water, and soon wither if exposed to the sun alone. When we have once grasped the way in which Nature works, there can be no difficulty in our understanding how, as may occur in chronic disease, the momentary disturbances (curative crises) called forth by the sun bath, may be counteracted immediately by cooling water baths. My water baths, already described in connection with sun baths, have a wonderfully curative effect.

One might imagine that the action of the sun upon the naked body would be much more intensive than upon the body when covered or dressed. This, however, is a great error. A glance at Nature suffices to convince us. Look at the vine, for instance: do not the grapes always seek protection under the leaves against the rays of the sun? They ripen best if everywhere guarded by the leaves; those which are exposed to the sun remain sour and small. The same is the case with cherry trees, if when the fruit ripens, the leaves have been all eaten by caterpillars. The fruit does not ripen better than otherwise would have been the case; on the contrary, the cherries wither up without ever attaining their full size. Every fruit requires leaves for its protection when ripening. The examples just cited from Nature, show us most clearly what a difference there is in effect between the direct and indirect influence of the sun. It is the alternate effect of sun and water on the human body that gives it the greatest vitality.

The action of the sun upon the uncovered head is injurious, all kinds of troubles arising from such exposure. If we keep the body covered with our clothes, the skin opens its pores readily, soon becomes moist and warm and begins to perspire. But the action is greatly increased, if we lay over the naked body a cover containing much water in bound condition. Exactly such a cover is formed by large green, succulent, fresh leaves.

It is well known that through black clothing the sun's rays act quite differently than through white. It is, therefore not a matter of indifference whether we use clothes, or cloths, or green juicy leaves as protection. Many years of observation in my establishment have convinced me that by far the best dispersive action is exercised on the morbid humors of the body, if the sun shines through green leaves. Sun baths, combined with my other remedial agents, will thus be found of extraordinary value, especially in cases of nodular deposits in the abdomen, in green sickness [hypochromic anemia], anemia, consumption and gout.

THE FRICTION HIP BATH

This is taken as follows: A bath of the form shown in Figure 4 [a sitz tub], is filled with water just so far as to reach to the thighs and navel. The water should be at 64° to 68° F / 18° to 20° C, and the bather, half sitting and

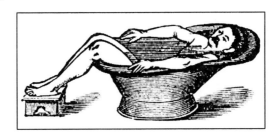

Figure 4

half reclining should then briskly and without stopping, rub the entire abdomen from the navel downwards and across the body with a coarse moderately wet cloth (jute, coarse linen). This should be continued until the body is well cooled down. At first five to ten minutes will suffice; afterwards the baths may be somewhat prolonged. For very weak persons and children, on the other hand, a few minutes are enough. It is highly important that the legs, feet and upper part of the body should not be cooled, as they usually suffer from want of blood, and should, therefore, be wrapped in a woolen blanket. After the friction hip bath, the body must immediately be warmed again, this best effected by exercise in the open air. In the case of patients who are seriously ill, or very delicate, warmth may be restored by their being put to bed, well covered up. Should warmth return too slowly, a body bandage may be used.

Such friction hip baths can be taken from once to thrice daily, and the duration and temperature likewise suited to the patient's condition. In many cases, friction sitz baths should be taken instead, or both baths may be taken.

THE FRICTION SITZ BATH

This is of special importance in diseases of women, and is taken in the following manner.

In the same bath as last mentioned, a foot stool, or a wooden seat as made by me, is set. Water is then poured in but only so much, that it rises to a level with the upper edge of the seat, leaving the top dry. The bather then sits down upon the dry seat, dips a coarse linen cloth (jute or a rough towel) into the water and begins gently to wash the genitals and abdomen, always bringing up as much water as possible with the cloth. It is important that only the external lips, and never the inner parts of the sexual organs, are washed; and they must not be roughly rubbed backwards and forwards, but only laved with as much water as can be brought up. Then the patient, or nurse, should gently rub the back up and down and crosswise, from the small of the back opposite the navel to the hips. Thus, it will be seen, the legs, feet and upper part of the body remain dry. Care should be taken to restore the warmth of the body again quickly, either by exercise or by additional wraps and cover. The baths should be discontinued during the periods. If, however, there should be abnormal menstruation, they can be continued during this time also; but only if given as specially prescribed by me in each individual case. The periods should not occupy more than from two to three days, or at most four; a more prolonged menstrual flow indicates an abnormal and morbid condition.

The water for these friction sitz baths should be at the temperature at which Nature supplies it, 50° to 60° F/ 10° to 16° C, though in special cases, water of a slightly higher temperature up to about 66° F/ 19° C may be used.

The bath may last from ten minutes to an hour, according to the age and condition of the patient. The room should be kept comfortably warm, especially in winter. The colder the water in these friction sitz baths, the better the result. But it should never be colder than the bather's hands can bear it. In the tropics and hot countries, it is not possible to get such cold water as here; but it can be taken as cold as it is to be had. There need be no fear as to the working [effectiveness] of the bath in such cases, for the relation between the temperature of the water and the temperature of the air in those warm countries, very nearly aggress with such relation here at home; so that the effect of the bath will be the same in both cases. This opinion has been confirmed in every way, by reports which I have received from tropical regions.

Where no hip bath is to be had, any washtub whatever can be employed for the friction sitz baths. It has only to be large enough for the reception of a stool or some other convenient seat, and contain at least from five to six gallons of water, reaching up to the edge of the seat. If too little water is taken for these baths, it soon grows warm, thus rendering the bath less effective. Soft water is preferable to fresh spring water. Where, however, only the latter is obtainable, it is well to let it stand a while, taking care that it does not get too warm.

In almost all better class families, similar baths are taken over a bidet, simply for the sake of cleanliness. Such cold water, however, is not used; nor is the bath taken for the same length of time, nor in the same manner as prescribed by me.

For males, the bath is arranged in the same way, and the extremity, that is, the extreme edge of the foreskin is washed in the cold water.

The bather, with the middle and forefinger, or the thumb and forefinger, of the left hand, draws the foreskin as far as possible over the tip of the glans penis, so that the latter is quite covered and protected against the rubbing. He then, without interruption, gently washes the extremity of the foreskin, thus held between the fingers, with a jute or linen cloth of the size of a handkerchief, held in the water in the right hand. It is very important to exactly follow these directions. Anyone, therefore, who does not feel sure whether he understands the correct manner of proceeding, is strongly advised to apply for special particulars, so as to save himself needless trouble and loss of time, perhaps even positive injury to his health.

In the case of the patients suffering from inflamed or gangrenous places in the interior of the body or where there is a change from chronic, latent disease to acute, the internal inflammation is very soon, frequently after the first bath, attracted downwards, reappearing in the spot rubbed, or in its immediate neighborhood. This is by no means an unfavorable symptom. In Part II of my complete work* in the chapter on cancer, I have treated it more in detail. There need be no anxiety on account of chafing; the baths should be continued as before, a rather softer cloth being used, if desired.

In many cases, a still quicker effect will be obtained by letting the water stand three fingers high above the seat. The water in such case should be from 63° to 73° F/17° to 23° C. The buttocks are then in the water; for the rest, the procedure is the same as before.

It may appear inexplicable to many, that just the particular part of the body mentioned, and no other, should be chosen as the place to apply these baths. But as a matter of fact, there is no other part so suitable for the purpose. In no other spot are there so many important nerve terminations. These are especially the branches of many spinal nerves, and of the nervous sympathicus, which, owing to their connection with the brain, render it possible in this way to exert an influence upon the nervous system. It is only at the genitals that the entire nervous system can be influenced. Here is, in a sense, the root of the whole tree of life. By washing in cold water, not only is the morbid internal heat diminished, but there is also a marked invigoration of the nerves; that is, the vitality of the whole body, down to the minutest part, is stimulated. Exceptions occur only where the nerve connection has been interrupted, for instance, by surgical operation.

Every reasonable person, not fearing a practical experiment, will admit that the friction sitz bath, in the form prescribed by me, fulfils all the conditions requisite for the restoration of the proper bodily functions.

---

*Louis Kuhne wrote *The New Science of Healing* in 1891 in German. By 1901, it had been translated into 25 languages. The first English translation was by Kenneth Romanes. In 1917, Benedict Lust translated it as *Neo-Naturopathy, A New Science of Healing.* —Ed.

It is to be remarked that the friction sitz bath, which has already brought aid to thousands, is intended only for the sick in health. Everyone who knows to what painful, as well as disagreeable and indecent operations the human body is very often subjected by orthodox medical science, will look upon the simple, yet surely curative, friction sitz baths with an unprejudiced eye. Least of all is prudery in place where it is a matter of benefiting the suffering. Upon completely healthy persons the friction sitz bath has no effect, and is moreover not recommended to such. They will find it tiresome, whereas the sick patient will often continue it longer than is required.

Here, it is also necessary to call attention to the continued efforts at equalization met with in Nature. These are not limited, as is often falsely imagined, to physical processes. They are also found in the regular change of temperature of the human body in relation to that of its surroundings. There is a change of temperature from within to without, from without to within, not incorrectly designated as an electric current. And as with the purely physical current, there must here be a certain tension. Now the higher this increases, as for instance, in the case of the body seized by fever, the more unbearable becomes the condition of the person, and the more intensive is the symptom of disease. Like a storm cloud with its sultry, uneasy oppression, so acts the encumbrance in the human body. Now what can be more natural and more rational than to bring about equalization? The higher temperature must be equalized with the lower; the surplus reduced to the normal. And the bridge, leading to this end, together with my other remedial agents, the friction sitz baths, which for the various reasons already explained, must of course only be taken with cold water. Their working is incomparable and in innumerable cases most effective. Where the desired result is not attained, it is because the body has lost its vitality.

If the body is loaded internally with morbid matter, so that it may be compared to a rusty machine, the debilitated digestion will no longer be able to procure sufficient vitality from the usual quantity of food to maintain the person in his former condition. Larger quantities of food are required than before, and as a rule particularly stimulating food, in order to keep him in condition to work. But in this case, naturally, the digestive powers will continue to decrease more and more.

If we wish again to raise the vitality of the body, we can only do so by the agency of some means which improves the digestion. The best means known to me, together with natural diet, are these cooling baths. They improve even the worst digestion (so long as this is capable of improvement at all), within a shorter time than any other remedy, and moreover act in a natural manner. Furthermore, these baths diminish the fever, caused by the friction of the morbid matter, to the normal, whereby further development of the disease is prevented. If we wished to change the steam rising from boiling water in a room—to take an example from daily life—back to its original form, water, the only way would be to reduce the temperature. It is the same with the morbid matter, that is, with every disease. Disease arises by reason of increased temperature in the body, and can only disappear if the opposite condition is produced, that is, by continued cooling and reduction of the excessive internal heat.

But exactly as a machine can only be properly driven from one point, faster or slower as the case may be, so it is with the human body. The vital power can only be properly influenced from one point—that which I have selected for the application of the friction sitz baths.

After this explanation, it will be plain to all how it is that I successfully treat diseases of the eyes and ears with the same remedy (adopted, of course, to the circumstances of each individual case) with which I, in other cases, cure scarlet fever, smallpox, cholera, etc. The vitality of the entire body is raised, and at the same time there is no possibility of one part being more excited than another, unless as stated above, nerve connections have been interrupted. How heightened vital power manifests itself, is, however, quite unknown to most people, and often precisely the opposite of that which the patient expected, occurs. For instance, it may happen that smokers after using these baths can no longer continue the use of tobacco and are consequently inclined to think that their stomachs have been weakened, whereas just the contrary is the fact. Previously their stomachs were too debilitated to resist the nicotine, whilst now they have regained the necessary vigor to rebel against the poison. Wherever the nerves are still capable of being strengthened by these baths, the system will always recover the power of expelling, by the natural secretory organs, the foreign matter which has gradually collected in it.

In addition to the friction sitz baths, earth (clay) bandages round the abdomen will be found most effective in decreasing the external heat and breaking up the morbid matter. Such bandages are also most beneficial in cases of direct injuries and sores.

No one should suppose, however, that these remedies (adapted to the circumstances of each individual case) will infallibly cure every patient. As I have already remarked, I can cure all disease but not all patients. For where the bodily vitality and therefore, the digestive power, is already broken down, these remedies will afford relief, such indeed as no other means will, but they cannot in such case effect a complete cure.

There are also severe cases where my baths must only be used with the greatest moderation, where often, indeed, they should be temporarily discontinued. In such serious cases it would appear inadvisable for patients themselves to proceed simply on the basis of these directions, without a more intimate acquaintance with my method. In such cases, it is better to apply for more complete details so that no ill effects may result from the application of the cure.

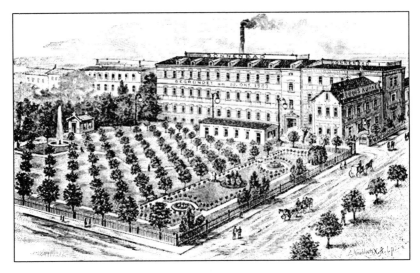

Louis Kuhne's clinic in Leipzig

Here, again, we must expect to find unity of cure, for the very reason that all forms of disease have one common origin.

Those parts of the body which are especially encumbered with fermenting matter, perspire with difficulty and the patient himself will experience the desire for greater heat at such places.

On leaving the steam bath, a friction hip bath at 68° to 81° F/20° to 27° C should be taken in order to cool down the body.

After the friction hip bath, it is necessary that the bather should again be warmed, so as to induce slight perspiration. Strong patients can attain this warmth by exercise in the open air, especially in the sun.

Bathing for the abdomen, which is especially adapted for use in obstinate abdominal complaints and in cases of chlorosis, menstrual disturbances and other female diseases is shown in Figure 2 [the sitting abdominal steam bath].

In many cases, especially in diseases of women, it is well, after the steam bath, to take a friction sitz bath. This, or the friction hip bath, must be continued so long until a feeling of coolness commences to be felt.

After the sun bath, a cooling friction hip bath, or friction sitz bath, as shown in illustrations, should be taken, to carry off the morbid matter which has been loosened.

The existence of all living beings on the earth, depends upon the alternate action of sun, water, air and earth.

The sun bath alone, without the subsequent water bath, would never enable us to attain the desired result. The water has the effect of raising the vitality of the body to increase which must be our first aim.

Many years of observation in my establishment have convinced me, that by far the best dispersive action is exercised on the morbid humors of the body, if the sun shines through green leaves.

The water should be at 64° to 68° F/18° to 20° C, and the bather, half sitting and half reclining should then briskly and without stopping, rub the entire abdomen from the navel downwards and across the body with a coarse moderately wet cloth (jute, coarse linen).

The water for these friction sitz baths should be at the temperature at which Nature supplies it, 50° to 60° F/10° to 16° C, though in special cases, water of a slightly higher temperature up to about 66° F/19° C may be used.

It is only at the genitals that the entire nervous system can be influenced. Here is, in a sense, the root of the whole tree of life.

If the body is loaded internally with morbid matter, so that it may be compared to a rusty machine, the debilitated digestion will no longer be able to procure sufficient vitality from the usual quantity of food to maintain the person in his former condition.

If we wish again to raise the vitality of the body, we can only do so by the agency of some means which improves the digestion. The best means known to me, together with natural diet, are these cooling baths.

Disease arises by reason of increased temperature in the body, and can only disappear if the opposite condition is produced, that is, by continued cooling and reduction of the excessive internal heat.

For instance, it may happen that smokers after using these baths can no longer continue the use of tobacco and are consequently inclined to think that their stomachs have been weakened, whereas just the contrary is the fact. Previously their stomachs were too debilitated to resist the nicotine, whilst now they have regained the necessary vigor to rebel against the poison.

In addition to the friction sitz baths, earth (clay) bandages round the abdomen, will be found most effective in decreasing the external heat and breaking up the morbid matter. Such bandages are also most beneficial in cases of direct injuries and sores.

As I have already remarked, I can cure all disease but not all patients. For where the bodily vitality and therefore, the digestive power, is already broken down, these remedies will afford relief, such indeed as no other means will, but they cannot in such case effect a complete cure.

1918

PRIESSNITZ, INTRODUCER OF HYDROTHERAPY
BENEDICT LUST

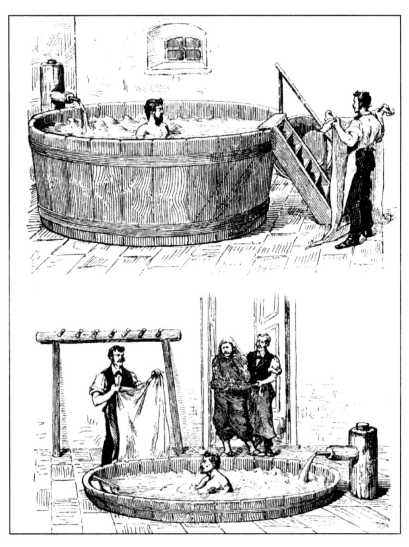

Vincent Priessnitz used large bath tubs (20 to 30 feet in circumference) for his patients. These cold baths followed immediately after a period of profuse sweating.

Priessnitz, Introducer Of Hydropathy

by Benedict Lust

Herald of Health and Naturopath, XXIII (3), 223-224. (1918)

All life is formed in water, and as though following the order of evolution, Nature Cure had its modern birth in the Water Cure. Although we have records of cures by the use of water at an earlier date, it was not until Vincenz Priessnitz opened his Water Cure institution in Gräefenberg, Austrian Silesia, in 1826 that the movement gained headway. Many regular physicians prior to this time had advocated the use of water, among them Dr. Theodore Hahn, who departed from life in 1773.

Hahn's greatest contribution to the progress of Water Cure was a little book on the subject, which fell into the hands of Sebastian Kneipp, and which gave Kneipp his first ideas on the thing that was later to make him the greatest natural physician of his day.

It is seldom that great discoveries or world-wide movements are instituted by learned men. The greatest things have the humblest beginnings. It is markedly true in this case.

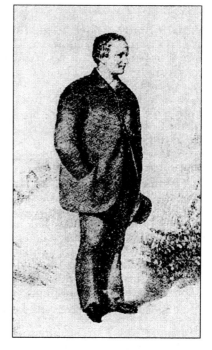

Born October 4th, 1799, Vincenz Priessnitz, of Gräefenberg, Silesia, founder of Hydrotherapy.

Priessnitz was a man of meager education. Being born October 4, 1799, the son of a poor, blind farmer, his responsibilities began at an early age. His education came through observation and experience. The story of his first experience with the Water Cure is told by Mrs. Louisa A. Nash:

> I remember staying with my grandmother and aunt in the first 'Hydropathic Institute' in England. It was started by Dr. Ellis, who, with his wife, had recovered from what the ordinary doctors considered an incurable malady at the Priessnitz 'Water Cure' in Gräefenberg.

They told me how Priessnitz, as a child, had cured a sore hand by using the out-door pump of his home town. "If water does it so much good, it shall have it all the time!" he determined. So he wetted his handkerchief, binding it on his hand.

The idea possessed him, "If water cured my hand, why shouldn't it cure other troubles?"

When he grew up, he started his 'Water Cure Establishment' at Gräefenberg to solve the problem. Patients flocked to him from all over Europe, so much so, that he found it hard to get sheds enough built to shelter them, or food sufficient to sustain them.

But even in Priessnitz' days there was a jealous medical profession—that great guardian of public health. Here was a man who made cures with water—a miracle worker. Surely, it could be nothing short of witchcraft—devil's work. Can't you see the same group 1900 years ago, denouncing the works of healing of the Master? Can't you hear their voices raised the loudest to demand his crucifixion? Why not—such a one robbed them of their living. Times have changed but little—they are reincarnated today. The spirit of intolerance breeds them over and over again.

They involved the authorities to close the institution of Priessnitz. They raided his place and wrecked it, searching for his secret. "Water Cure? Nonsense. This man has some secret substance, and we mean to find it." They ripped out his tubs, hoping to lay bare the mystery in the linings. They cut up all his sponges, towels, cloths and sheets, but the mystery was not revealed. Priessnitz was forbidden entrance to his sanitarium—the seal of the state was placed on his door.

Priessnitz led his patients and sympathizers to the public square and made a speech. "Do not be troubled," he said. "If they forbid us here, we will go to the open country, to the fields, the woods and the streams—there Nature shall heal you."

But Gräefenberg woke up. Priessnitz was its biggest business asset. He was attracting thousands of people to the town annually. These people had to be fed, clothed, housed; that meant business. Priessnitz had literally put Gräefenberg on the map, and Gräefenberg was not slow to recognize that business would slump without Priessnitz, so Priessnitz was reinstated.

The Priessnitz system is almost universally practiced today, and the Priessnitz bandage or compress has place even in the orthodox system of medicine. His principle, expressed in his own words, is: "Not the cold but the body heat, produced by the reaction to cold water, is the healing factor."

And if, after the war, you should visit Gräefenberg, the statue of Vincenz Priessnitz will greet you in the public square.

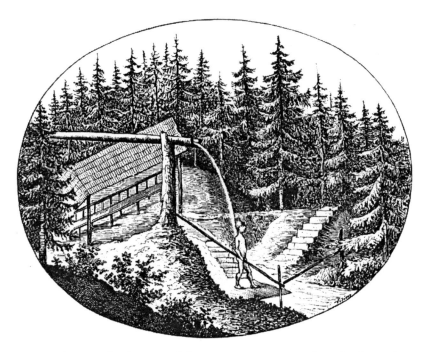

Patients who came for therapy with Priessnitz were encouraged to take the outdoor douches found scattered throughout the forests at Gräefenberg. The water in these douches came from cold mountainous streams. The height of the water fell from 10 to 20 feet.

Although we have records of cures by the use of water at an earlier date, it was not until Vincenz Priessnitz opened his Water Cure institution in Gräefenberg, Austrian Silesia, in 1826, that the movement gained headway.

Hahn's greatest contribution to the progress of Water Cure was a little book on the subject, which fell into the hands of Sebastian Kneipp, and which gave Kneipp his first ideas on the thing that was later to make him the greatest natural physician of his day.

But even in Priessnitz' days there was a jealous medical profession—that great guardian of public health. Here was a man who made cures with water—a miracle worker. Surely, it could be nothing short of witchcraft—devil's work.

They ripped out his tubs, hoping to lay bare the mystery in the linings. They cut up all his sponges, towels, cloths and sheets, but the mystery was not revealed.

In his [Priessnitz's] own words, "Not the cold but the body heat, produced by the reaction to cold water, is the healing factor."

1919

NATURE'S CURE FOR DISEASE
DR. LORNE A. SUMMERS

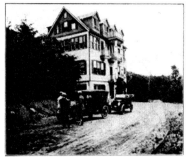
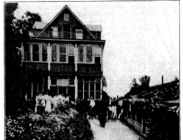
Louisa and Benedict Lust built two Yungborns in the USA. The first one was established in Butler, New Jersey, and the second was in Tangerine, Florida.

Nature's Cure For Disease

by Dr. Lorne A. Summers, Director of Armour Gymnasium

Herald of Health and Naturopath, XXIV (8), 343-345. (1919)

Nature's cure by water is one of the best remedies for stomach and bowel disorders so prevalent in summer. The cold application to the abdomen is the means of quick relief from over activity of the bowels. When we find over activity of the intestines, it is also found that the musculature of the bowels are in an over-relaxed condition. When the cold application is applied, contraction takes place and the organs are brought back to normal. If this procedure is preceded by a hot enema (temperature of water 105° F/40.6° C) better results will be obtained, as sometimes we find a large amount of poisonous material in the intestines and this should be thoroughly eliminated before any contraction takes place. It is well to follow this by an alternate hot and cold application to the abdomen for fifteen to twenty minutes, as this will promote a normal circulation to the bowels caused by the alternate contraction and relaxation of the muscles, thereby bringing and supplying fresh blood to the part affected.

The Warm Bath Before Retiring

The best method by which to relax the body and soothe the nervous system is by a warm bath taken just before retiring, which will relieve any irritation by assisting in the elimination of fatigue poisons. To take this bath, fill the tub up to the overflow with water at a temperature of 105° F/40.6° C; after being in the water a couple of minutes turn on the cold water and cool the bath down to 95° F/35° C, and then remain in the water for about ten to twenty minutes, then dry thoroughly and go to bed. Many have found this bath, called the neutral bath, a valuable remedy in the case of insomnia. The neutral bath before retiring is also very valuable in reducing high blood pressure.

It has been shown by many observers that the internal use of water powerfully stimulates the tissue change, both anabolism (building up) and catabolism (breaking down) being greatly increased. There is usually a great increase in building up than in breaking down, so that a person using water freely usually gains weight. It is for this reason that persons suffering from obesity should drink as little fluid as is necessary to keep the body in health. Water drinking gives nature an abundant supply of the great cleansing agent which washes the tissues free from impurities and thereby assists the vital functions of the body. The amount of water to be taken depends upon the condition of the patient and the effect desired. For example, a dyspeptic whose power of absorption is very slow should take small quantities of water at frequent intervals and sip it slowly. In fact, it is well for the ordinary person to take water at frequent intervals in smaller amounts rather than drink an excess amount to make up for the deficiency. Care should be taken not to take too large a quantity of water after a meal.

Those who are suffering from inactivity of the bowels have found great relief in drinking two or three glasses of water in the morning before breakfast. It is needless to say that every effort should be made to see that the water is as pure as possible. Many people have cultivated the habit of drinking ice water and it is a very dangerous habit as it seriously interferes with the digestive process; and if continued for any length of time, it is apt to result in stomach trouble. Water drinking is one of the best remedies for people suffering from the effects of inactivity of the skin and kidneys. Although until recently many physicians disagreed on the advisability of using water in fever cases, it is now commonly agreed upon that the use of cold water, with the addition of fruit juice, is a very valuable means of lowering temperature.

A Time-Honored Curative Agent

Sunlight, as a natural curative agent, has been known as far back as the earliest times by savages and wild animals who probably were led to use this rational agency by natural instinct. The ancient Greeks who were admired by all lovers of physical development were strong believers in the great benefit derived from sunlight. In the time of Hippocrates, the sun bath was part of the daily routine and was religiously followed as a mode of purification of the body.

There are numerous evidences that the sun bath was not only known among the ancients, but was used by them to considerable extent. Plutarch tells us that Diogenes, the renowned Athenian Cynic, was in his old age accustomed to lying in the sunshine for the purpose of restoring his energies, a custom which according to Pliny, was common in Greece. It is known that the custom of sun bathing was common amongst the Romans. Hippocrates prescribed the sun bath for chills. Many other evidences could be stated regarding the value the ancients put on the use of the sun bath.

When Sunlight Is Denied

The value of sunlight in the maintenance and restoration of health, although well recognized, is seldom appreciated by the average American. The important relation of sunlight to health is shown in the effect produced upon plants as well as animals by depriving them of this influence of sunlight. In caves and other places excluded from the light, plants do not grow to their natural development. The same is true of animals.

In the deep valleys among the Alps of Switzerland the sun shines only a few hours each day and in consequence, the inhabitants suffer from skin and other diseases which result from poor nutrition. It has also been found that a large number of the males are idiots. However, upon going up the mountain side and visiting the inhabitants who live in the sunshine, a much better physical and mental development is found, although they follow the same habits of life as their fellows who live in the valley. When the afflicted people of the valley are carried up the mountain and receive the sunlight, they make rapid improvement.

The value of sunlight in the treatment of tuberculosis has attained great renown. It is known that the sun's rays produce a chemical effect upon the diseased tissue in the lungs and are able to destroy the tubercular bacilli.

So that we may understand the value of sunlight, it probably would be well for us to consider its composition and effect upon the human body. The solar spectrum is the spectrum of the sun or any source of light resembling the sun in spectral composition. The solar light contains seven visible kinds of light, i.e., seven varieties of energy capable of affecting the retina of the human eye. These visible rays of the spectrum are red, orange, yellow, green, blue, indigo and violet. These seven varieties are shown when sunlight is refracted by moisture in the atmosphere after a shower in the form of what is commonly known as the rainbow. There are other forms of light that are not perceived by the human eye. These invisible rays are found on either side of the visible spectrum and to indicate their respective location with reference to the red and violent fields of the spectrum are called infrared and ultra-violet rays.

The spectral rays have three distinct functions, that is, heat production, light radiation and chemical action. Heat is produced principally by the infrared, red and orange rays. Light is generated mainly by the yellow and green rays, while the blue, indigo and violet and especially the ultra-violet rays are chemical in their action.

The heat rays stimulate, promote oxidation, accelerate and increase metabolism (building up and breaking down), encourage absorption. It also has the power to relieve pain and is valuable as a sedative.

CHEMICAL RAYS GERMICIDAL IN ACTION

The chemical rays are the most valuable from the therapeutic standpoint. They are germicidal in their action, as no germs can exist after being exposed for any length of time to the sun's rays. The chemical rays powerfully stimulate the process of organic development, especially by their affinity for oxygen. They affect the process of restoration and circulation by influencing the consumption of oxygen and increasing the quality and quantity of the blood.

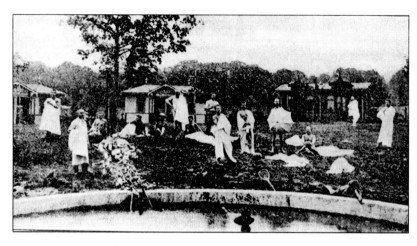

Separate areas were designated for men and women for their air and sun baths at Benedict and Louisa Lust's Yungborn at Butler, New Jersey.

The value of sunlight for the sick has gradually become recognized in hospital practice, as records show a larger percent of recoveries in rooms which are built so as to take advantage of all sunlight, than the recoveries made from rooms which are not so constructed. The powerful influence which the sun has upon the skin is shown by the great increase in pigmentation, which is commonly known as a tan. This is produced by free exposure to the sun and air and results in an increased activity of the cutaneous tissue.

The sun bath may be taken by exposing either the entire or a portion of the body to the rays of the sun, or can be protected by a single covering of white muslin. In taking the bath it is well to have the head protected from the effects of the sun as this may produce unpleasant symptoms. Like all other forms of natural curative agencies, this should be started gradually and gradually increased. Many people have experienced severe burns owing to the fact that they tried to tan their skin in shorter time than was practical. Therefore, it is well to start by exposing the skin for a short time only and gradually increase the length of time as the skin becomes accustomed to the sun's rays. In this way, the skin will gradually assume a tan, and no burning sensation will be experienced.

Ample opportunity is afforded everybody during the summer to take advantage of this wonderful natural curative power. The numerous bathing beaches and summer resorts can provide many places where this bath can be taken and in selecting a bathing suit it would be well to have the material consist of a light colored cloth, such as gray, as in this way the light rays are absorbed and the heat rays reflected, whereas if the suit consists of a dark cloth, the light rays are reflected and the heat rays absorbed.

Those people who have homes or who are living at a place where a portion of the yard can be screened off by canvas on all four sides and the top remain open, can take this bath to good advantage.

It is well to follow this by an alternate hot and cold application to the abdomen for fifteen to twenty minutes, as this will promote a normal circulation to the bowels caused by the alternate contraction and relaxation of the muscles, thereby bringing and supplying fresh blood to the part affected.

The best method by which to relax the body and soothe the nervous system is by a warm bath taken just before retiring, which will relieve any irritation by assisting in the elimination of fatigue poisons.

Many have found this bath, called the neutral bath a valuable remedy in the case of insomnia. The neutral bath before retiring is also very valuable in reducing high blood pressure.

Many people have cultivated the habit of drinking ice water and it is a very dangerous habit as it seriously interferes with the digestive process; and if continued for any length of time, it is apt to result in stomach trouble.

The value of sunlight for the sick has gradually become recognized in hospital practice, as records show a larger percent of recoveries in rooms which are built so as to take advantage of all sunlight, than the recoveries made from rooms which are not so constructed.

The sun bath may be taken by exposing either the entire or a portion of the body to the rays of the sun, or can be protected by a single covering of white muslin.

1920

THE COLD BATH
Dr. Lorne A. Summers

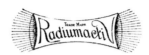
New bath powder concoctions replaced the properties of cold water.

The Cold Bath*

by Dr. Lorne A. Summers, Director of the Armour Gymnasium

Herald of Health and Naturopath, XXV (5), 286-288. (1920)

Natural forces consist essentially in the application of prophylactic measures; that is, the employment of means which are capable of maintaining a normal individual in a state of health. It may be stated that by the employment of these physiologic methods which are most effective in the restoration of the sick, the individual will be maintained in good health.

However applicable the principle may be to other therapeutic means, experience has shown most positively that the cold bath, while one of the most powerful tonics and most efficient of restoratives, is at the same time one of the most valuable of all known prophylactic or hygienic measures. The cold bath acts powerfully upon the sympathetic nervous system, which is the great regulator of nutrition. It likewise affords a gymnastic means for the vasomotor system of nerves and centers, and develops by exercise the contractile activity of the small blood vessels.

Effects Of A Cold Bath

Cold water, in common parlance, hardens the skin; technically we would say it increases the vital resistance of the skin. If habitually employed, the cold bath protects against taking cold, not by closing the pores but by increasing the activity of the cutaneous circulation and developing the vital resistance of the body in general, and especially the ability of the body to reheat the skin after it has been chilled by exposure or cold applications.

Through the influence of the cold bath upon the sympathetic nervous system, all the processes of nutrition and assimilation are quickened. The amount of hydrochloric acid produced by the glands of the stomach is increased, as the result of which the appetite and digestion are improved, and the stomach being provided with a better quality of gastric juice is better prepared to protect itself against injury from intruding microbes. Modern research has shown that typhoid fever germs, cholera germs, and in fact all varieties of germs are killed by coming in contact with healthy gastric juice. Hence, the daily cold bath, by maintaining a sound digestion as well as by increasing the general vital resistance of the body, serves as a most valuable protection against infectious disorders.

One of the most interesting effects of the cold bath is the increased number of blood corpuscles found in the surface vessels after the establish-

---

The original title of this article was "Nature's Cure for Disease." —Ed.

ment of the reaction which follows these cold applications. The blood is the means by which oxygen is conveyed to the tissues, and carbonic acid gas to the lungs, where it is discharged from the body. Certain of the blood cells are also useful in destroying the germs which may find their way into the blood vessels, and in removing dead and useless particles of various sorts.

It is thus apparent that the number of corpuscles contained in the blood is a matter of the greatest importance in relation to the degree of vital resistance, or the ability of the body to maintain itself in health under adverse circumstances or against the destructive influences of disease-producing causes.

Experiments made on the body after a cold water bath have shown that the blood distribution has been increased thirty to fifty percent. This means that all tissues will have a better blood supply to carry off waste material and fight any germs that may enter.

The minutest little cell, the frailest filament of tissues, no matter how far removed from the great centers of life, receives its due share of nutriment through the medium of the blood. The blood is referred to as a great railway system. For while the blood carries to each tissue material for the repairing of losses sustained in its work, for the building up of its structure, it takes in exchange for the new material which it supplies the old worn-out poisonous material, the waste, the rubbish of the tissue, thus securing a constant change of matter. This change is essential to life. In fact, the intensity of life depends upon the rapidity of the change. The more rapid the change of material in the body through the medium of the blood, that is, the more rapidly old material is carried away and new material deposited in its place, the higher the degree of vital activity, the more rapidly the wheels of life turn, the greater the amount of work done, the more one really lives. It may be said that the body is a living form, a mold, through which a stream of life flows. It is also interesting to note the fact that the increased rate of change does not hasten the wearing out of the body, but rather delays it, for deterioration of the body takes place much more rapidly during diminished activity than when all the organs are in use, because of the stagnation and accumulation of the poisonous wastes which necessarily accompany slow tissue activity and change, and thus interfere with the rebuilding of the tissue and cause disease.

A BATTLEFIELD IN MINIATURE

On a microscopic examination of the blood, we find it made up of minute bodies of various sizes and shapes known as the blood cells or corpuscles. The smaller ones are the most numerous. They have the shape of flattened, biconcave discs, and are of a faint amber color. These are the oxygen carriers of the blood. As they are swept along in the blood current to and fro between the lungs and the tissue, they transport in one direction from the lungs to the tissues the vitalizing, life-giving oxygen, and on the return trip carry the poisonous material which is brought to the lungs to be thrown off. This is the reason why it is so important that the body receive a constant supply of fresh air so that oxygen may be supplied to the lungs.

The large ones are spherical in shape, transparent and have a jelly-like consistency; they float in the blood stream or creep along the inner surface of the vessel. Often they may be seen passing straight through the walls of the tissue. These cells are constantly in motion, changing their form continually by reaching out a process called a "foot"; first in one direction, then in another, stretching themselves out in worm-like shapes, again gathering themselves together in small, jelly-like masses. Each cell seems to have a will of its own and to be possessed of a peculiar intelligence, whereby it is unerringly led to the place where it is needed. When these wonderful body defenders come to the area where the germs are present, they proceed at once to swallow them. If the germs are few in number they may be in this way destroyed, for the white cells not only swallow them, but digest them. If the number is great, however, the cells sacrifice themselves in the effort to destroy the germs, taking in a larger number than they are able to digest and destroy.

Some secret influence, which the scientists cannot understand and do not undertake to explain, brings white cells hastening to the scene of conflict from all parts of the body until the number accumulated may be so great as to greatly distend the parts. It is in this way that a boil or an abscess is formed, and the so-called pus which is discharged consists of these white cells which have left the blood and have laid down their lives in the defense of the body, just as the soldiers of today are laying down their lives in defense of their country.

Keeping The Body Guard Strong

The white cells constitute the most important defense of the body. They keep the blood channel free from germs and other poisonous substances. These are facts which seem to indicate that after capturing the germs which enter the circulation, they transport them to the spleen, which thus serves as a sort of headquarters in the field of battle for these body guards which are continually moving up and down the channels of the body destroying invaders and conveying them to a place where they can do no harm.

With the microscope one may see the blood cells of a sick person with malaria attacked by minute animal organisms, which, developing within the body, produce poisonous substances, which give rise to chills and fever. These parasites feed upon the red cells, sometimes destroying them with immense rapidity. The white cells, if present in sufficient numbers, are able to capture and destroy the malarial parasites before they have done their work of mischief, thus preventing the usual consequences of exposure to malarial fever. It is thus clear that it is of the highest importance that one's white cells should be in good fighting condition, that they may have the power to resist and destroy the germs which enter the blood in various ways.

The white cells to be kept in good fighting condition must be kept active. This is one of the ways in which the cold bath increases the resisting power of the body, and rallies the blood cells, so to speak, calling them out from various parts of the body and preparing them to fight with vigor the battles which must be waged every moment in defense of the body.

The cold bath acts powerfully upon the sympathetic nervous system, which is the great regulator of nutrition. It likewise affords a gymnastic means for the vasomotor system of nerves and centers, and develops by exercise the contractile activity of the small blood vessels.

If habitually employed, the cold bath protects against taking cold, not by closing the pores but by increasing the activity of the cutaneous circulation and developing the vital resistance of the body in general, and especially the ability of the body to reheat the skin after it has been chilled by exposure or cold applications.

Hence, the daily cold bath, by maintaining a sound digestion as well as by increasing the general vital resistance of the body, serves as a most valuable protection against infectious disorders.

Experiments made on the body after a cold water bath has shown that the blood distribution has been increased thirty to fifty percent. This means that all tissues will have a better blood supply to carry off waste material and fight any germs that may enter.

The more rapid the change of material in the body through the medium of the blood, that is, the more rapidly old material is carried away and new material deposited in its place, the higher the degree of vital activity, the more rapidly the wheels of life turn, the greater the amount of work done, the more one really lives.

It is thus clear that it is of the highest importance that one's white cells should be in good fighting condition, that they may have the power to resist and destroy the germs which enter the blood in various ways.

This is one of the ways in which the cold bath increases the resisting power of the body, and rallies the blood cells, so to speak, calling them out from various parts of the body and preparing them to fight with vigor the battles which must be waged every moment in defense of the body.

This advertisement appeared in the issues of *Herald of Health and Naturopath* in 1921. As a modality, we can see that Hydrotherapy, modeled after Kneipp, Kuhne, Just, Rikli, and Bilz, followed Dietetics in importance.

1921

The Development Of Hydrotherapy Since Priessnitz
Robert C. Biéri, N.D.

Naturopathy In Practice
William Freeman Havard, N.D.

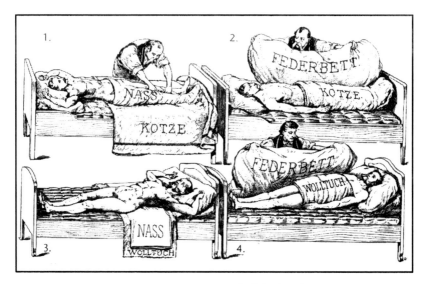

The Priessnitz compress using thick feather duvets

THE DEVELOPMENT OF HYDROTHERAPY SINCE PRIESSNITZ

by Robert C. Biéri, N.D.

Herald of Health and Naturopath, XXVI (5), 223-224. (1921)

Vincenz Priessnitz (1799-1851), a farmer of Gräefenberg, Upper Silesia, Austria, began his public career on his father's farm. Whatever adverse criticism may in the past have existed, it is now generally agreed that Priessnitz must be ranked among the world's leading pioneers of Hydrotherapy.

How could a farmer's boy attain such fame? His biographers tell us that young Priessnitz was sickly as a child, studious and observant as a youth, and a giant as a man in his untiring labor, his clear thinking, and his American-like spirit of enterprise. His possession of such qualities answers our question, and explains why the quiet, rustic homestead of the elder Priessnitz became a buzzing center of humans, flocking there in ever increasing numbers, to leave their bodily afflictions behind them, and return with a heart brim full of love and enthusiasm for Priessnitz and his Water Cure.

This huge stimulant, emanating from Gräefenberg by Priessnitz, gave Hydrotherapy its running start. His family drew people of every rank from many countries. Medical men were conspicuous by their numbers, some being attracted by curiosity, others by the hope of finding cures for the incurables. Like all other movements, however, the one so brilliantly started by Priessnitz could never have attained such great popularity, had it not been fostered and energized by many brilliant pupils and admirers.

In the years 1756-1805, Dr. James Currie of Liverpool had worked out a system similar to the one of Priessnitz, and published observations in the book entitled, *Medical Reports on the Effects of Water, Cold and Warm, as a Remedy in Fevers and other Diseases.* This work, translated into German and Bohemian in 1807 by Michaelis, became very popular, and the profession soon realized the great importance of Hydrotherapy. Indeed, the movement spread at once like a leaven all over Europe. For example, Kuhne, Rikli, and particularly the followers of Priessnitz. Johann S. Hahn's writings had meanwhile created much enthusiasm among his countrymen; societies were being formed everywhere to promote the medicinal and dietetic use of water. Much was being written in those days. Some of these writings, however, were no classics. Fanaticism, ignorance, and personal animosity obscured greatly the beauty and importance of the new movement.

In this whirlpool of dissonances, Priessnitz found a real friend. Professor Oertel of Ausbach collected the best works on Hydrotherapy of that period and published them in 1842. This was a masterstroke for the cause of Priessnitz. It standardized Hydrotherapy on its scientific feet, and the rising Priessnitz found in Professor Oertel a zealous advocate and doubtless a splendid instructor, also.

For the next ten years nothing of importance happened. Many records were meanwhile being published from the Priessnitz establishment at Gräefenberg.* These found their way all over Europe, and a few came even to our shores. Most of their little tracts were favorable to the claims of Priessnitz and many were eulogies in their estimate of his genius and penetration.

Captain Claridge introduced Hydrotherapy into England in 1840, his writings and lectures, and later those of Sir W. Erasmus Wilson (1809-1884), James Gully (1808-1886), and Edward Johnson, making numerous converts, and filling the establishments opened in many places. In Germany, France and America, hydriatic sanatoria multiplied with great rapidity.

During that period many Water Cure celebrities made their bow to the world. Among them we find men as heroes like Father Sebastian Kneipp of Wörishofen fame, Dr. Lahmann, Friedrich Bilz, Beni-Barde, Ernest Brand of Berlin (1826-1897), Theodore von Juergnsen of Kiel, Karl Liebermeister of Basel, and many others. Antagonism ran high between the old practice of medicine and the new art. Unsparing condemnation was heaped by each on the other, and many legal prosecutions were instituted. All these, however, served but to make the names of Priessnitz, Hahn, Rikli, and Kneipp dearer to the masses, and made their new science stand higher in public estimation.

It was about the year 1794 that the first American physician, Dr. Benjamin Rush of Philadelphia, began using water in fever cases. Then came Dr. Lockette and John Bell, whose work on *Baths* is a classic of its kind.**

Men like Thayer, Kellogg, Baruch, Breitenbach, Lindlahr and Lust have all contributed nobly towards the real advance of Hydrotherapy.

However, no lecture, review, book, treatise or compendium on Water Cure is complete, or can in any way be authoritative without giving honor to the man who is justly called the Father of Modern Hydrotherapy. The monumental work which elevated Water Cure once and for all above suspicion, and placed it beyond the scope of charlatanry is the life work of Wilhelm Winternitz. Medical men of all ranks, Naturopaths of all creeds, Chiropractors of all nations, hats off to a grand old man: Wilhelm Winternitz.

------

*Such men as Drs. Joel Shew, Francis Graeter, Charles Schieferdecker and many others wrote prolifically on the work of Priessnitz. —*Ed.*

**John Bell published, *Baths*, in 1850 in Philadelphia. It was one of the earliest comprehensive books on the subject published in America. A copy of Bell's book can be found in NUNM's Rare Book room, thanks to the generous donation by Dr. André Saine. —*Ed.*

The writer prides himself upon having been a pupil of Winternitz. His system, which means all there is in Hydrotherapy, is being taught in the school. Theory and practice, by lectures and demonstrations are equally divided between the various classes. It has been the writer's aim to make this subject to the pupils free from the pedantic and partisan and instead fill the minds with accurate knowledge and the hearts with enthusiasm.

Whatever adverse criticism may in the past have existed, it is now generally agreed that Priessnitz must be ranked among the world's leading pioneers of Hydrotherapy.

In the years 1756-1805, Dr. James Currie of Liverpool had worked out a system similar to the one of Priessnitz, and published observations in the book entitled, Medical Reports on the Effects of Water, Cold and Warm, as a Remedy in Fevers and other Diseases.

In this whirlpool of dissonances, Priessnitz found a real friend. Professor Oertel of Ausbach collected the best works on Hydrotherapy of that period and published them in 1842.

Antagonism ran high between the old practice of medicine and the new art. Unsparing condemnation was heaped by each on the other, and many legal prosecutions were instituted.

All these, however, served but to make the names of Priessnitz, Hahn, Rikli, and Kneipp dearer to the masses, and made their new science stand higher in public estimation.

Men like Thayer, Kellogg, Baruch, Breitenbach, Lindlahr and Lust have all contributed nobly towards the real advance of Hydrotherapy.

The monumental work which elevated Water Cure once and for all above suspicion, and placed it beyond the scope of charlatanry is the life work of Wilhelm Winternitz.

NATUROPATHY IN PRACTICE

by William Freeman Havard, N.D.
Herald of Health and Naturopath, XXVI (7), 325-326. (1921)

THE TREATMENT OF ACUTE DISEASES

THE ABLUTION BATH

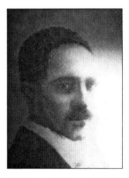

William F. Havard, N.D.

The patient should have a daily refreshing bath. This is best given in the morning before the bed linen is changed. Roll back the covers from the foot of the bed until the patient's legs are exposed to the knees. Moisten a washcloth or sponge with tepid water, and beginning at the feet bathe the patient's lower legs. Dry with a soft towel and finish by gently rubbing with the hands, stroking from the foot towards the knee. Follow the same procedure on the thighs, the abdomen, arms and chest, using fresh water for each part. Last of all, bathe the face and have the patient wash the mouth with cold water to which a little lemon juice has been added.

If packs are being used, this ablution may be given after the removal of the pack.

SPECIAL TREATMENTS

Contrary to the popular conception, the treatment in acute disease is not directed to the reduction of fever, or at least should not be. Fever is the indicator of the body's activity. The fluctuations in temperature tell the observer how the patient is progressing. If the temperature falls suddenly to below normal it means vital exhaustion and is a very grave sign. The treatment is directed towards the elimination of toxins. The fever subsides naturally when all irritating poisons have been oxidized and thrown out from the body. These matters are taken care of by increased respiration, increased circulation, increased skin and kidney action. The objects of rational treatment then is to maintain circulation and assist elimination. Water is our greatest aid towards these accomplishments.

THE COLD WET PACK

Heat and moisture applied to the surface of the body increase the activity of the skin, thereby causing the elimination of much poison through porous activity. Therefore, wet packs are valuable in reducing inflammations and swellings, preventing congestion and normalizing circulation.

The method of Priessnitz still holds first rank. It consists of first wrapping the body or a part in wet linen and over this several thicknesses of flannel or woolen blanket.

The Full Pack

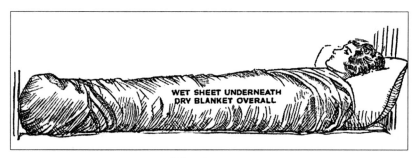

WET SHEET UNDERNEATH
DRY BLANKET OVERALL

The full pack or compress

This is sometimes referred to as the sheet pack. Spread three blankets, one on top of the other, on the bed. Over these spread a sheet which has been dipped in cool water and wrung out. Lay the patient on the sheet and wrap it thoroughly around him so that only the head remains uncovered. Tuck it in well between the arms and the body and between the legs. Draw the blankets, one at a time, over the body until the patient is encased like an Egyptian mummy with only the head protruding from the pack. Every part of the pack must fit snugly so that there is no opportunity for a circulation of air between the pack and the body. A damp cool cloth may be applied to the head while the patient is in the pack or the patient's face may be bathed frequently with cool water. Take the patient's temperature every fifteen or twenty minutes and when it has dropped two degrees, remove the pack, sponge the body and allow the patient to rest.

The full pack is indicated in all cases where there is a high degree of toxicity or where there is high fever. The higher the fever, the better the patient reacts to the pack. In so much as it has a tendency to induce profuse perspiration and lower the blood pressure, it is weakening and should not be applied for too long a time nor too frequently. Let the fever and the condition of the skin be your guides. When the fever rises and the skin feels hot and dry and the patient begins to get restless, apply the pack. Once or twice a day is usually sufficient in severe cases.

The patient will often continue to perspire after being removed from a full pack if the body is sponged with cool water, or where the patient can stand it if a cold ablution is given, and the patient immediately placed in bed without drying and covered with blankets. The full packs are sometimes alternated with part packs; i.e. after a sufficient rest one of the following packs may be used.

THE HALF PACK

This is sometimes referred to as the body pack or trunk pack. In this case, the wet sheet is folded so as to cover the trunk of the body, from under the arms to the hips. For the outer, woolen covering it is best to use strips of old blankets or light weight blankets folded to the convenient size. The body pack is indicated in cases of inflammations and congestions in the abdomen or chest or in cases where the fever is low (101° to 102° F/38.3° to 38.9° C). It may also be used as an alternate for the full pack where the fever is persistently high.

LOCAL PACKS

Abdominal packs, chest packs, leg packs, arm packs, throat packs, hip packs, and shoulder packs are local packs that are applied to the parts as indicated to alleviate local injuries, swelling or inflammations.

THE "T" PACK

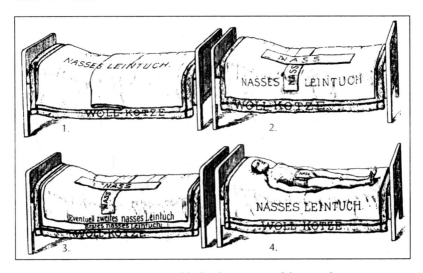

Priessnitz is responsible for the creation of the T pack.

The "T" pack or pelvic pack consists of a pack covering the lower abdomen and an extra strip which is fastened to the circular bandage in front, drawn around between the legs and fastened again to the circular bandage in the back.

HOT WET PACKS OR FOMENTATIONS

Several thicknesses of flannel cloth wrung out of very hot water and applied over the site of inflammation or congestion may be used to advantage in pneumonia, appendicitis and other conditions of like character. Hot fomentations should only be applied for short periods, five to fifteen minutes, but may be renewed frequently.

DRY HEAT

This form of application is best made with an electric lamp. It is useful wherever there is severe local congestion. The application may be continued longer than the hot fomentation. In pneumonia the therapeutic lamp may be used for one half to one hour at a time. This is also valuable in pleurisy, general or localized peritonitis and inflammatory rheumatism.

MANUAL AND MECHANICAL TREATMENT

The greatest relief may be given to the circulation in congested areas by gently pressing and manipulating the lymphatic glands and vessels that drain the affected parts. Groups of these structures can be reached in the neck, the arm pits and the groins. In disorders like grippe and typhoid fever, where the tissues over the entire body ache and are sore, a very light stroking and kneading of the legs, arms and neck, always working toward the heart, will give the patient considerable relief and permit him to rest.

Spinal treatment may be employed very successfully to rest the patient. It should consist of what is known as Neuropathic inhibition, and is applied by making gentle, continuous pressure with the tips of the fingers on either side of the spinous processes of the vertebrae. With the patient resting on the back, slip your hands beneath him until the end of the fingers touch the vertebrae. Make gentle pressure with the finger tips along the side of the spine nearest to you. Beginning down near the sacrum, hold each area which your hands cover for three to five minutes, then slip the hands upward to the next contact. When finished with one side of the spine, go around to the other side of the bed and treat the other side in the same manner. This will have a wonderfully quieting effect and will often induce perspiration. It will prove restful to the patient and induce sleep.

Contrary to the popular conception, the treatment in acute disease is not directed to the reduction of fever, or at least should not be. Fever is the indicator of the body's activity.

The fever subsides naturally when all irritating poisons have been oxidized and thrown out from the body.

The objects of rational treatment then is to maintain circulation and assist elimination. Water is our greatest aid towards these accomplishments.

The method of Priessnitz still holds first rank. It consists of first wrapping the body or a part in wet linen and over this several thicknesses of flannel or woolen blanket.

Spread three blankets, one on top of the other, on the bed. Over these spread a sheet which has been dipped in cool water and wrung out.

The full pack is indicated in all cases where there is a high degree of toxicity or where there is high fever. The higher the fever the better the patient reacts to the pack.

Let the fever and the condition of the skin be your guides. When the fever rises and the skin feels hot and dry and the patient begins to get restless, apply the pack.

The body pack is indicated in cases of inflammations and congestions in the abdomen or chest or in cases where the fever is low (101° to 102° F/38.3° to 38.9° C).

The greatest relief may be given to the circulation in congested areas by gently pressing and manipulating the lymphatic glands and vessels that drain the affected parts.

1922

THE HOT WATER CURE

BENEDICT LUST, N.D., M.D..

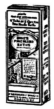
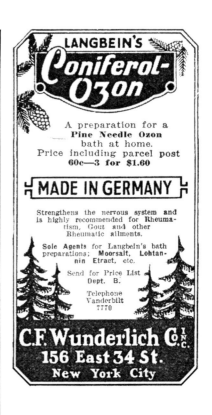
Pine needle baths were used to alleviate rheumatism. Kneipp would pick the pine needles to be used fresh in the therapeutic bath.

THE HOT WATER CURE

by Benedict Lust, N.D., M.D.

Herald of Health and Naturopath, XXVII (7), 317-323. (1922)

THE JAPANESE BATHS, A NEW REGENERATION SYSTEM

The use of water for bathing can be followed back to prehistoric ages and among the rules laid down by Moses and Zoroaster for religious customs we find some in regards to bathing. In the sixteenth century before Christ, Moses in his hygienic rules for the Jews ordered bathing as remedy against all kinds of disease and hemorrhages and commanded the cleansing of the body by bathing. 500 years later, Zoroaster did the same and the Indians, Egyptians and Persians considered bathing a sacred duty. At the time of Alexander the Great (320 B.C.), warm free public baths were already established. In 250 B.C., Archimedes built a ship furnished with water supply and warm baths.

All Hellenic schools were provided with bathing establishments and Hippocrates, the father of medical science, attached great value to bathing. From Greece, the culture of bathing spread to Italy and soon the smallest Roman city had a bathing house.

Of this tremendous movement of public hygiene, Christendom, alas, did not take any notice in its instructions, perhaps considering it as a matter of course. In the year 36, Emperor Augustus established 170 public baths for the free use of the people. In the year 300 A.D., there were 800 public baths in Rome, besides fourteen immense hot baths (*Termae*) in each one of which thousands could bathe at the same time. The gigantic remnants of the hot baths of Dioclotian and Garacalla give the spectator even today an idea of the immensity of these bathing places.

But all the classical splendor and grandeur was trampled down by barbarians who had no idea about art and hygiene.

The only country in which the art of bathing has taken permanent and solid roots is Japan, where sufficient bathing establishments for all classes of the people are provided in every part of the country.

Anyone who considers how many germs of diseases gather on our skin and which can be swept away by a thorough bathing, will understand that frequent bathing is a necessity. Professor Lassar, a famous skin specialist says that the bathing question is a question of scientific hygiene, the last secret of which will be: so much nourishment to substitute strength and so much protection against dirt. The questions for solving the problem of public hygiene therefore are: "Which nourishment for human beings is the cheapest and healthiest?" and "Which are the best means to keep our bodies internally and externally clean?"

Considering the second question I have found that our modern physicians do not understand the importance of bathing at all, or anyhow not sufficiently. For them the bath only serves the purpose of cleansing and refreshing.

I claim that a bath, especially a hot bath, like the Japanese take it, not only cleans the body externally, but also internally; not only sweeps away the germs which have fastened to the body externally, but also acts against diseases of the internal organs and especially of the blood, and also acts as preventative.

Now as our scientific medical lights pay so very little attention to bath culture, let us laymen try to investigate what value bathing could have and which effect bathing can have on our bodies.

There are three reasons for taking a bath. First, for the sake of cleanliness. It is obvious that the body in a full bath can be cleansed better from the oily substances which penetrate the millions of pores of the skin and the dust gathered there, than by simply washing, by which procedure not all parts of the body can be reached.

A bath is also taken to get refreshment and comfort. For instance, how refreshing is it if in the hot summertime we can dive into a cool bath. These two kinds of baths do not need any further explanation as to their value. They rather belong to the province of luxury; one can do without them and substitute ablution.

But the third form of bathing is entirely different: the health bath! The understanding and consideration of the bath as remedy, as a health builder, almost have been lost since the decline of the Roman Empire. Even in medical circles the importance of full baths in cases of sickness (except fever) has not entered the minds of these gentlemen of science and therapeutics. Only in hospitals, baths are prescribed but mainly on account of cleanliness but otherwise the writing out of prescriptions is preferred. What value a full water bath has in general, only a very few realize.

Of course, there are physicians who prescribe baths for their patients, if the patients are wealthy and desire to go to a fashionable bathing resort. But to tell patients with limited means to take a hot bath in the tub at home—that is not done. And when it once happens that a physician prescribes a bath, the patient is a child who has fever, and every thinking mother knows that much. To prescribe a bath as a remedy by internal diseases. "Nonsense", says the learned doctor.

Let me illustrate a law of physical penetration. If a dirty garment is washed, it is saturated with clean water which penetrates the texture of the garment and the substances of dirt, salt, gases, etc., are conveyed to the clean water which then is becoming dirty. If this procedure is repeated often enough, the water finally will stay clear, which denotes, that the garment is perfectly clean.

If a human body is put into water, it is subject to the same physical law as a garment in the water. Through the skin and the pores a reciprocal action of the fluid of the body, which consists of seventy percent of water, and the water surrounding the body, takes place. As the body [fluids] are heavily loaded with salt and gases, while the bathing water is pure, a brisk equalization of the salt and gases in the body through the skin into the water takes place. Just like hot water is more effective in washing a garment than cold water, a fact that every housewife knows, so a hot bath is more effective in cleansing the body externally and internally.

The next question I will try to answer is, how a health bath has to be. In the first place, the water must be as pure as possible, which is, however, a matter of course. The main point is the temperature.

A river or sea bath should only be taken in the summertime, when the water has a temperature of 19° C /66° F*. These baths, which I have called luxury baths, are of great importance to health for the reason that the bather on account of the difference between the warmth of the water and the blood feels the necessity of brisk exercises in the water in order to substitute the loss of warmth through the cooling down by developing internal warmth, which exercises muscles that are not much used. At the same time, the lungs are strained to increased activity and inhale pure air, explains that according to the tests of an American physiologist that the swim sport is the healthiest of all sports. Therefore, if we could have swimming baths in the river regularly throughout the whole year, it would be a great blessing but that cannot be in the northern countries. Therefore, in larger cities swimming pools are established for winter and summer. But not all people live in great cities and not everyone can swim, and many prefer a bath at home.

And now arises the important question: which temperature has the home bath to have to make it a hygienic valuable health bath for the ailing and healthy? The opinion, and unjustified prejudice prevails—except in Japan—that full baths must not be taken with a higher temperature than that of the blood, 100° F/38° C. I say unjustified prejudice, because it has been proven by the Japanese that baths at a temperature above 100° F/38° C are not only not harmful, but highly beneficial. I myself have proven this by a 15 year practice.

I have arrived at the following conclusion: the warmth of the blood is 100° F/38° C. If I bathe below 100° F/38° C my body cools. If I take a bath above 100° F/38° C, my body takes on warmth!

In this lies the whole secret, the value of the right temperature of a full bath.

The slogan of the Hydropathics always has been: "Cold, cold, cold!"

---

*Benedict Lust cites Reaumur temperature units throughout this article which I have taken the liberty to convert to Fahrenheit and Celsius. —*Ed.*

The hot blood must be cooled down, so that after the bath it reacts so much more, gets so much warmer." It cannot be denied, that the champions of the cold Water Cure, especially Rev. Sebastian Kneipp, had remarkable results in some cases. It is an open question if these results would not have been greater with hot baths.

But it seems that a strong countercurrent against the cold water cures has set in, and many Naturopaths prescribe warm treatments. If we observe our domestic animals, we will find that a sick one never lays down at a cold place but hunts the warm one, near the stove or in the sun. For warmth is life.

THE JAPANESE FULL BATH

In 1894, I read in a newspaper an article about "Japanese Baths" in which it said that the Japanese take a bath daily with a temperature of 50° C/122° F.

I was very much surprised and it seemed almost unbelievable to me that anybody should be able to stand a bath with a temperature of 50° C/122° F. Because once I had tried a bath with a temperature of over 37.5° C/99.5° F, but I could not stand it and had to turn on the cold water. I now considered that the Roman and Russian baths have a temperature of 50° C/122° F and even 62° C/145° F degrees and also that at Wiebaden, Baden-Baden and other places, baths are taken which have a temperature of 44° C/111° F. But the beneficial effects of the baths at these health resorts is attributed not to the high temperature, but to the salt and radio-activity contained in the water. I never have added salt of any kind to the water; on the contrary, in my opinion hot baths are far better without salts, because it will be more penetrating.

Also, I am of the opinion that the hot baths, Roman, Russian and Japanese, have one good characteristic quality in common, and that is that they put the body in a state of an artificial fever, increase the temperature of the blood, and thereby dissolve waste matter and force it out through the skin.

How important the skin is as secretive organ is shown by the fact that it contains 2,000,000 pores and that, if three-quarters of these pores are clogged, the man must die.

If now such a porous skin with a temperature of 37.5° C/99.5° F comes in contact with a bath with less than 37.5° C/99.5° F the pores naturally will contract and the secretion of the skin is partly obstructed. On the other hand, a bath with a temperature of more than 37.5° C/99.5° F, the pores are enlarged and the process of secretion is more energetic.

MY EXPERIENCE WITH JAPANESE BATHS

After I had gathered and considered all information of the Japanese bath obtainable, I decided to try one myself. I went into a bath with a temperature of 44° C/111° F. When I went in, my breath nearly stopped. I had a sensation which I never had before, neither in a bath nor otherwise. I felt as if something were throttling me. If I moved only a little, I felt as if something was hitting me. When I kept motionless, it was bearable. I had an awful sensation of anguish, but I withstood it.

When today, after 28 years, I think of my first Japanese bath and realize how easy it is now for me to take one and that I long for it even, I have to laugh at my fear when I took that first one. After about ten minutes, I felt palpitation of the heart, the expected artificial fever came. Before the bath, my pulse was 88, now I counted 132 in a minute. Perspiration was streaming down my head. A fever in regular form! Finally the sensation in my head caused me to reach for a sprinkling can with cold water and poured some of it on my head.

Yes, that was it, what always had been missing at the Japanese baths. That is the reason that the Japanese after five or ten minutes leave the bath because their heads start to revolt and because they do not use any antidote; that is, cold water on the head. This cold shower on the head while in the Japanese bath, gives them the real hygienic character! It is this precaution which I deem absolutely necessary when taking a Japanese bath!

When the first drops of cold water struck my head, all anguish disappeared and a sensation of ecstasy and feeling of comfort ran through me.

I felt that I was face to face with a great hygienic event, the importance of which must be extraordinary, must be, if the effect on other persons should prove to be the same. I tried it out and it was a success. I had discovered a great factor in Hydropractic.

I found that a temperature of 44° C/111° F must be the limit of a Japanese bath. I tried one with 46° C/115° F but although I constantly held the sprinkling can over my head, the cold shower did not take effect, I could not stand it and when after about three-quarters of an hour in the bath, the veins on my head and neck were swollen, my pulse was 160, for nearly an hour beads of perspiration ran down my forehead and my face looked like a ripe tomato. I felt weak and had the sensation as if I were just recovering from a heavy illness. But the next morning I felt well as ever. But I never again took a Japanese bath with a temperature higher than 44° C/111° F.

Of course, with Russian, Roman or electric baths with a temperature of 46° C/115° F are entirely different, they are easy. That a 46° C/115° F water bath has such a tremendous effect on the body proves that water irritates the skin far more thoroughly than air, light and steam of the same temperature.

Another very strong objection against Japanese baths I had to invalidate was the obvious objection that such hot baths would weaken, enervate, and in wintertime would easily attract a cold. I tried it out myself. During several winters after a one hour 44° C/111° F bath, I took an extended walk, dressed lightly, without overcoat and without socks, vest and hat. And I never even had a trace of a cold. I am perfectly convinced that Japanese baths do not weaken; on the contrary, they harden the body decidedly and give more power of resistance against colds. And that is quite natural.

In a bath below 37.5° C/99.5° F, the body gives from its warmth to the water. The loss of warmth is also loss of strength and power of resistance against the inclemency of the weather. In a bath below blood heat, the body cools down and a cold is easily attracted if the body is exposed to a still colder temperature of the air. Except the body is strong enough to react and produce warmth enough to restore the quantity of warmth given to the water. Most bodies, especially those ailing, have not this power of resistance and the only way to protect against catching a cold immediately is, to take right after leaving the bath some gymnastic exercises.

On the other hand if a bath of over 37.5° C/99.5° F is taken, the body receives warmth from the surrounding water. Where warmth is developed, power increases, in this case vital power, power of resistance against the inclemency's of the weather. In such a bath the body has gathered a surplus of of warmth, which now can be given to the cold outer air.

To find out the effects of a Japanese bath of my kind when taken longer than one hour, I took one for three hours at 44° C/111° F , and the effect was the same as by a one hour bath, only that I had three times more thirst.

After I had tried out the Japanese baths in every way, I recommended them to my acquaintances and they too got the best results.

As I now during a period of 25 years have prescribed Japanese baths for over 500 sick persons and all have been benefited by same, I deem it my duty to make public my knowledge about this important part of Naturopathy that the general public may benefit by these Japanese baths.

HOW TO TAKE JAPANESE BATHS

Healthy adults I would advise to take for the first months a bath every week, then for three months twice a week, then for six months every other day, and thereafter every day. Perhaps the everyday bath can be shortened to half an hour, but a full hour is better.*

Some might think a daily bath is overdoing it. My answer is that the real enjoyment and benefit of a Japanese bath as I prescribe it will be only gained by and by. Besides, "daily" is not exactly to be taken literally. But I am convinced that a daily bath can become a cherished habit like eating and drinking. And the benefit of daily bathing everyone will find out for himself.

The temperature of a Japanese bath has to be 44° C/111° F. The best time to take the bath is after supper, just before going to bed. The duration of a Japanese bath should be an hour, but also ought to depend upon the mood of the bather. If he feels after half an hour that he should leave the bath, he should do so, but he should try if possible to stay in for an hour which with time he will find is not so long.

Bathing right after a full meal should be avoided. The bather should try to keep away all worrying thoughts while in the bath.

The bath itself is taken after the following rules. After the thermometer shows, that the water has a temperature of 44° C/111° F, enter the bathtub quickly and lay down that the water reaches up to the chin. Keep quiet and do not move much, because if hot water is stirred, it irritates the skin more as when it is quiet. If a bather should for some reason feel uneasy or uncomfortable, he should raise his arms and upper body for a little while above the water, and the discomfort soon will disappear.

For a person afflicted with heart disease, it is advisable to make the temperature of the bath only 39° C/102° F, or to take only a half bath, the water to reach no further than to the hips.

Those who cannot tolerate a full bath should during the first few months take only a three-quarter bath, the water reaching as far as the nipples.

If the head gets too hot, sit up and put the head under the cold shower. The necessity of a shower usually is felt already after five minutes and repeats itself every five or ten minutes. Each time a short shower should be taken.

In the middle of the bath, that is after 15 or 30 minutes, leave the bathtub and take a short air bath, by walking wet and without any wrap, up and down in the bathroom. As soon as the body cools down, reenter the bathtub. These air baths in the midst of the Japanese baths are necessary, to give the pulse a chance to go back to normal. This air bath is just as necessary as the shower.

---

*Hot tubs today certainly mimic the Japanese hot bath. —Ed.

For children, that is babies up to the time they take solid foodstuffs should take a bath at a temperature of 39° C/102° F, starting with a bath of five minutes duration which by and by can be prolonged to 15 minutes. Instead of a cold shower on the head, one with lukewarm water should be applied. After the bath the child should, wet as it is, be wrapped into flannels and then let the child sleep as long as he/she may, or if the child does not go to sleep, leave the child wrapped for 15 minutes in flannels; then dress it properly. These baths should be given every morning. A strong and healthy child can stand a daily bath of half an hour with a temperature of 44° C/111° F. Such baths will prevent many ills, to which children are subjected.

Old people, not anymore free from dizziness, should take baths of the same duration and temperature as the children. They should start with one bath a week with a temperature of 39° C/102° F for half an hour and by and by increase the temperature to 44° C/111° F and the duration to one hour.

It is difficult to give fixed rules for people how to take the Japanese bath. Nervous persons should begin with half an hour bath of 39° C/102° F, while those less nervous can start with 41° C/106° F.

To all healthy people I can recommend the Japanese bath as a very effective preventative against diseases of all kinds, and also especially against calcinations of the arteries, the general disease of old age. I am convinced that everybody, who takes regularly every week at least one Japanese bath, will prolong his life by preventing calcinations of the arteries.

In cases where an arm or leg is paralyzed and it is impossible to take a full bath, a part bath is to be taken. The paralyzed arm or leg must be put at least once a day, twice is better, in a bath with a temperature of 44° C/111° F and must be kept there at least one hour, but a duration of two, three of four hours is of more benefit. Especially for gout, these part baths of long duration are an effective remedy. If a part bath is taken for four hours, the arm or leg should be taken out of the water every hour and for fifteen minutes kept in a flannel wrapping. After the bath, a long, woolen stocking should be put over the limb and be kept there till the limb is entirely dry.

The Japanese bath also can be taken as a hip bath for persons suffering with abdominal trouble. They are very beneficial for the intestines, kidney, spleen, stomach, piles and genital organs. They are taken in a seating position, the water reaching to the hips.

Of great beneficial effect are also the hot showers. They can be taken while in the full bath, or without. Applied to the neck they are a remedy for carbuncle, rheumatic pains, and hardening of the muscles of the neck.

Hot showers on the larynx are of great benefit for persons who exert their voices: singers, actors, teachers, etc. Also by swollen tonsils hot showers have a healing effect.

To cultivate a clear, healthy, rosy skin, free from wrinkles, I recommend to wash and rub the face and neck and breast every morning thoroughly with hot water that is water with a temperature of 44° C/111° F. If however, a person takes every day a Japanese full bath, the washing of the face with hot water is superfluous, because the full bath sends part of the blood to the head and keeps the skin from getting wrinkled.

To make the effect of the here described baths still stronger, I recommend to massage the skin while taking the five minute air bath when half through with the Japanese bath.

The following is a list of diseases by which in my experience the Japanese baths have been especially beneficial and curative: emaciation, asthma, anemia, neuralgia, bronchitis, abscess of intestines and stomach, diabetes, epileptic cramps, dandruff, goiter, sexual diseases, tumor on the ovaries, rheumatism, very great nervousness, decline of vigor, liver trouble, spasm of the stomach, rigid muscles, spasms of the kidney, mercury poisoning, stiff joints, paralytic stroke, syphilis, etc.

For diseases of the heart I recommend Japanese baths with a temperature of 39° C/102° F degrees, though if the heart is not too weak, a temperature of 44° C/111° F can safely be taken.

The Japanese baths are also a very good remedy to bring persons who seldom perspire—a sign of calcinations of the arteries—to perspire easily.

Prof. Harless, a famous physician, who lived in Bonn in 1830's, said: "Give me the means to create artificially a mild fever, and I will cure most incurable diseases."

I am convinced to have found such means in my Japanese baths, which create such artificial fevers. I am convinced that Japanese baths, if they ever become a universal habit, will be a great blessing for humanity.

In the year 300 A.D., there were 800 public baths in Rome, besides 14 immense hot baths (Termae) in each one of which thousands could bath at the same time.

The understanding and consideration of the bath as remedy, as a health builder, almost have been lost since the decline of the Roman Empire.

Just like hot water is more effective in washing a garment than cold water, a fact that every housewife knows, so a hot bath is more effective in cleansing the body externally and internally.

The slogan of the Hydropathics always has been: "Cold, cold, cold!" The hot blood must be cooled down, so that after the bath it reacts so much more, gets so much warmer."

Also I am of the opinion, that the hot baths, Roman, Russian and Japanese baths, have one good characteristic quality in common, and that is, that they put the body in a state of an artificial fever, increase the temperature of the blood and thereby dissolve waste matter and force it out through the skin.

This cold shower on the head while in the Japanese bath, gives them the real hygienic character! It is this precaution which I deem absolutely necessary when taking a Japanese bath!

For a person afflicted with heart disease, it is advisable to make the temperature of the bath only 39° C/102° F, or to take only a half bath, the water to reach no further than to the hips

The temperature of a Japanese bath has to be 44° C/111° F.

I am convinced that everybody, who takes regularly every week at least one Japanese bath, will prolong his life by preventing calcinations of the arteries.

Prof. Harless, a famous physician, who lived in Bonn in 1830's, said: "Give me the means to create artificially a mild fever, and I will cure the most of the incurable diseases."

1923

The Wonderful Value Of The Neutral Bath
Dr. M. Ferrin

—··—

The Blood Washing Method
William Freeman Havard, N.D..

—··—

Hydro-Therapeutical Comments
Author Unknown

The blood washing method was discovered by accident by a young man, Christos Parasco, who remained in a hot shower for up to eight hours at a time. Benedict Lust, convinced of its miraculous ability to clean the blood, took it up in practice. The two men collaborated to reveal the wonders of the therapy.

The Wonderful Value Of The Neutral Bath

by Dr. M. Ferrin, A.N.A. Member

Naturopath, XXVIII (7), 317-319. (1923)

I n the United States the neutral bath is rather new. Most people have never even heard of it. It is so valuable in purifying the system of poisons that a complete description of this kind of bath will be given.

In the first place the writer wishes to state that these baths last from three hours to three days. The bath tub is made comfortable to lie in by doubling old quilts several times and placing in the tub. Always select padding that will not fade, of course.

The person who is afflicted lies in the bath tub with the body covered with water, blood heat; in other words, 98.6° F/37° C. It is absolutely necessary to have a thermometer to go by, as the water must not go below the body heat, for it might chill, and it must not go above the heat of the body for it might have a weakening effect.

It requires an attendant to look after the fire which heats the water and to watch the thermometer. The water must run in continuously and be allowed to run out at the overflow pipe.

To think of lying in the bath tub for three, six, nine or twelve hours seems long, but after a few of these baths are over and you find yourself giving three cheers for your renewed efficiency; you soon forget the inconvenience. Lying in a bath tub on soft bed clothes for six hours and knowing that you are actually doing something to promote your health is no worse than lying in bed for six hours with the consciousness that you are no nearer recovery than when you took your bed. Do not feel sorry for yourself at all, and do not consider that you are wasting time by taking an occasional neutral bath.

The Principle

Here is the principle on which the neutral bath works: first, allow me to remind you that there are relaxing foods and there are contracting foods, and people generally are eating a predominance of the latter class. Therefore, their muscles are terribly contracted, particularly is this the case in the thighs. The large thigh muscles in most people are in pitiable condition; they are generally as hard as a piece of stove wood.

Now we breathe through our muscles as well as through our skin and lungs. With the muscles in such a contracted condition that they are almost mummified, and of course, no oxygen passes through the muscles to purify them. As a result, much of the poison that should be continually escaping from the body is retained. Therefore, the long soak so softens and relaxes the larger muscles of the body that the patient notices a singular relief and a gradual disappearance of his troubles, no matter what they may be.

AFTER THREE HOURS

After three hours in the tub every hour is golden, for in the first three hours the water penetrates the internal organs in a manner floating them and relieving much pressure on each other.

The liver is wonderfully purified in six to nine hours, and some of the most encrusted bowels are softened. The effete matter is enabled, owing to its softened condition, to pass on to the lower bowel, so that it may be evacuated. The gall stones many times soften and pass away with ease, thus saving a painful and expensive operation. Who would dare complain at a half dozen nine-hour neutral baths if he could escape an operation for gall stones?

Many times the water turns perfectly yellow and brown during the fifth hour, and the odor is so offensive it is difficult for the attendant to stay in the bath room.

WHY ALL THIS?

Why is all of this? Where does it come from? Why, right out of the body, and that is just what has been the matter with you all the time you were pale—literally crowded full of toxins—and by your ignorant eating habits kept increasing this awful condition. You thought you were sick; you were just dirty. "Cleanliness is next to Godliness", we often hear, but how few people ever get the real conception of what cleanliness is? Just one neutral bath would be a revelation to them.

No matter what you have the matter with you, cancer, hardening of the liver, gall stones, nervousness, etc., a few neutral baths will probably make a new man or woman out of you. You can then start life all over with a clean body and the delightful consciousness that you have actually done something for yourself. Most sick folks just lie in bed or sit around and let their earthly house just burn down.

A SURPRISING FACT!

It is surprising how many people are quite content to accept the verdict of "incurable"! That caps the climax! Life is practically over with them and they visualize coffins and can hear the hearse wheels on the gravel in the street. My! How little fight there is in some people? "Give Up" is their middle name.

When you conceive the idea that disease is spelled F-I-L-T-H and when you get up and dust around a little and get a pure body, you will be amazed at your feelings!

Some people start out by taking a two or three-hour neutral bath for the psychological effect it will have on them—if they are still alive they will take another one in a day or so much longer. Sometimes two neutral baths a week are sufficient. Always keep a cold cloth on the forehead and rest for some time on the bed after you are dried off.

You Are Minus The Poison!

If you feel weak after a few of these baths, do not be surprised, for you have lost the poison which was the stimulant that kept you going. Some people feel weak after they leave off coffee the first morning. Why? They have just left off that much poison and they miss it. In a few mornings, however, they get along well without their coffee. So, in losing the bodily poisons in the neutral bath, you are likely to feel like some great support is gone from you, and so it has, but you do not want your life to be built upon stimulations which come from toxins.

No wonder so many people die young. We generally think of a man of forty-five as a middle aged gentleman. The writer looks at many fifteen and twenty years of age as middle aged people, for when they are thirty or forty, they will have passed out.

People who are filled with poison and do not understand the wonderful cleaning and purifying effects of the neutral bath are losing their teeth at twenty, their hair at thirty, their stomachs at forty, their kidneys at fifty, and their lives at sixty!

If there could be a little window in the abdomen, so that as we pass along the street everybody could take a peep, what an awful demand there would be for window shades!

Water In, Poison Out!

All these filthy conditions are improved in the neutral bath by the processes known as exosmosis and osmosis—a going in of pure water and a coming out of the body impurities.

There are sometimes specific directions in certain cases such as arthritis (one of the fourteen kinds of rheumatism). Anyone interested in the purification of his body from rheumatism, asthma or tuberculosis, should write for directions. During the long bath no food should be taken, of course, except fruit or vegetable juices—better refrain from eating anything.

It is also valuable to take a good enema first before getting into the tub to take a neutral bath. Trouble? Yes, it is trouble—everything that is worthwhile is trouble.

The Japanese Are The Cleanest People

There are much less sickness and disease among some of the heathen than there is in America. The little brother of the East, the Japanese, has the credit of being the cleanest person in the world. He has from three to five baths per day. If he works in a factory, he is permitted a shower of five minutes in the middle of the morning and also a shower bath in the middle of the afternoon. He already has had a bath upon arising and he will enjoy one upon going to bed. He believes in health and cleanliness and the Americans do not.

One can be in the midst of hundreds of workmen in Japan and not smell the first suggestion of perspiration. The American workman many times has his one Saturday night bath and that satisfies him.

Even the houses of ill fame in Japan are daily watched by medical examiners, and any woman that shows symptoms of disease is put out of business for weeks or months, if necessary, so that the Japanese youths may not be contaminated. What about our own American youths? They rush on, contracting the most loathsome diseases, and no precaution is exercised by those in authority. The neutral bath in venereal disease works wonders, as it does with any other disease.

The writer cannot say too much in favor of the neutral bath!

Laundering Our Blood

When a woman has a real dirty shirt of her husband's, what does she do with it? She puts it to soak and leaves it sometimes all day and all night before she attempts to wash it. So, if we will use the same good sense about a filthy interior and be put to soak, the results will be marvelous.

It is stated that after one has been thoroughly "soaked" through and through, that the addition of three to four pounds of Epsom salts dumped into the bath tub will remove enlarged joints if the patient will remain in the water thirty or forty minutes longer. Sometimes even a two-hour bath in warm Epsom salts water works wonders in the removal of surplus carbon from the body. Some people declare that in their case this simple process has worked miracles in their bodies.

Pine Needles Or Hay Seed

Many people find great help in losing their asthma, rheumatism, catarrh, and nervousness if a peck of pine needles is put in the water of the neutral bath to greatly aid in elimination. When pine needles cannot be obtained, clover hay may be used—all these things have a tendency to neutralize body acids, thus leaving the body in a pure, sweet, clean condition, and hence free from disease. It is truly the case that DIRT, INWARD FILTH, and DISEASE ARE SYNONYMOUS TERMS!

Thousands of people in Germany and England have found out this secret of muscle purification and are happy. Indeed, it is quite an old German and English custom.

In the United States the neutral bath is rather new.

In the first place the writer wishes to state that these baths last from three hours to three days. The bath tub is made comfortable to lie in by doubling old quilts several times and placing in the tub.

Lying in a bath tub on soft bed clothes for six hours and knowing that you are actually doing something to promote your health, is no worse than lying in bed for six hours with the consciousness that you are no nearer recovery than when you took you took your bed. Do not feel sorry for yourself at all, and do not consider that you are wasting time by taking an occasional neutral bath.

Sometimes two neutral baths a week are sufficient. Always keep a cold cloth on the forehead and rest for some time on the bed after you are dried off.

So, in losing the bodily poisons in the neutral bath, you are likely to feel like some great support is gone from you, and so it has, but you do not want your life to be built upon stimulations which come from toxins.

It is stated that after one has been thoroughly "soaked" through and through, that the addition of three to four pounds of Epsom salts dumped into the bath tub will remove enlarged joints if the patient will remain in the water thirty or forty minutes longer.

Many people find great help in losing their asthma, rheumatism, catarrh, nervousness, that a peck of pine needles put in the water of the neutral bath greatly aids in elimination.

The Blood Washing Method

by Dr. Benedict Lust

Naturopath, XXVIII (10), 521-526. (1923)

> A restorative and creative revelation for ideal perfection
> Motto: "Glorify, and bear God in your body."
> —St. Paul

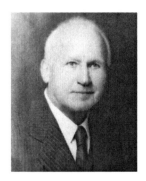

Benedict Lust

The subject of this communication is the most vital subject in all the world; it deals with the possible and sure and true transformation of the 80, 100, 60 or 50 year old person in every way, while being in possession of the wonderful experiences of the 100 years. This statement should not bring any unpleasant excitement to anybody, but comfort and joy to everybody, and the gratitude belongs only to our Lord. Old age does not exist. But sometimes like it exists, and it is noticed that bright old people always declare that their heart is as young as ever. This, in fact, explains that there is something which drives them and keeps them away from youth and life, but their thoughts are the same as ever before.

It will be admitted that every person in the world has the right to be young. Youth is a natural source of good will. Now, this may seem to come from an unexpected source and way, but in fact it does not. The discoverer of the method below has been an athlete in general from childhood.* He is a self-educated man and a very profound student of Nature. He has been very successfully his own doctor, and now with this method he has uncovered deceit and learned the secret of Nature. Thanks, God. This method is practical, easy and so simple that if the hows and whys and wherefores are not explained first, it would not be able to attract the attention and interest and the realization of the reader.

To explain the method, we must first find out of what old age really is. Old age is the worn out, run down, weak and unhealthy state and appearance of the whole body. Second, what is it that causes old age? Old age is caused by a chemically analyzed, lifeless matter in the flesh, stuck to the flesh, and growing into the flesh every day in the year for not being met with practical opposition, just as the dust would penetrate and grow into

---

*Christos Parasco is the actual inventor of the "blood washing method". He shared his discovery with Benedict Lust who adopted it into his naturopathic curriculum and in his clinical practice.. —Ed.

a brown sponge, changing its color to grey making it a nest of unhealthy microbes if the sponge is left in a damp place and out of the way of an air current. Now, this lifeless matter grows upon the body automatically through unavoidable carelessness, because it exists everywhere, including the air, the liquids and the food. It goes into the body, stays there and grows because no successful way is used to drive it out. Also, ignoring the correct way of breathing, drinking, eating, sleeping, working, playing and on the other hand, worrying, excitement, exhaustion and exposure, and all the wrong ways assist this lifeless matter to deprive the blood of its strength and its purity. Sooner or later the blood will be unable to produce any opposition to the growth of this lifeless matter, which keeps on growing, till around the first 20 years it causes the growth of the body to stop gradually and then it begins to be felt by producing in the body various weaknesses and inefficiencies, thus discouraging the mind, and as if by mystery, making the mind thinking that the body begins to grow old. Thus the mind is doing injustice to the body and is beginning to put various barriers between the body and life, while terribly neglecting it. All the while this lifeless matter continues to grow until it becomes an invincible enemy of life, producing old age, so that in the later years it completely dominates the body, takes possession of it and drives away martyred life.

To rid the body of the lifeless matter must not be done by any other way except by washing it out from the flesh with pure water; but none of the known ways of washing the body can do such cleaning. The lifeless matter cannot be washed away in one hour or two or ten, but it takes about as much time as it would for a big burn or a wound upon the aged body to heal, and if any of the known ways were used, sooner or later the system would get exhausted and would badly discourage the mind. The body gets quickly exhausted by the known ways because it is at the same time overtaken from everywhere either by too much heat or by too much cold, too much vapor or lack of pure air for breathing, or by the lack of the free and joyful ways exhausting the nervous system. In other words, by the absence of the right way of washing, without which the lifeless matter cannot be reached; also terrible and fatal exhaustion would follow if attempted to resist the required time with the known ways.

But here is the method by which the lifeless matter can be taken away from the body, so the body will again become young and will stay young. In our especially constructed and patented shower bath, the continuously shooting and showering water has the virtue to harmlessly penetrate the flesh and to produce stimulant-electricity, with the aid of which the water molds and shakes the flesh, dissolves and washes away the lifeless matter, thus enabling the blood to overcome it and to thoroughly supply the relieved flesh and all parts of the body with new life, like the water fills up the sponge. In this special shower bath, the temperature of the water can be changed and regulated at will and accordingly to the pleasure with our patented regulator, to suit the various and periodically changing temperature of the body. These changes happen because some parts of the body and of the flesh are more sensitive than others and they become a little more harmlessly uncomfortable, because all parts have been treated with the same, the whole system affecting power, and consequently changes of temperature of the body occur. While hopeless exhaustion would follow if the whole body was to be treated at once from all sides in this shower bath, with this method one part of the body at a time is to be treated. In the meantime, the other parts are resting and enjoying the charming benefits of the treated parts and making up for it. Then the next part is treated, while the one already treated makes up tenfold. By treating all parts this way, a feeling of great relief and a very pleasant sensation are created. Following this method, the body can stand the shower bath the full required time, and instead of getting exhausted it acquires every minute more strength and more power of resistance, a feeling of joy and happiness; in other words, youth.

The treatment is as follows: put up this special shower head to a height from 8 to 14 feet and let the hot water fall upon a cork matting, wood crating, air-mattress or just a porcelain or tile floor, where on the body, with extended arms and legs, head and feet, can comfortably spread out or may assume any other position. Start by showering the lower parts of the body, the lower joints, the knees, then going upwards all over the body, front, back and sides, from the toes up to the top of the head, then the same showering all over again and again, or according to the pleasure. Forty percent of the showering more or less is to be applied upon and around the stomach and the intestines, also upon the sexual parts, the rectum and surroundings, and all over the most sensitive parts of the body.

Also plenty of showering must be applied upon all parts which during the many years have acquired an old look, but not much showering to be applied to the chest and ears on the first three hours of the eight hour unit. The temperature of the bath room must be mild and comfortable and it must be without vapors; the air must be pure and wholesome. During the treatment no food of any kind should be taken, but soft warm water as much as desired, as it helps very much the cleansing of the internal body. During the treatment everyone will be able to stand the shower bath individually for himself and will be convinced and will realize that he is able to stand it, and in fact, will enjoy very much the hot water for long hours. Instead of getting pneumonia or rheumatism, as some people may imagine, this treatment will drive away these diseases forever from them, and they will realize and will become convinced that with the help of this method they will not have to submit someday to old age and to its misfortunes, but they will thank God for this blessing. After the shower, no towel should be used to dry the body, but the water should be gently rubbed from the body with one's own hands until the body is well dried by the cool air.

After the bath the one who is treated ought to take a rest for 45 minutes. Then, whether the call of Nature has been answered or not, an internal bath should be taken with a regular syringe and with pure heated water. This application promotes greatly the process of cleaning. Any time after this, vegetarian food may be taken if it is wholesome, fresh and finely chopped, to save much valuable energy of the stomach, or if it is liquidated in the form of a vegetable soup or vegetable cream soup, so much the better. After the meal rest comfortably for two hours. The rest of the time may be utilized according to pleasure, but it must be enjoyable. Sleeping in bed at night should be kept up not less than ten hours, whether sleep comes or not. This is one of the most important factors of this treatment. Also, let it be known that the shower for rejuvenating should be applied each time at least for eight hours. Internally take every night with one-third glass of water "Inner-Clean" or eat one-half teaspoonful with each meal. Follow Ehret's Mucusless Diet, as outlined in Ehret's *Specific Healing and Body Renewing Eating System.* You may read or do something else of the sort which is interesting and enjoyable to you. After this do some physical exercise for 15 minutes, but not so strenuously to cause perspiration. Every part of the body should be exercised. Therewith the treatment ends, except with possible modification in special cases. Otherwise for staying young, healthy and efficient, follow strictly the natural method of living as so wonderfully explained in detail and so easy to follow by Adolf Just's book, *Return to Nature.*

This true and real natural common-sense treatment for rejuvenating must necessarily last about twice as many days as it requires for the healing of a large wound upon the aged body, and according to the age and the percentage of the existing quantity of lifeless matter upon the body, more days are required for older people than for the younger. In order to regulate your daily habits and to practice the natural life for permanent youth, the highest efficiency and happiness, follow the methods of Louis Kuhne, Adolf Just, Sebastian Kneipp, Friedrich Bilz, Arnold Ehret, and August Engelhardt. Read and follow also Dr. Benedict Lust's ten *Health and Success Lessons,* the so-called Vitalisme Series.

Technic of The Blood-Washing Method

(Use always our Special Patented Shower Head as otherwise you will not have real results.)

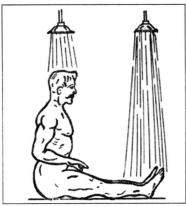

Figure 1.

Shower top of head only a minute when starting or when feeling dizzy, with cool water. Always put a plug of cotton in your ears to prevent inflammation. Shower face, sides and back of head longer, especially over ears in congestion. Feet from every angle repeatedly. Shower every part of the body at least 1 to 30 minutes at one place or as long as agreeable and repeat.

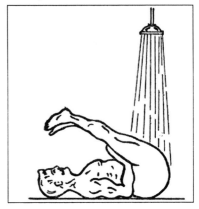

Figure 3.

Shower lower abdomen and thighs, pelvic region for a long time. Turn over and shower all of back from neck to heels thoroughly, also sides, then raise legs and let shower strike over rectum, lower back, groins and inside the legs.

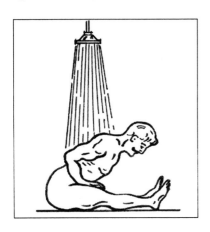

Figure 2.

Shower back and neck in sitting and lying position, also sides of arms and shoulders for a long time. Repeat.

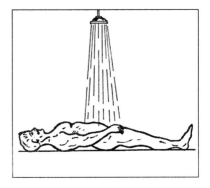

Figure 4.

Shower over chest, abdomen, sex organs, legs and feet repeatedly for a long time. Turn to right and left sides and shower for a long time all the way up to shoulders.

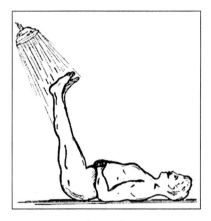

Figure 5.

Shower soles of feet: Repeat several times during duration of shower bath. Hold up feet for shower and soles while in front and back position.

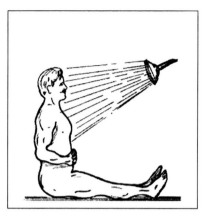

Figure 7.

Chest: Head in front. Neck also from sides and back. Not long over lungs. Always hold an object or shield over nose, mouth and eyes to prevent irritation and breathing difficulties from spray or respiratory organs.

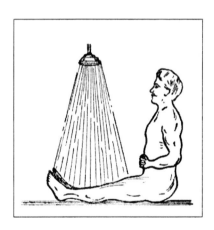

Figure 6.

Thighs and Knees: Front, back and sides and insides.

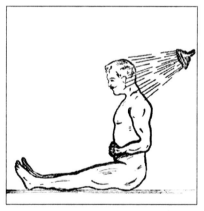

Figure 8.

Sitting position showing shower coming down on shoulders and ears, sides of head in back and neck.

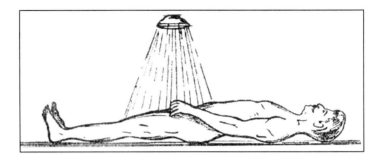

Figure 9.

Sexual region and pelvic center. Turn also to sides in sitting or lying positions.

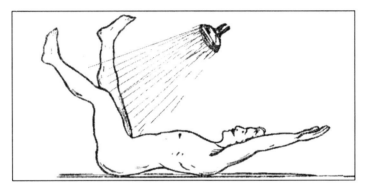

Figure 10.

Interior of legs, sexual organs. Apply also from sides, front and back.

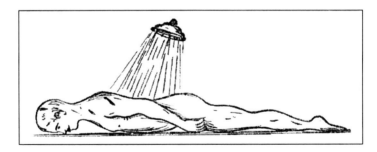

Figure 11.

Pelvic region of kidneys. Apply also on right and left sides.

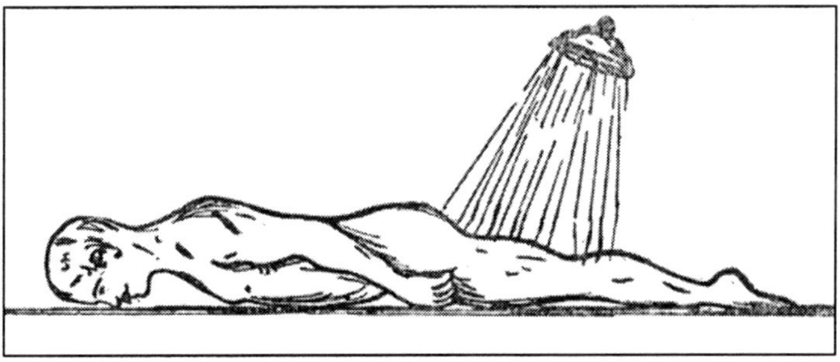

Figure 12.

Back of legs.

To rid the body of the lifeless matter must not be done by any other way except by washing it out from the flesh with pure water; but none of the known ways of washing the body can do such cleaning.

The treatment is as follows: put up this special shower head to a height from 8 to 14 feet and let the hot water fall upon a cork matting, wood crating, air-mattress or just a porcelain or tile floor, where on the body, with extended arms and legs, head and feet, can comfortably spread out or may assume any other position.

Forty percent of the showering more or less is to be applied upon and around the stomach and the intestines, also upon the sexual parts, the rectum and surroundings, and all over the most sensitive parts of the body.

Also, let it be known that the shower for rejuvenating should be applied each time at least for eight hours. Internally take every night with one-third glass of water "Inner-Clean" or eat one-half teaspoonful with each meal. Follow Ehret's Mucusless Diet, as outlined in Ehret's Specific Healing and Body Renewing Eating System.

Otherwise for staying young, healthy and efficient follow strictly the natural method of living as so wonderfully explained in detail and so easy to follow by Adolf Just's book, Return to Nature.

Hydro-Therapeutical Comments

by Unknown Author
(Translation Made By The "Naturopath")

Naturopath, XXVIII (12), 736-739. (1923)

The following remarks in regard to the hydropathic treatment may be appropriate, although they bring nothing new, but only revive or rescue from oblivion some old facts. In respect to the curative application of water, so much was done in the last century that it would be impossible to say much that is new about it. Also, the times are gone when water was considered a panacea, and therefore every assistance to therapeutics was believed to be valueless if not even harmful. But our younger generation of naturopathic physicians are thinking more biologically and are willing to look for the good wherever it can be found. They do not hesitate to accept diagnostic and therapeutic measures from practicing laymen, their aim being greatest success with least accompanying harmfulness. For every fair-minded medical man is bound to admit that we have had and that there are still among us born physicians who educationally went their own way which led them past the official colleges.

In the course of time the practical physician has learned to distinguish the limits of water's medical qualities. He has come to the conclusion that while in some cases water offers a radical remedy, in most of the diseases it is useful as an excellent medium to arouse and to assist Nature's curative power. Unfortunately, for the medical science, there still are thousands of water fanatics who refuse to believe in the wonderful curative powers of herbs and of the vegetable diet. I know some of these "water rats," who, in their old age, tortured by pain, had to humble and to force themselves to call on the hated mixer.

My statement will only confine itself to such applications of water which can be employed in the home even of the most indigent patient.

Where good water from a well or from a water-service is at hand, it is advisable to drink of it heartily. Of course, drinking too much water is just as injurious as drinking too much beer. It dilutes the gastric juices and dilates the stomach walls. The other day I had to regularly pump out a patient whose lower stomach extremity was situated between the navel and the pubic bone. Such men must be considered worse than animals.

In case of feverish diseases (also in all infectious diseases), it is advisable to prescribe sufficient quantities of fresh well-water which with benefit to the patient is to be soured by the addition of some lemon or lime juice. Especially if the urine is concentrated and is taking on a red-yellowish tint, the offering of water must not be a sparing one. Do not act like the relatives of one of my typhoid patients, whom I found at my first visit nearly dying with thirst because, on account of his thin stools, his family had not dared to give him a drop of water in spite of his suppliant entreaties. If only people would let themselves oftener be influenced by instinct instead of by some reasoning, which in too many cases is lacking of the simplest logic. Reservation in regard to the drinking of water is only a necessity in the case of anemic patients suffering from obesity, as well as in cases of heart disease, which rule is based on the languid blood circulation of such patents. On the other hand, it is wise to recommend to people suffering from obesity, who still have a strong heart action, to drink water copiously. In such cases, the drinking of even excess quantities often has beneficial results.

The waters of the medicinal springs I have to leave aside as they need a separate discussion. Also, the public baths, in general, I have to pass over, as these institutions are not everywhere at hand and where they still exist they are in demand no more than former times. I noticed the other day four gentlemen, evidently belonging to the best society, who after inspecting the price list attached to the door of a public bath, turned away from it. Another sorry example of our social conditions!

For my purpose, I only can take into consideration hip baths and foot baths. The cold hip baths are in the first place prescribed for the derivation of the blood from the chest and the head.* In such case we have, though, to act very carefully as anemic women in consequence of the compensatory anemia of the brain incline to dizziness and fainting spells. On the other hand, a short cold hip bath is an excellent soporiferous remedy for mentally overworked people. But also in this respect it is necessary to individualize, and it would be wrong to give in too great zealousness a cold hip bath to an apoplectic patient afflicted with congestions, as it may cause his instantaneous death. The effect of such procedure ought to be realized, as it chiefly concerns the vasomotor sphere. The blood vessels of the abdomen, as is well known, if sufficiently dilated, are able to receive a large part of the blood of the human body. From the cold hip bath, first of all results during the first minutes a reflective dilation of the blood vessels of the head as well as of the lower extremities. Upon this a reaction sets in in the form of an increase in the volume of the abdominal vessels. If this effect should turn out in rather forcible manner, it may cause in case of brittleness of the vessels, a disruption.

I shall not fail to mention an excellent application of the therapeutic treatment which unfortunately begins to fall into oblivion—presumably in consequence of exaggerated bacillus delusions. I refer to cold hip baths to be applied after childbirth and in case of metrorrhagia.

---

*The terminology for physiological mechanisms is captured in words that have become obsolete. "Derivation" refers to reduction of congestion in an area of the body by applying cold and / or hot water applications to move blood elsewhere, causing dilation of blood vessels of the distal area. —Ed.

About ten minutes after the delivery the patient ought to be treated with a cold hip bath, the water to be of 10° to 12° C/50° to 54° F. The patient is to be rubbed vigorously by the midwife at the loins and at the abdomen, to be put back after ten minutes into the warmed bed and to be laid on a woolen cloth, to be rubbed dry with it. After such procedure, the women feel surprisingly well and the expulsion of the placenta also passes off much quicker and without the need of any artificial help. This method combines at the same time a cleansing of the female genital organs, as it physiologically could not be effected any better.

The same procedure is well applied in cases of atonic metrorrhea. In such a case, the effect is also generally very beneficial as the musculature of the uterus begins to contract immediately, stypticity following later on. This method, of course, will fail in cases of larger arterial hemorrhage; like they will occur after operations with the help of instruments although rarely.

The method of applying cold hip baths, first recommended by a German physician, Medizinalrat Dr. Pingler of Koenigsstein, for the period following childbirth, deserves widest dissemination, even if the ergot treatment should become somewhat neglected as a result of it.

Hot hip baths are to be recommended in cases of colic-like pains in the abdomen and as cure for dysmenorrhea. They may also be applied for reabsorption of inveterated exudations, although inventive warming apparatus are generally of better service in such cases. The time for applying such baths ought not be exceed 15 to 20 minutes; neither must it be neglected to have a pitcher with hot water on hand to add some more of it to the bath.

While the hip baths have the effect to derivate the blood to the splanchnic sphere, the foot baths have the effect to increase the volume of the vascular system in the calves and in the feet. For coldness of the feet the application of short, cold foot baths is very serviceable. Nervous patients must be prepared for the foot bath by properly rubbing and washing their feet, and in many cases this procedure must be repeated for weeks. After a foot bath the patient ought to take a walk, if he does not prefer to seek his bed. It is to be noted that the foot bath for warming up the feet must be of the short duration of only a few minutes, while the same procedure for derivating purposes eventually can be continued for 20 minutes. From the foot baths intended for foot warming, a quick and good result is not to be expected. Much more certain is the good effect in respect to the lungs; besides, such baths offer the only remedy to impart to the feet the same temperature as that of the body.

Before passing over from the baths for parts of the body to the wet packings, I have to mention one kind of water application which I have found in case of pneumonia to be of excellent service. Such patients are from three to nine times daily to be chafed vigorously with wet towels and then to be rubbed dry, or a better result is obtained, in some cases, if the wet body is wrapped in a warmed woolen cloth. The dry rubbing must not last longer than about one minute. Patients with a slight attack of pneumonia will benefit themselves if they daily make own use of such cold rubbing in the morning as well as at night, and especially by rubbing the upper part of the body.

The method of cold rubbing is also serviceable as a good diagnostic indicator of the patient's state of vitality. In case a collapse is imminent, a superficial washing of the forearm will soon give a hint which cannot be mistaken. If the skin only slowly begins to take on a reddish color, if the high temperature falls in a conspicuous and rapid manner, such symptoms prove that the patient's vital energies are near the freezing point. Hot packs are then of valuable service. In the case of aged people, the cold rubbings are to be applied with great caution.

The ultimate purpose of all these hydrotherapeutic measures, like those of a different nature, for instance, bloodletting, is to create new activity of the remaining vital energies, and in the case of senile people these powers are consumed much quicker than in the case of stronger individuals. The wet packing are finding a much more general application. This method is made use of in a great number of acute diseases. The main rule is that with the help of these packing, perspiration must not be forced. The patient must be unwrapped immediately if high temperature makes him restless and uneasy. But when the patient in his sleep begins to perspire easily and without incitement, he should not be disturbed as long as he feels comfortable. If he is sleeping, he must not be roused. A quick sponge bath of the unwrapped body with vinegar-water will, in most cases, be felt as very comforting, as by this method the relaxed skin recovers its former tension. At the conclusion of this dissertation I shall explain a theory—nearly unknown to medical science—about the effect of cold water, which deserves to have a great future, although its originator is a lay doctor.

That in high fever cases cold water is to be used for the packing is self-evident. I cannot understand why some Hydrotherapists absolutely decline to use chilled water. Also in this regard, it is a necessity to individualize and while it has to be admitted that packings with the use of fresh well-water effectuate a stronger reaction, on the other hand it is evident that this method demands a stronger constitution which will not be found in every case. Concerning the number of packings, a strict rule cannot be laid down. It would not be advisable to apply more than seven packing within 24 hours.

Finally, I have to say something in regard to lavaments [enemas]. For stool regulation they must not be too voluminous. In most cases, half a liter of warm water will be sufficient. To use this treatment successfully, that is, to again accustom the bowels to stronger action, such warm water injections ought to be administered for four weeks daily, using the same quantity at the same temperature and—what is especially noteworthy—always at the same time of the day. It is wrong to expect a stool from each of such treatments, as only a daily stimulation of the intestinal organs is intended. The clyster is, therefore, not to be put aside altogether.

Cold water injections (1 liter at 15° C/59° F) produce increased peristalsis of the small intestines, and in many cases they bring on a more profuse secretion of bile. In the first place, they are to be applied in the case of jeterus [jaundice], but they also are very serviceable at occurring disarrangements in the upper section of the small intestines.

Herewith, I have drawn a partial picture of our Hydrotherapy in the sick room and I hope not only to have offered some valuable suggestions to many laymen, but also to some physicians.

In closing, I will give a short sketch of the water action theory as originated by Wachtelborn—a born physician. It is based on the ancient wisdom which is also drawing nearer to our modern science that the smallest particle of everything that is alive as well of everything that apparently is lifeless is in a constant vibration. These vibrations produce in our body positive and negative currents, and our health or illness is based on the harmony or the dissonance of these life-currents. In the case of high fever, for instance, the positive life-magnetic vibrations are strongly predominant and will only exhaust themselves in death, if not the energies vibrating negatively in their struggle to regain a balance are supported from outside. For such purpose there is at our disposal in the negatively acting cold water an excellent remedy, whose application to the overheated body neutralized the excess of positive currents. In a separate article I again will refer to this medical theory, and I will try to give a prospective view what the future may have in store for it. In the meantime, I earnestly recommend the reading of Wachtelborn's book, *The Medical Science and the Law of the Epidemics*, to all unprejudiced physicians and laymen.

In the course of time, the practical physician has learned to distinguish the limits of water's medical qualities. He has come to the conclusion that while in some cases water offers a radical remedy, in most of the diseases it is useful as an excellent medium to arouse and to assist Nature's curative power.

The cold hip baths are in the first place prescribed for the derivation of the blood from the chest and the head.

On the other hand, a short cold hip bath is an excellent soporiferous remedy for mentally overworked people. But also in this respect it is necessary to individualize, and it would be wrong to give in too great zealousness a cold hip bath to an apoplectic patient afflicted with congestions, as it may cause his instantaneous death.

The blood vessels of the abdomen, as is well known, if sufficiently dilated, are able to receive a large part of the blood of the human body. From the cold hip bath first of all results during the first minutes a reflective dilation of the blood vessels of the head as well as of the lower extremities.

About ten minutes after the delivery the patient ought to be treated with a cold hip bath, the water to be of 10° to 12° C / 50° to 54° F. The patient is to be rubbed vigorously by the midwife at the loins and at the abdomen, to be put back after ten minutes into the warmed bed and to be laid on a woolen cloth, to be rubbed dry with it. After such procedure the woman feel surprisingly well, and the expulsion of the placenta also passes off much quicker and without the need of any artificial help.

While the hip baths have the effect to derivate the blood to the splanchnic sphere, the foot baths have the effect to increase the volume of the vascular system in the calves and in the feet.

It is to be noted that the foot bath for warming up the feet must be of the short duration of only a few minutes, while the same procedure for derivating purposes eventually can be continued for 20 minutes.

The dry rubbing must not last longer than about one minute. Patients with a slight attack of pneumonia will benefit themselves if they daily make own use of such cold rubbing in the morning as well as at night, and especially by rubbing the upper part of the body.

Benedict Lust compiled a Home Course comprising of ten lessons on Vitalism and Nature Cure.

Glossary

Each of the various hydrotherapy application's methodology can be found on the page/s indicated. When there are numerous pages cited, this means that there are different versions by different Hydrotherapists.

Abdominal compress [81, 223] has several variations, i.e. cold, warm using herbal decoctions, or vinegar and water. A wet cloth folded creating layers depending upon the vitality of the patient is placed over the abdomen.

Ablution [227, 246, 277, 446] is simply a washing of the body done with the hands, a washcloth, a bath mitt or a sponge with the benefit of applying friction as a means of completing another hydrotherapy application.

Affusion is a washing of the body by pouring water from a vessel, such as a bucket or large pitcher.

Air baths taken outside or in the comfort of one's home in front of an open window were taken preferably wearing no clothing.

Alternate warm/hot and cold bath [96] is a sequence of baths beginning with a warm bath for ten minutes that is immediately followed with a short one minute cold bath. Repeated three times.

Back douche or gush [314] is cold water administered either by a watering can or a hose to the back.

Bandage [220] implies a wet cold compress to a body part that is entirely wrapped around the body and covered with a dry blanket in a similar manner of wrapping.

Lower bandage [221] a wet sheet wrapped around the body from the axilla to the feet.

Short bandage [221, 260] or pack [326] is a wet piece of linen or cotton, wrung out and wrapped around the body three to five times. The short pack extends from the axilla to the hips or knees.

Baths [225] taken in a bath tub varied in the amount of water and temperature. See full and half baths.

Bare foot walking [271] was used long before Kneipp to help harden and strengthen the body's constitution.

Bed steam bath [116] is a three-quarter or full pack with one hot bottle wrapped in a wet towel applied to the feet, two of such bottles outside to the calves, and two bottles to the thighs. First, the body has to be wrapped in a wet sheet, then the hot bottles have to be placed, then the woolen blanket has to be enveloped round the whole. Three hot bottles on average are sufficient. Duration of the bed steam bath is from one to three hours.

Blood washing method [472, 474] was a prolonged shower, often lasting as long as eight hours. The height of the showerhead is from 8 to 14 feet and water is hot. The patient starts showering the lower parts of the body, the lower joints, the knees, then going upwards all over the body, front, back and sides, from the toes up to the top of the head, then the same showering all over again and again for eight hours.

Compress [222] uses a piece of cotton or linen dipped in cold water and wrung out before applying to the body. The wet compress is then covered with a dry blanket or similar material.

Cooling packs [306] used to lower fevers employed tepid water a few degrees lower than the body temperature.

Depletion: the reduction of congestion anywhere in the body.

Derivation: the reduction of congestion by moving the excess blood elsewhere by using hot or cold water application for such purpose.

Douche [199] was adopted by Lust to describe the gushes that Kneipp devised for the various parts of the body. Originally, Priessnitz used douches which were flowing water from cold mountainous streams falling a distance of 10 to 20 feet.

Epsom salt baths [377] assist in the elimination of uric acid.

Fluxion: cold water applications increase the movement or flow of blood in a particular part of the body.

Fomentation [168] is one of the most efficient means of applying heat in the case of pain by using hot moist compresses applied to the body.

Foot bath [91] is taken in cold water for the purpose of diverting blood from the head and upper body to the feet. Foot baths are excellent for insomnia and increasing blood flow to cold feet. Warm foot baths [91-93] use various herbal decoctions.

Friction [305] is a dry friction rub of the body using either a soft bristled brush, friction glove or a towel to stimulate the skin prior a cold water procedure.

Friction hip bath [411] was devised by Kuhne and a sitz tub was filled with cold water to the patient's umbilicus. Using a coarse cloth, the abdomen and sexual organs are briskly rubbed.

Friction sitz bath [411] was especially helpful for women. The patient sits on a dry stool placed in a tub of water. Using friction and rubbing, cold water is used during this treatment.

Full pack [447] is also known as the wet sheet pack.

Gushes [111, 224] were the signature water application developed by Sebastian Kneipp by using a simple garden watering can to pour water on different parts of the body. In time, the gush was often called a douche.

Half baths [120, 225, 248] short cold water bath lasting from one to three minutes with water reaching the umbilicus. Benefits include strengthened digestion, convalesce, hardening, etc.

Half pack [448] is a wet sheet pack that covers the trunk of the body from the arms to the hips. It is also called the short bandage.

Hardening the constitution employed various methods, such as walking barefoot, ablutions, affusions, and baths.

Hay flowers [92, 123, 219, 258, 342] were made into a decoction that was used in baths, such as the foot bath compresses such as the short compress or Spanish mantle, and vapor baths.

Heating Compress is a cold compress with wool coverings to induce heat production in the body.

Herbal baths [92, 219] are prepared with warm water infused with decoctions or extracts of herbs, such as hay flower, oat straw, shavegrass [Equisetum], and other herbs.

Hip douche [311] is a modification of the knee gush and water is poured onto the feet and continues to the hip.

Hot spinal fomentation [307] was used by Bernarr Macfadden to stimulate the nervous system via the spinal cord.

Injection is an enema or a vaginal douche.

Internal bath [306] is an enema.

Japanese hot bath [459] are extremely hot baths of 50° C/122° F which Benedict Lust modified with lower temperatures of 44° C/111° F.

Knee gush [113, 139. 224, 239, 247] was Kneipp's signature treatment which he administered using a garden watering can. Water is streamed onto the body forming a layer of water like a sheet of glass. The knee gush begins at the feet and ends at the knees.

Lower bandage [221] a wet sheet wrapped around the body from the axilla to the feet.

Lightening gush or douche [115, 247] required an experienced practitioner to administer. Water is applied to the whole body using a pressurized hose to deliver the cold water using a whipping action.

Natural bath [185] was created by Adolf Just after observing animals in the wild take their baths. A natural bath is taken in a shallow bath tub containing three to six inches of water and bather sits in the water using friction and rubbing of water onto their pelvic area.

Natural Method of Healing is a term that implies the work of Friedrich Bilz who was a follower of Kneipp's water cure methods.

Nauheim bath [385, 403] is a carbon dioxide bath that is effective for the treatment of congestive heart disease. Still used in many medical spas around the world.

Neutral bath [427, 465] is taken in water that is at body temperature, and water temperatures varies from 92° to 98° F/33° to 37° C. The temperature of the water is neutral meaning that the body loses heat at the same rate that its muscles create heat. No net loss of body heat. A neutral bath is considered a panacea for insomnia.

Non-stimulating diet consists of fruits, vegetables, cereals, whole wheat bread, fruit juice, milk. Excluded are alcohol, caffeinated drinks, beef broth, meat, and smoking.

Oat straw [82, 92, 120, 219, 223, 258] made into a decoction was used in baths such as the foot baths, compresses and vapor baths.

Packs [258] is another name for a bandage or a wrap. Wet cloth is wrapped around a body part or the whole body.

Priessnitz abdominal bandage [357] is a small and effective bandage wrapped around the abdomen.

Reaction: cold water applied to skin will result in blanching of the skin followed by hyperemia. At the first sign of hyperemia, the cold water application is terminated.

Retrostasis: the movement of blood from the peripheral circulation; example, the skin to the blood vessels of the interior or core organs.

Revulsion: the mobilization of blood flow from one area to another with the use of cold or hot water or both used alternatively.

Revulsive compresses is the application of hot fomentations followed by cold compresses for the purpose of producing mild fluxion in an area.

Russian bath: Hot vapor or steam at temperatures varying from 105° to 145° F/41° to 63° C for 10 to 20 minutes. The body is showered with hot water and gradually cooled.

Salt bath [91] used salt combined with wood ashes to warm water for a foot bath.

Salt rub or glow [399] is a friction rub of the whole body using salt.

Sauerkraut poultice [262] is a poultice using sauerkraut externally on the skin to heal wounds, ulcers, lumbago and headaches.

Scotch douche is a pressurized douche that is administered by a bath attendant. The temperature of the water alternates between hot [100° to 110° F/38° to 43°C] and cold water [60° to 80° F/16° to 27° C].

Shavegrass [Equisetum arvense] decoctions were used in many of the warm water applications.

Shawl bandage [221, 261] uses a square linen clothe that is folded into a triangular shape which is dipped into cold water, wrung out and placed over the chest.

Short bandage [222, 260] or a pack [326] is a wet piece of linen or cotton, wrung out and wrapped around the body three to five times. The short bandage extends from the axilla to the knees. Over the wet cloth, a dry woolen blanket to securely wrapped around to prevent evaporation and increase body warmth.

Sitz bath [375, 381, 400] is taken by immersing the hips and pelvic area into a tub containing either cold, warm or hot water.

Spanish mantle [119, 221, 259] consists of a long shirt made of coarse linen dipped into cold water, wrung out and put on like a night shirt. Woolen blankets are wrapped over the patient. The duration of the Spanish mantle is one to two hours. Indicated for gout, kidney stones, smallpox, typhus, fever, catarrh and mucus.

Steam bath [405] was devised by Louis Kuhne to be used at the beginning of a water cure protocol. The steam bath was used to warm up weak and debilitated patients before the cold water application.

Stimulating compress is a term coined by Friedrich Bilz to name a cold compress that stimulates heat production in the body by increasing blood flow to the surface of the body.

Temperature: The classification of water temperature varied between Hydrotherapists. Here is a chart with different water temperatures used in Hydrotherapy:

Hydrotherapist	Very Cold	Cold	Cool	Tepid	Neutral	Warm	Hot	Very Hot
F E Bilz (1898) (Bilz, 1898, 1942)		43-54° F/ 6-12° C	55-65° F/ 12-18° C	77-88° F/ 25-31° C		88-110°F/ 31-43°C		
J H Kellogg (1903) (Kellogg, 1903, 100)	32-55° F/ 0-13° C	55-65° F/ 13-18° C	65-80° F/ 13-27° C	80-92° F/ 27-33° C	92-95°F/ 33-35°C	92-96°F/ 33-36°C	98-104°F/ 37-40°C	>104°F/ 40°C
C Pope (Pope, 1909, 22)	34-55° F/ 1-13° C	55-65° F/ 13-18° C	65-80° F/ 13-27° C	80-92° F/ 27-33° C	92-96°F/ 33-36°C	96-98°F/ 36-37°C	98-104°F/ 37-40°C	>104°F/ 40°C
G H Abbott (Abbott, 1914, 38)	32-55° F/ 0-13° C	55-70° F/ 13-21° C	70-80° F/ 21-27° C	80-92° F/ 27-33° C	94-97°F/ 33-36°C	92°-100° F/ 33°-38° C	100-104°F/ 38-40°C	>104°F/ 40°C
C Schultz (Schultz, 1914, 348)	32-54° F/ 0-12°C	55-70° F/ 13-21° C	70-80° F/ 21-27° C	80-92° / 27-33° C	94°-97° F/ 34°-36° C	92°-100° F/ 33°-38° C	92-100°F/ 37-38°C	>104°F/ 40°C
RM Le Quesne & M Granville (Le Quesne et al., 1936, 28)		<65° F/ 18° C	65-75°F/ 13-24° C	75-92° / 24-33° C	92-97°F/ 33-36°C		98-104°F/ 37-40°C	>104°F/ 40°C

Throat compress [175, 194, 248, 344] is wet compress applied to the throat and removed or renewed once the compress is heated.

T pack [448] consists of a lower abdomen pack with an extra strip which is drawn between the legs.

Turkish bath: a hot air bath for the purpose of inducing perspiration, often in a room designed for this purpose. Massage is given during the hot air bath which is then followed by a cool shower.

Vapor bath [122, 219] is a hot steam bath applied to the feet, or head or other parts of the body using hot water or herbal extracts.

T pack [448] consists of a lower abdomen pack with an extra strip which is drawn between the legs.

Turkish bath: a hot air bath for the purpose of inducing perspiration, often in a room designed for this purpose. Massage is given during the hot air bath which is then followed by a cool shower.

Under compress [223] covers the area from the cervical spine extending to the entire spine. Compresses are folded into different thicknesses depending upon the strength of the patient.

Upper gush or douche [112, 223, 310] is applied with either a watering can or a hose to the upper back and shoulders.

Upper compress [223] is a compress placed on the chest and abdomen.

Vapor bath [122, 219] is a hot steam bath applied to the feet, or head or other parts of the body using hot water or herbal extracts.

Vinegar [82, 220, 227, 258] is used in many water application that include wet socks, cold ablution and packs to stimulate heat production in the body.

Walking in water or water treading [73] is walking in cold water. Begin with water ankle deep for one minute and increase the depth of water and the duration of time in the water. One must continue to walk while in the water.

Wet sheet packs or wraps [260, 326, 343, 402] is a wet cold or tepid sheet wrapped around the body followed by two or more layers of blankets wrapped over the wet sheet.

Wet shirt [221] is another form of a modified wet sheet application. Variations include the use of salt water.

Wet sheet packs or wraps [260, 326, 343, 402] is a wet cold or tepid sheet wrapped around the body followed by two or more layers of blankets wrapped over the wet sheet.

Wet socks [220, 262, 360] are usually worn with a covering pair of dry wool socks to bed to alleviate chronic cold feet, insomnia, lower fever, and fatigue.

REFERENCES

Abbott, G. K. (1912). *Elements of Hydrotherapy for Nurses*, Review and Herald Publishing Assn., Washington, D.C., 275 pp.

Baruch, S. (1892). *The Uses of Water in Modern Medicine*, George S. Davis, Detroit, 228 pp.

Baruch, S. (1898). *The Principles and Practice of Hydrotherapy*, William Wood and Company, 1st edition, 435 pp.

Baruch, S. (1920). *An Epitome of Hydrotherapy for Physicians, Architects and Nurses*, W.B. Saunder Company, Philadelphia, 205 pp.

Baruch, S. (1916). The Nauheim bath. *Herald of Health and Naturopath*, XXI (8), 532-536.

Bauergmund, Dr. (1908). How should Kneipp's treatment be taken? *The Naturopath and Herald of Health*, IX (3), 69-76.

Baumgarten, A. (1903). Drinking cold water. *The Naturopath and Herald of Health*, IV (3), 48-51.

Baumgarten, A. (1903). Water applications. *The Naturopath and Herald of Health*, IV (5), 124-128.

Baumgarten, A. (1903). On the different effects of cold water. *The Naturopath and Herald of Health*, IV (7), 184-185.

Baumgarten, A. (1904). The knee douche. *The Naturopath and Herald of Health*, V (1), 7-10.

Baumgarten, A. (1909). *Die Kneipp'sche Hydrotherapie*, Buchdruckerei Und Verlags, Anstalt, Wörishofen, 895 pp.

Biéri, R. (1910). The water cure in gay Paris. *The Naturopath and Herald of Health*, XV (9), 517-521.

Biéri, R. (1921). The development of hydrotherapy since Priessnitz. *Herald of Health and Naturopath*, XXVI (5), 223-224.

Bilz, F. E. (1901). The Kneipp cure. *The Kneipp Water Cure Monthly*, II (8), 211-213.

Bilz, F. E. (1901). Bad Health. *The Kneipp Water Cure Monthly*, II (11), 287-291.

Boyle, W., Saine, A. (1988). *Lectures in Naturopathic Hydrotherapy*, Eclectic Medical Publications, Sandy, Oregon, 235 pp.

Buttgenbach, F. J. (1912). An unknown, inexpensive and yet effective sweat bath. *The Naturopath and Herald of Health*, XVII (8), 522-523.

Dieffenbach, W. H. (1909). *Hydrotherapy, a brief summary of the practical value of water in disease*. Rebman Company, New York.

Ferrin, M. (1923). The wonderful value of the neutral bath. *Naturopath*, XXVIII (7), 317-319.

Gröfere, Gusgabe. (1897). Pater Kneipp, iein Leben und iein Wirten, Kempten Publishers.

Habel, M. (1911). The vinegar [Vinegar]. *The Naturopath and Herald of Health*, XVI (5), 294-295.

Hartmann, T. (1905). The cold water treatment. *The Naturopath and Herald of Health*, VI (7), 178-179.

Hartmann, T. (1905). The cold water treatment in general, [the compresses]. *The Naturopath and Herald of Health*, VI (12), 372-378.

Havard, W. F. (1921). Naturopathy in practice. *Herald of Health and Naturopath*, XXVI (7), 325-326.

Hinsdale, G. (1910). *Hydrotherapy, a Work on Hydrotherapy in General, its Application to Special Affections, the Technic or Processes Employed and the Use of Waters Internally*, W. B. Saunders Company, Philadelphia, 466 pp.

Hoegen, J. A. (1916). Hydrotherapy, various applications, [sitz baths]. *Herald of Health and Naturopath*, XXI (7), 468-469.

Hoegen, J. A. (1917). Hydrotherapy. *Herald of Health and Naturopath*, XXII (5), 311-316.

Judd, C. E. (1909). Hydrotherapy. *The Naturopath and Herald of Health*, XIV (7), 411-414.

Just, A. (1901). The natural bath. *The Kneipp Water Cure Monthly*, II (11), 315-317.

Kellogg, J. H. (1901). *Rational Hydrotherapy*, F. A. Davis Company Publishers, Philadelphia, 1193 pp.

Kneipp, S. (1897). Water applications. *Amerikanischen Kneipp Blätter*, II (15), 186-187.

Kneipp, S. (1897). Water applications, [Snow walking]. *Amerikanischen Kneipp Blätter*, II (21), 279-281.

Kneipp, S. (1897). Wet sheets. *Amerikanischen Kneipp Blätter*, II (22), 310-311.

Kneipp, S. (1898). Ablutions. *Amerikanischen Kneipp Blätter*, III (13), 115-117.

Kneipp, S. (1898). Water applications, [ice and bleeding]. *Amerikanischen Kneipp Blätter*, III (14), 126-127.

Kneipp, S. (1898). Water applications, foot baths. *Amerikanischen Kneipp Blätter*, III (15), 137.

Kneipp, S. (1898). Warm full baths. *Amerikanischen Kneipp Blätter*, III (20), 193-194.

Kneipp, S. (1902). Kneipp's apotheca. *The Naturopath and Herald of Health*, III (9), 384-386.

Kneipp, S. (1909). Kneipp's cold water douches. *The Naturopath and Herald of Health*, XIV (8), 492-499.

Kuhne, L. (1917). My remedial agents. *Herald of Health and Naturopath*, XXII (6), 359-368.

Lindlahr, H. (1923). The new blood wash treatment. *Naturopath*, 28(10), 527-530.

Luepke, J. (1911). Systematic bathing, a preservative of health. *The Naturopath and Herald of Health*, XVI (2), 103-104.

Lust, B. (1900). A brief history of Natural Healing. *The Kneipp Water Cure Monthly*, I (1), 2-5.

Lust, B. (1900). The Kneipp gushes or pours. *The Kneipp Water Cure Monthly*, I (1), 6-7.

Lust, B. (1900). The Spanish mantle. *The Kneipp Water Cure Monthly*, I (3), 36-38.

Lust, B. (1900). Natural healing in America, I. *The Kneipp Water Cure Monthly*, I (4), 55-56.

Lust, B. (1900). Kneipp as author. *The Kneipp Water Cure Monthly*, I (5), 67.

Lust, B. (1900). Natural healing in America, II. *The Kneipp Water Cure Monthly*, I (5), 79.

Lust, B. (1900). Kneipp and his system. The Kneipp Water Cure Monthly, I (7), 112.

Lust, B. (1901). Fomentations. *The Kneipp Water Cure Monthly*, II (9), 241.

Lust, B. (1901). Baths and the water cure. *The Kneipp Water Cure Monthly*, II (9), 241.

Lust, B. (1902). The neck bandage. *The Naturopath and Herald of Health*, III (12), 493-494.

Lust, B. (1903). Health incarnate, [Hydropathy, hydrotherapy, water cure]. *The Naturopath and Herald of Health*, IV (10), 286-287.

Lust, B. (1903). Means of hardening for children and adults. *The Naturopath and Herald of Health*, IV (11), 313-322.

Lust, B. (1904). Health incarnate. *The Naturopath and Herald of Health*, V (7), 4-7.

Lust, B. (1904). Father Kneipp and his methods. *The Naturopath and Herald of Health*, V (1), 145-149.

Lust, B. (1905). Hardening. *The Naturopath and Herald of Health*, VI (1), 19-21.

Lust, B. (1905). Does hydrotherapy require reform? *The Naturopath and Herald of Health*, VI (3), 70-71.

Lust, B. (1906). The effect of Kneipp's treatment on diseases. *The Naturopath and Herald of Health*, VII (2), 74-75.

Lust, B. (1907). The importance of ablutions in natural healing. *The Naturopath and Herald of Health*, VIII (9), 261-262.

Lust, B. (1910). The treatment of acute diseases. *The Naturopath and Herald of Health*, XV (2), 85-86.

Lust, B. (1913). The Priessnitz or abdominal bandage. *The Naturopath and Herald of Health*, XVIII (9), 617-618.

Lust, B. (1913). Wet socks. *The Naturopath and Herald of Health*, XVIII (9), 770.

Lust, B. (1914). How to use water to cure chronic cold feet. *The Naturopath and Herald of Health*, XIX (9), 570.

Lust, B. (1914). Magnesia sulphate or Epsom salts bath. *The Naturopath and Herald of Health*, XX (7).

Lust, B. (1917). Preface. *Neo-Naturopathy, the New Science of Healing*, Benedict Lust Publisher, Butler, New Jersey. 291 pp.

Lust, B. (1918). Priessnitz, introducer of hydropathy. *Herald of Health and Naturopath*, XXIII (3), 223-224.

Lust, B. (1922). The hot water cure. *Herald of Health and Naturopath*, XXVII (7), 317-323.

Lust, B. (1923). The blood washing method. *Naturopath*, XXVIII (10), 521-526.

Lust, L. (1911). Water cure, water applications. *The Naturopath and Herald of Health*, XVI (4), 231, 233.

Metcalfe, R. (1898). *Life of Vincent Priessnitz, Founder of Hydropathy*. Metcalfe's London Hydro. Ltd, Richmond Hill, Surrey.

Metcalfe, R. (1900). Letter to editor. *The Kneipp Water Cure Monthly*, I (10), 187.

Metcalfe, R. (1901). Vincent Priessnitz. *The Kneipp Water Cure Monthly*, II (8), 218-220.

Pope, C. (1909). *Practical Hydrotherapy, a Manual for Students and Practitioners*, Cincinnati Medical Book Company, 646 pp.

Reinhold, A. F. (1900). Professor Reinhold praises the cold water cure. *The Kneipp Water Cure Monthly*, I (11), 206.

Schultz, C. (1914). Hydrotherapy or water cure. *The Naturopath and Herald of Health*, XIX (6), 345-349.

Staden, L. (1900). Hydropathic medical adviser. *The Kneipp Water Cure Monthly*, I (1), 14.

Staden, L. (1901). Naturopathic adviser. *The Kneipp Water Cure Monthly*, II (6), 170.

Stroebele, L. (1899). Mountain air resort, Bellevue, Butler, New Jersey, *Amerikanischen Kneipp Blätter*, IV (6), 141.

Strueh, C. (1915). Sitz baths. *The Naturopath and Herald of Health*, XX (4), 215.

Summers, L. A. (1919). Nature's cure for disease. *Herald of Health and Naturopath*, XXIV (8), 343-345.

Summers, L. A. (1920). Nature's cure for disease, II. *Herald of Health and Naturopath*, XXV (7), 286-288.

Tally, A. N. (1898). Kneipp cure institutes in America. *Amerikanischen Kneipp Blätter*, III (22 & 23), 227-228.

(Unknown author). (1921). Hydro therapeutic comments. *Naturopath*, XXVIII (12). 736-739.

Winternitz, L. (1909). Is Kneipp's hydrotherapeutic treatments unscientific? *The Naturopath and Herald of Health*, XIV (4), 221-223.

INDEX

A

Abdomen, 21, 52, 54, 56, 123-124, 160, 168, 174, 185, 277, 291, 357, 382, 398, 400-401, 427, 474, 479; bandage, 52, 151-153, 329, 357-359, 361, 415, 448; compress, 81-82, 152, 185, 222-223, 272-273; douche, 178, 311-312; massage, 222, 263, 278, 305, 381, 411, 480; steam bath, 407-408

Ablution, 34, 48, 67-68, 93, 96-98, 163, 205, 217-219, 227, 231, 246, 272-273, 277-280, 306, 325, 342, 352, 446-447; vinegar, 227

Abscess, 176-177, 180, 272, 291, 437, 461

Acute Disease/s, 11, 21, 48, 50, 59, 101, 126, 142, 172-173, 215, 272-273, 306-308, 325, 342-344, 357, 381-383, 399, 401, 413, 446, 481

Affusion, 22, 44, 157-159, 162-163, 165, 170, 179-180, 329, 332, 388

Air, 157, 170, 186, 196, 205-206, 216, 246, 271, 287, 289, 304, 342, 369, 389, 409, 471; bath, 36, 47, 106, 305, 308, 340, 430, 458-461; cure, 38, 141; exposure, 35, 70, 72, 74, 80-82, 96, 177, 247-248, 258-259, 261, 287, 290, 326, 358, 447; fresh, 72, 74, 95, 100, 105-106, 117-119, 139, 152, 168, 173-174, 176, 177-180, 185, 208, 211, 235, 294, 305, 307, 319, 343-344, 407, 411, 437, 455, 471

Allopath/y, 12, 26, 30, 59, 244, 255, 319

Alcohol, 149, 152, 186-187, 203, 262, 272, 292, 345-346, 357, 387

Aloe, 152

Amerikanischen Kneipp Blätter, 16, 25, 34, 37, 110, 380

Analgesic, 331

Anemia, 101, 170, 333, 339-341, 411, 461, 479

Anise, 160

Antibiotics, 63

Antifebrin, 272

Anti-inflammatory, 330-331

Antipyrin, 272

Appendicitis, 40, 151, 306-307, 370, 381, 401, 449

Appetite, 59, 158, 200-201, 208, 292, 319, 435; loss of, 201, 265, 287, 292-293, 333, 339-340

Apoplexy, 54, 286, 375

Arteries, 205, 387

Arteriosclerosis, 54, 334, 375, 403, 460-461

Ashes, 36, 91

Assimilation, 101, 233, 235, 247, 285, 287-289, 293, 435

Asthma, 37, 101, 112-113, 116-117, 334, 369, 461, 467-468

Auscultate, 22, 158

Austria, 141, 157, 249, 320, 421, 443

B

Back, 158, 175-176, 223, 278, 448; douche, 37, 50, 111, 113-114, 116, 224-225, 247, 256; gush, 265, 313-317, 319; pain, 81, 159

Bandage/s, 31, 42-43, 45, 67, 81, 121, 217, 304, 330, 332, 442, 448; abdominal, 52, 151-153, 329, 357-359, 361, 415, 448; clay, 52, 346, 415; foot, 220, 361; full, see wet sheet; lower, 221; neck, 43, 151, 194-196, 220, 248; shawl, 221; short [three-quarter], 47, 51, 118, 222, 326

Barefoot, 45, 73, 151, 158, 175,

INDEX OF NAMES

About the Editor, NUNM, NUNM Press

Sussanna Czeranko, ND, BBE, is a 1994 graduate of CCNM (Toronto). She is a licensed ND in Oregon. In the last twenty-two years, she has developed an extensive armamentarium of traditional naturopathic therapies for her patients. Especially interested in balneotherapy, botanical medicine, breathing and nutrition, she is a frequent international presenter and workshop leader. She is a monthly Contributing Editor (Nature Cure—Past Pearls) for NDNR and a Contributing Writer for the Foundations of Naturopathic Medicine Project. Dr. Czeranko founded *The Breathing Academy* and along with Dr. Karis Tressel *The Nature-Cure Academy*, both of which provide training and practicums for Naturopathic doctors, the former in the scientific model of Buteyko breathing therapy, and the latter in traditional Naturopathic modalities. Dr. Czeranko also founded *Manitou Waters Clinic, Spa and Health Education Centre* in Saskatchewan, Canada, on the shores of a pristine, highly mineralized northern lake.

NUNM (National University of Natural Medicine, Portland, Oregon) was founded in 1956 as National College of Naturopathic Medicine (NCNM). It transitioned to university status in June 2016. NUNM is home to the longest serving, accredited clinical doctorate naturopathic program in North America and to numerous accredited graduate research programs and undergraduate programs. NUNM's program mix also includes one of the country's most unique clinical doctorates in Classical Chinese Medicine.

NUNM Press publishes distinctive titles that enrich the history, clinical practice, and contemporary significance of natural medicine traditions. The rare book collection on natural medicine at NUNM is the largest and most complete of its kind in North America and is the primary source for this landmark series— *In Their Own Words*—which brings to life and timely relevance the very best of early naturopathic literature.

The Hevert Collection: *IN THEIR OWN WORDS*
A Twelve-book Series

ORIGINS of Naturopathic Medicine

PHILOSOPHY of Naturopathic Medicine

DIETETICS of Naturopathic Medicine

PRINCIPLES of Naturopathic Medicine

PRACTICE of Naturopathic Medicine

VACCINATION and Naturopathic Medicine

PHYSICAL CULTURE in Naturopathic Medicine

HERBS in Naturopathic Medicine

MENTAL CULTURE in Naturopathic Medicine

HYDROTHERAPY in Naturopathic Medicine

CLINICAL PEARLS of Naturopathic Medicine, Vol. I

CLINICAL PEARLS of Naturopathic Medicine, Vol. II

From the NUNM Rare Book Collection On Natural Medicine.
Published By NUNM Press, Portland, Oregon.

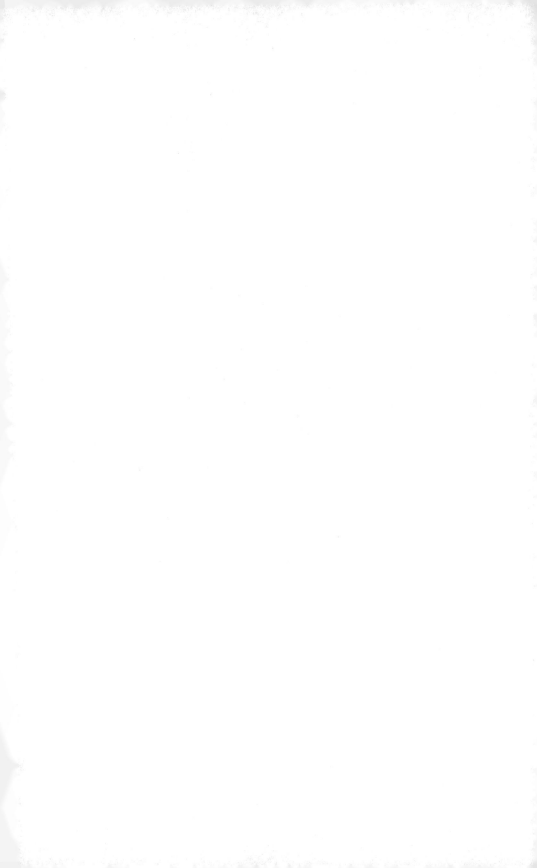